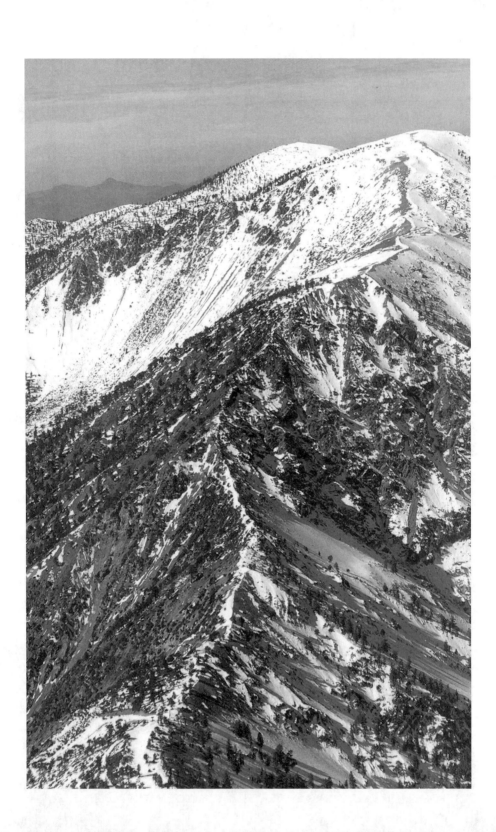

101 HIKES

in Southern California

Exploring Mountains, Seashore, and Desert

Third Edition

Jerry Schad and David Money Harris

 WILDERNESS PRESS ... *on the trail since 1967*

In memory of Jerry Schad, 1949–2011

101 Hikes in Southern California

1st EDITION 1996
2nd EDITION 2005
3rd EDITION 2013

Copyright © 1996, 2005, and 2013 by Jerry Schad and David Money Harris
Cover photos copyright © 2013 by David Money Harris
Interior photos: Jerry Schad and David Money Harris
Maps: Jerry Schad, David Money Harris, and Steve Jones
Cover and interior design: Larry B. Van Dyke
Editor: Laura Shauger

ISBN 978-0-89997-716-4; eISBN 978-0-89997-717-1

Manufactured in the United States of America

Published by: **Wilderness Press**
                c/o Keen Communications
                PO Box 43673
                Birmingham, AL 35243
                (800) 443-7227; FAX (205) 326-1012
                www.wildernesspress.com

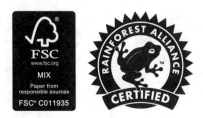

Visit our website for a complete listing of our books and for ordering information.

Distributed by Publishers Group West

Cover photos: Palm Canyon (Hike 51)

Frontispiece: Devil's Backbone (Hike 32)

SAFETY NOTICE: Although Wilderness Press and the author have made every attempt to ensure that the information in this book is accurate at press time, they are not responsible for any loss, damage, injury, or inconvenience that may occur to anyone while using this book. You are responsible for your own safety and health. The fact that a trail is described in this book does not mean that it will be safe for you. Be aware that trail conditions can change from day to day. Always check local conditions and know your own limitations.

Preface

Just beyond the limits of Southern California's ever-spreading urban sprawl lies a world apart. In snippets of open space here and in sprawling wilderness areas there, California's primeval landscape survives more or less untarnished. In hundreds of hidden places just over the urban horizon (and sometimes within the cities themselves), you can still find nature's radiant beauty unfettered—or at least not too seriously compromised—by human intervention.

Our purpose in writing this book is to entice you to explore some of these hidden places. In the pages ahead you will find updated versions of trips previously published in Jerry Schad's *Afoot & Afield* series of guidebooks on Los Angeles, Orange, and San Diego Counties, plus additional trips from eastern Ventura County, western San Bernardino County, and western Riverside County—a total of 101 hikes described in detail. The overview map on pages x–xi reveals how the majority of hikes chosen for this book cluster around the major urban areas of Los Angeles, Orange County, and San Diego. As a result, no matter where you live within Southern California, you can likely access 50 or more of these hikes in less than a two-hour drive.

Users of the *Afoot & Afield* books will already be familiar with the format and layout of this book. Each hike description includes a capsulized summary. Each trip is plotted on an easy-to-read sketch map. Photos of scenery and interesting features on or near the trails are sprinkled throughout the book.

The book was originally written by Jerry Schad, the grandmaster of Southern California hiking guidebooks. Unequaled in his knowledge of the region's wild places and in enviable physical condition, Jerry was abruptly diagnosed with kidney cancer in 2011 and passed away in the same year. At his request, I have revised this book to keep it up to date with changing conditions. I have endeavored to retain Jerry's lively writing and insightful descriptions while reflecting recent changes, rendering the driving directions as unambiguous as possible, and adding GPS coordinates for the trailheads.

I physically walked every trail in this book to ensure that the information contained herein is up to date. Based on this fieldwork, I have replaced 17 of the hikes covered in the second edition with outstanding substitutes. Seven of these hikes were closed or rendered inaccessible by fire. Two had access issues due to private property. The road to one had deteriorated to the point that it was impassable by stock four-wheel-drive vehicles. The others had become brushy, poorly defined, or simply less interesting than nearby trails. I have enjoyed all of the hikes in this book and hope you will enjoy them too.

I would like to thank the team at Wilderness Press for making this book possible. My editor, Molly Merkle, envisioned the new edition. Laura Shauger's exceptional copyediting has made the book clearer and more consistent. Amber Henderson skillfully assembled the pieces into the final layout. The remaining errors are my own.

Roads, trailheads, and trails continue to change every year. You can keep me apprised of recent developments and/or changes by writing me in care of Wilderness Press at info@wildernesspress.com. Your comments will be appreciated.

David Money Harris
Upland, California
June 2013

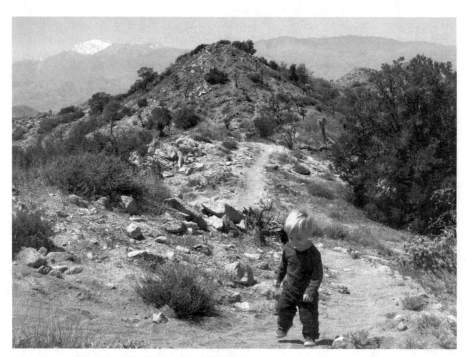

San Gorgonio from Joshua Tree National Park (Hike 44)

Contents

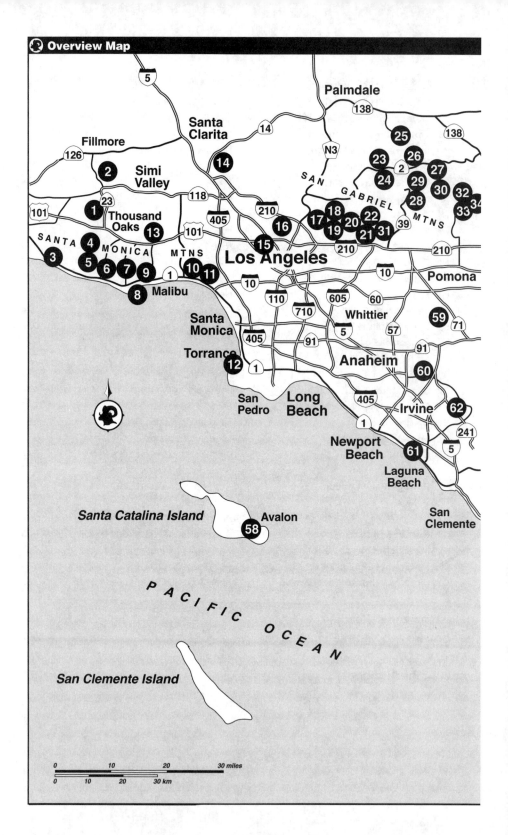

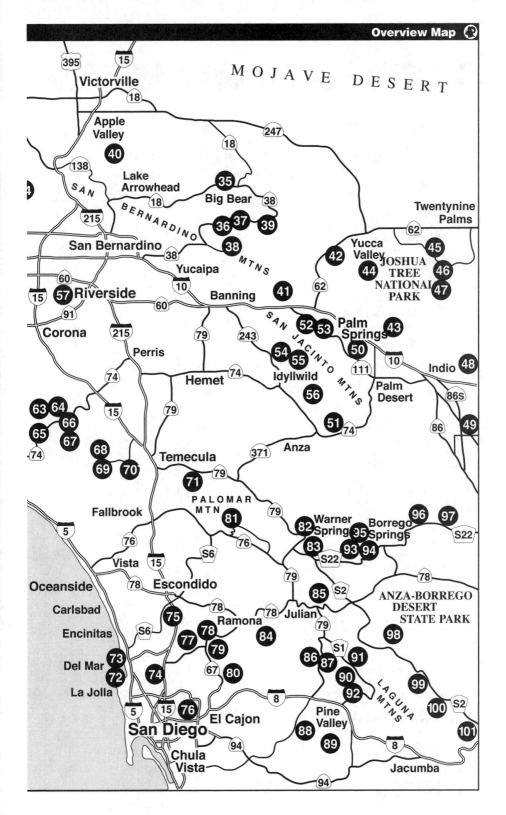

MOJAVE DESERT

395 15 Victorville
18
Apple Valley
40
138 Lake Arrowhead
SAN 18
35 Big Bear 38
BERNARDINO 36 37 39
215 38
San Bernardino 38 MTNS
Yucaipa
60 10
15 57 Riverside Banning
Corona 60
215
Perris 79 243
74
Hemet 74
79
63 64 15 79
66
65 67
74
68 Temecula
69 70 371 Anza

247
18
Twentynine Palms
62
Yucca 45
42 Valley
44 JOSHUA 46
TREE
NATIONAL 47
PARK
41 62
SAN 52 53 Palm 43
JACINTO Springs
54 50
55 111 10 Indio 48
Idyllwild Palm 86S
56 Desert
86
51 74 49

71
PALOMAR
MTN
81 79
Fallbrook
5 76 76
Vista 15 S6
Oceanside 78 Escondido
Carlsbad 78
75 Ramona
Encinitas S6 77 78
73 79
Del Mar 72 74 67 80
La Jolla
5 15 76 El Cajon
San Diego 94
Chula 94
Vista

Warner 96 97
82 Springs 95 Borrego
83 93 94 Springs S22
S22
78
ANZA-BORREGO
85 S2 DESERT
STATE PARK
78 Julian
79 98
86 87 91 S1
90 LAGUNA
92 99
M
T 100 S2
N
S 101
Pine
88 Valley
89 8
Jacumba

OVERVIEW OF HIKES

NO.	HIKE	DISTANCE (in miles)	ELEVATION GAIN (in feet)	TRAIL TYPE	DOGS ALLOWED	GOOD FOR KIDS	MTN. BIKING	BACKPACKING
1	Paradise Falls	2.7	400	Loop	✓	✓		
2	Happy Camp Canyon	11	1,300	Loop			✓	
3	La Jolla Valley Loop	11	1,950	Loop				✓
4	Sandstone Peak	6	1,400	Loop	✓			
5	The Grotto	2.8	650	Out-and-back	✓	✓		
6	Charmlee Wilderness Park	2.8	500	Loop	✓	✓		
7	Zuma Canyon	9	1,700	Loop				
8	Point Dume to Paradise Cove	2.1	200	Out-and-back		✓		
9	Solstice Canyon	2.4	350	Out-and-back	✓	✓		
10	Temescal Canyon	2.8	850	Loop		✓		
11	Will Rogers Park	2.0	350	Loop	✓	✓	✓	
12	Malaga Cove to Bluff Cove	2.0	200	Loop		✓		
13	Cheeseboro and Palo Comado	10	1,200	Loop	✓		✓	
14	Placerita Canyon	5.0	700	Out-and-back	✓	✓		
15	Mount Lee	3.2	750	Out-and-back	✓	✓	✓	
16	Verdugo Mountains	6	1,500	Loop	✓		✓	
17	Mount Wilson	15	4,800	Out-and-back	✓			
18	Down the Arroyo Seco	10	-2,600	Out-and-back				✓
19	Mount Lowe	3.2	500	Out-and-back	✓	✓		
20	Mount Lowe Railway	11	2,800	Loop	✓			✓
21	Eaton Canyon	3.4	400	Out-and-back	✓	✓		
22	Santa Anita Canyon Loop	9	2,300	Loop	✓			✓
23	Cooper Canyon Falls	3.2	800	Out-and-back	✓	✓		
24	Mount Waterman Trail	8	1,400	Out-and-back	✓			✓
25	Devil's Punchbowl	1.4	300	Loop	✓	✓		

OVERVIEW OF HIKES

NO.	HIKE	DISTANCE (in miles)	ELEVATION GAIN (in feet)	TRAIL TYPE	DOGS ALLOWED	GOOD FOR KIDS	MTN. BIKING	BACKPACKING
26	Mount Williamson	4.4	1,600	↗	🐕			🚶
27	Mount Baden-Powell Traverse	9	2,400	↗	🐕			🚶
28	Lewis Falls	0.8	300	↗	🐕	🧒		
29	Mount Islip	8	2,400	↻	🐕			🚶
30	Down the East Fork	16	-4,800	↗	🐕			🚶
31	Fish Canyon Falls	3.8	600	↗	🐕	🧒		
32	Old Baldy	6	2,300	↗	🐕			🚶
33	Cucamonga Peak	12	4,300	↗	🐕			🚶
34	The Three T's	13	5,000	↗	🐕			🚶
35	Cougar Crest Trail	4.4	600	↗	🐕	🧒		
36	Forsee Creek Trail	13	3,700	↗	🐕			🚶
37	Dollar Lake	13	2,700	↗	🐕			🚶
38	San Gorgonio Mountain	16	5,700	↗	🐕			🚶
39	Aspen Grove	1.8	350	↗	🐕	🧒		
40	Deep Creek	3.8	950	↗	🐕			
41	Whitewater Canyon	4.0	400	↗	🐕	🧒		🚶
42	Big Morongo Canyon	1–3	50–300	↻		🧒		
43	Pushwalla Palms	6.5	1,000	↻				
44	Black Rock Panorama Loop	6.5	1,200	↻				
45	Wonderland of Rocks	6	200	↗				
46	Ryan Mountain	2.8	1,000	↗		🧒		
47	Lost Horse Mine	4.2	500	↗		🧒		
48	Lost Palms Oasis	7.5	700	↗				
49	Ladder Canyon	4.3	750	↻		🧒		
50	Murray Hill	7	1,700	↗				

OVERVIEW OF HIKES

NO.	HIKE	DISTANCE (in miles)	ELEVATION GAIN (in feet)	TRAIL TYPE	DOGS ALLOWED	GOOD FOR KIDS	MTN. BIKING	BACKPACKING
51	Pines to Palms	15	-3,500	↗				🚶
52	San Jacinto Peak (easy)	11	2,600	↗				🚶
53	San Jacinto Peak (hard)	20	10,600	↗				🚶
54	San Jacinto Peak (middle)	15	4400	↗				🚶
55	Tahquitz Peak	7	2,000	↗	🐕			🚶
56	Antsell Rock	4.2	2,300	↗				
57	Mount Rubidoux	3.3	450	↗	🐕	🧍	⊛	
58	Lone Tree Point on Catalina	6	1,800	↗		🧍		
59	Hills for Everyone	4.5	1,000	↺		🧍		
60	Santiago Oaks Regional Park	1–3	100–400	↺	🐕	🧍	⊛	
61	El Moro Canyon	6	900	↗			⊛	
62	Whiting Ranch	4.4	500	↗		🧍	⊛	
63	Santiago Peak	16	3,950	↗	🐕			
64	Trabuco Canyon Loop	10	2,700	↺	🐕			
65	Bell Canyon Loop	3.3	400	↺		🧍		
66	San Juan Loop Trail	2.1	350	↺	🐕	🧍	⊛	
67	Sitton Peak	9.5	2,150	↗	🐕			🚶
68	Tenaja Falls	1.4	300	↗	🐕	🧍		🚶
69	Tenaja Canyon	7	1,100	↗	🐕			🚶
70	Santa Rosa Plateau	6	650	↺		🧍		
71	Dripping Springs Trail	14	2,900	↗	🐕			🚶
72	La Jolla Shores	5.0	Flat	↗				
73	Torrey Pines State Reserve	up to 4	100–600	↺		🧍		
74	Los Penasquitos Canyon	6	300	↺	🐕	🧍	⊛	
75	Bernardo Mountain	7	1,000	↗	🐕		⊛	
76	Cowles Mountain	2.8	950	↗	🐕	🧍		

OVERVIEW OF HIKES

NO.	HIKE	DISTANCE (in miles)	ELEVATION GAIN (in feet)	TRAIL TYPE	DOGS ALLOWED	GOOD FOR KIDS	MTN. BIKING	BACKPACKING
77	Blue Sky Ecological Reserve	5.0	800	↗	🐕	🚶		
78	Woodson Mountain	6	1,500	↻	🐕	🚶		
79	Iron Mountain	6	1,200	↗	🐕	🚶	⚙	
80	El Capitan Open Space Preserve	12	4,000	↗	🐕		⚙	
81	Doane Valley	3.0	300	↻		🚶		
82	Agua Caliente Creek	8	900	↗	🐕			🎒
83	Eagle Rock	6	700	↗	🐕	🚶		
84	Cedar Creek Falls	5.5	1,000	↗		🚶		
85	Volcan Mountain	3.2–5.0	900–1,300	↗	🐕	🚶		
86	Cuyamaca Peak	5.5	1,650	↗	🐕		⚙	
87	Stonewall Peak	4.5	850	↗		🚶		
88	Horsethief Canyon	3.2	500	↗	🐕	🚶		🎒
89	Corte Madera Mountain	7	1,750	↗	🐕			🎒
90	Noble Canyon Trail	10	-2,500	↗	🐕		⚙	🎒
91	Garnet Peak	2.4	500	↗	🐕	🚶		
92	Sunset Trail	7	700	↻	🐕	🚶		
93	Culp Valley	1.7	300	↻		🚶		
94	Hellhole Canyon	5.0	900	↗		🚶		🎒
95	Borrego Palm Canyon	2.9	450	↗		🚶		
96	Villager Peak	13	5,000	↗				🎒
97	Calcite Mine	4.2	800	↻		🚶	⚙	
98	Ghost Mountain	1.2	450	↗		🚶		
99	Moonlight Canyon Loop	1.5	350	↻		🚶		
100	Mountain Palm Springs	2.1	350	↻		🚶		
101	Mortero Palms to Goat Canyon	6	2,400	↗				🎒

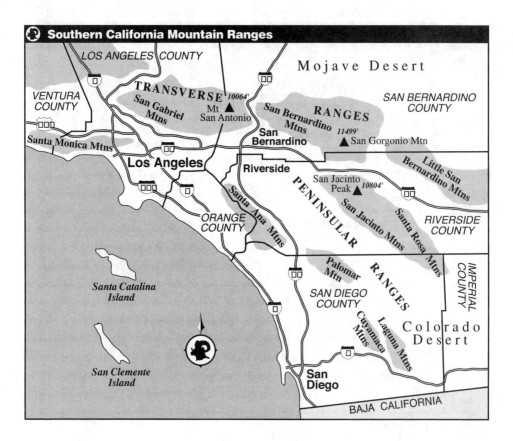

Southern California Mountain Ranges

LOS ANGELES COUNTY

Mojave Desert

VENTURA COUNTY

TRANSVERSE *10064'*

San Gabriel Mtns

Mt ▲ San Antonio

San Bernardino Mtns *11499'*

RANGES

SAN BERNARDINO COUNTY

Santa Monica Mtns

San Bernardino

▲ San Gorgonio Mtn

Los Angeles

Riverside

San Jacinto Peak ▲ *10804'*

Little San Bernardino Mtns

PENINSULAR

RIVERSIDE COUNTY

ORANGE COUNTY

Santa Ana Mtns

San Jacinto Mtns

Santa Rosa Mtns

Santa Catalina Island

RANGES

IMPERIAL COUNTY

Palomar Mtn

SAN DIEGO COUNTY

Colorado Desert

San Clemente Island

Cuyamaca Mtns

Laguna Mtns

San Diego

BAJA CALIFORNIA

Southern California's Wilderness Rim

SOUTHERN CALIFORNIA SITS astride one of Earth's most significant structural features—the San Andreas Fault. For more than 10 million years, earth movements along the San Andreas and neighboring faults have shaped the dramatic topography evident throughout the region today. The very complexity of the shape of the land has spawned a variety of localized climates. In turn, the varied climates, along with the diverse topography and geology, have resulted in a remarkably plentiful and diverse array of plant and animal life.

Living on the active edge of a continent has advantages and disadvantages that cannot be untangled. Like the proverbial silver lining in a dark cloud, the rumpled beauty of our youthful, ever-changing coastline, mountains, and desert redresses the ever-present threat of earthquakes, fires, and floods. Because much of Southern California is physically rugged, not all of it has succumbed to the plow or the bulldozer. When you've had the pleasure of hiking beside a crystal-clear mountain stream minutes from downtown L.A. or cooling off in the spray of a cottonwood-fringed waterfall just beyond suburban San Diego, you'll realize that not many regions in the world offer so great a variety of natural pleasures to a population of many millions.

Let us, in the next couple of pages, briefly explore the principal wild and semiwild natural areas bordering Southern California's coastal plain. When linked together, these natural areas form a broad, curving crescent around Southern California's urban population—now more than 20 million strong. About 90% of the hikes found in this book fall into this unpopulated or sparsely populated crescent.

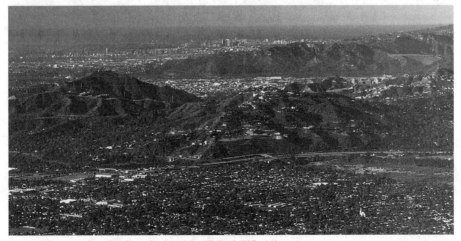

Los Angeles on a clear day from the Sam Merrill Trail (Hike 20)

1

The Santa Monica Mountains

We start with the Santa Monica Mountains, which rise abruptly from the Pacific shoreline west of (or up the coast from) Los Angeles. They, along with the San Gabriel and San Bernardino Mountains, are part of the Transverse Ranges, so named because they trend east-west and stand crosswise to the usual northwest-southeast grain of nearly every other major mountain range in California. This anomaly, it is thought, is largely due to compression along the San Andreas Fault. There is a kink in the San Andreas Fault north of Los Angeles where the fault, running southeast from the San Francisco Bay Area, jogs east for a while before resuming its course toward the southeast. Compression against this kink has caused the land south of it to crumple and wrinkle upward. The devastating January 1994 Northridge earthquake was just one small episode in the slow but fitful uplift of the Transverse Ranges.

Compared to other Southern California ranges, the Santa Monicas are modest in size—barely more than 3,000 feet high—but their rise from the sea is dramatic.

They are a shaggy-looking range, clothed in tough, drought-resistant vegetation that falls into two principal categories: coastal sage scrub and chaparral. The *coastal sage scrub* plant community lies mostly below 2,000 feet in elevation, on primarily south-facing slopes in the Santa Monica Mountains and elsewhere in the coastal ranges of Southern California. Characterized by various aromatic sages (California sagebrush, black sage, and white sage) along with buckwheat, laurel sumac, lemonade berry shrubs, and prickly pear cactus, sage scrub is fast disappearing in the Santa Monicas and elsewhere as urbanization encroaches on it. Much of the sage-scrub vegetation is dormant and dead-looking during the warmer half of the year but green and aromatic during the cool, wet half.

The *chaparral* plant community is commonly found between 1,000 and 5,000 feet in elevation—almost anywhere there's a slope that hasn't burned recently. Chaparral needs more moisture than sage scrub, so in the Santa Monicas it's often found on the shadier, north-facing slopes and other spots protected from the full glare of the sun. The dominant chaparral plants include chamise, scrub oak,

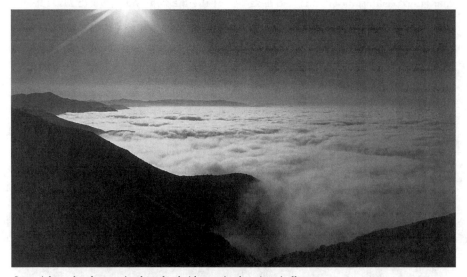

Late-night and early-morning low clouds (the marine layer) typically cover Southern California's coastline during spring and summer.

manzanita, toyon, mountain mahogany, and various forms of ceanothus (wild lilac). Yuccas, known for their spectacular candle-shaped blooms, often frequent the chaparral zones. The chaparral plants are tough and intricately branched evergreen shrubs with deep root systems that help the plants survive during the long, hot summers. Chaparral is sometimes called elfin forest—a good description of a mature stand. Without benefit of a trail, travel through mature chaparral, which is often 15 feet high and incredibly dense from the ground up, is almost impossible.

A touch of the *southern oak woodland* and *riparian woodland* communities is present in the Santa Monicas and sparsely distributed nearly everywhere else in coastal Southern California. The Santa Monica Mountains include the southernmost stands of the valley oak, a massive, spreading tree that is as much a symbol of the Golden State as are the redwoods farther north. The southern oak woodland is very parklike in appearance, especially in the spring when attended by new growth of grass and wildflowers. Riparian (streamside) vegetation includes trees such as willows, sycamores, and alders that thrive wherever water flows year-round—typically along the bottom of the larger canyons. Strolling through the riot of growth in riparian zones is the nearest thing to a jungle experience you can have in arid Southern California. Both types of habitat have declined all over California as a result of urbanization and agricultural development, and the attendant exploitation of water resources.

Wildfire plays a dominant role in the ecology of the Santa Monica Mountains, and indeed almost everywhere else in coastal Southern California. Sage scrub and chaparral vegetation readily renews itself after fire. Before modern times wildfires would incinerate most hillsides every 5–15 years, and thick stands of chaparral seldom developed. Over the past century, however, the active prevention and suppression of fires has led to longer growth

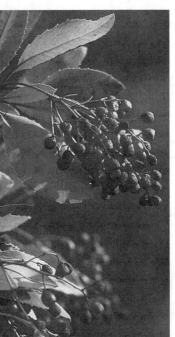

Toyon (California holly, the "holly" of Hollywood) is a common chaparral plant.

cycles and abnormally large accumulations of deadwood. Once started, today's wildfires in chaparral zones are often difficult or impossible to control.

From Malibu east into L.A.'s west side, the Santa Monicas are steadily filling up with custom houses and subdivisions, all of which are in jeopardy from firestorms during the dry summer and fall seasons. Large and small wildfires will forever torment those who seek to establish permanent residence here.

Today the Santa Monicas are a patchwork quilt of private lands (many already built upon or slated for future development) and public lands, protected from urban development by inclusion within

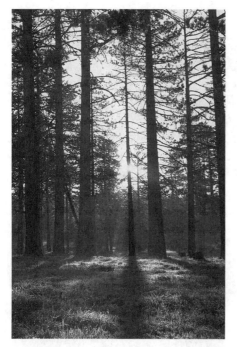

Jeffrey pines in the Laguna Mountains

Santa Monica Mountains National Recreation Area, a unit of the national park system.

The San Gabriel Mountains

Turning our attention farther north and east, we find the San Gabriel Mountains, another segment of the east-west-trending Transverse Ranges. Behind the south ramparts of the San Gabriels, whose chaparraled slopes rise sheer from the Los Angeles Basin and the San Gabriel Valley, stands a series of high peaks, the tallest of which—Old Baldy, also known as Mt. San Antonio—exceeds 10,000 feet in elevation. Yawning gorges slash into the range, in one place offering more than a mile of vertical relief between canyon bottom and adjacent ridge.

Geologists figure that the San Gabriels are being squeezed horizontally about a tenth of an inch each year, and being thrust upward much more rapidly than that. Caught in this tectonic frenzy, the San Gabriel Mountains are surging upward as fast as any mountain range on the planet. They are also disintegrating at a spectacular rate. Although the San Gabriels consist mainly of durable granitic rocks, much like those in the sturdy Sierra Nevada, the San Gabriel rocks have been through a tectonic meat grinder. The tops of the San Gabriels are fairly rounded, but their slopes are often appallingly steep and unstable. An average of 7 tons of material disappears from each acre of the front face each year, most of it coming to rest behind debris barriers and dams in the L.A. Basin below.

The San Gabriel Mountains themselves are relatively young as upthrust units—only a few million years old. This is not true of the ages of most of the rocks that compose them. Some rocks exposed here are representative of the oldest found on the Pacific Coast—more than 600 million years old.

Botanically, parts of the San Gabriel Mountains are extremely attractive, especially in zones above 4,000 feet that receive enough precipitation. There the *coniferous forest,* which has two phases in Southern California, thrives. The yellow pine phase includes conifers such as bigcone Douglas-fir, ponderosa pine, Jeffrey pine, sugar pine, incense-cedar, and white fir, and forms tall, open forest. These species are often intermixed with live oaks, California bay (bay laurel), and scattered chaparral shrubs such as manzanita and mountain mahogany. Higher than about 8,000 feet, in the lodgepole pine phase, lodgepole pine, white fir, and limber pine are the prevailing trees. These trees, somewhat shorter and more weather-beaten than those below, exist in small, sometimes dense stands, interspersed with such shrubs as chinquapin, snowbrush, and manzanita.

Excluding relatively small parcels of private land, the bulk of the higher San Gabriel Mountains lies within Angeles

National Forest. Hundreds of square miles of wilderness or near wilderness in the San Gabriels are available within easy reach of millions of L.A. residents.

The 2009 Station Fire devastated the western portion of the San Gabriel Mountains, charring more than 160,000 acres. More than three years later, many affected areas remain closed to aid recovery, while others are open but will be scarred for decades.

The San Bernardino Mountains

Farther east, across the low gap of Cajon Pass, the Transverse Ranges soar again as the San Bernardino Mountains. With Lake Arrowhead, Big Bear Lake, and winter ski areas, the mid-elevations of the San Bernardinos (5,000–8,000 feet in elevation) draw millions of day-trippers and vacationers annually. Hikers and backpackers can explore the 10,000-foot-plus peaks of the San Gorgonio Wilderness, including 11,500-foot San Gorgonio Mountain itself—Southern California's high point. There it is possible to ascend through the yellow-pine and lodgepole belts to treeline and above.

As in the San Gabriel Mountains, islands of private land in the San Bernardinos are surrounded by large sections of national forest. San Bernardino National Forest encompasses much of the San Bernardino Mountains, as well as the San Jacinto and Santa Rosa Mountains to the south.

The most dramatic change taking place in the high mountains of Southern California—especially the San Bernardinos —is a massive die-off of coniferous trees. The high-elevation areas in Southern California have been receiving less precipitation in recent decades. A string of very dry years beginning in 1998–99 triggered an acute infestation of bark beetles, which eventually resulted in sudden death for millions of drought-stressed pine, fir, and cedar trees. Wildfires in October 2003 and 2007 destroyed millions of these dead and dying trees, and many others are being removed by logging operations in an overall effort to thin the forest to attain a more healthy level of tree density.

The Mojave Desert

North and east of the San Gabriel and San Bernardino Mountains lies the vast, arid sweep of the Mojave Desert, a zone only partly included in this book. The Mojave, sometimes known as the high desert for its generally high average elevation, becomes far less populated and more diverse in its natural features as we move toward eastern California. A few of the hikes in this book explore the transitional region between high mountain and high desert.

There, at elevations of 3,000–5,000 feet, thrives the *pinyon-juniper woodland*,

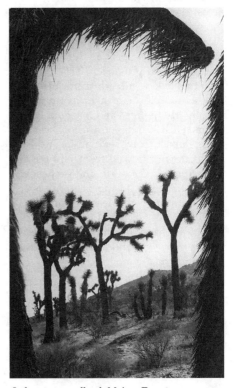

Joshua tree woodland, Mojave Desert

largely characterized by the rather stunted looking one-leaf pinyon pine and the California juniper. Large sections of the Mojave, again in the elevation range of about 3,000–5,000 feet, are dominated by *Joshua tree woodland*. Here the indicator plant is an outsized member of the yucca family—the Joshua tree. Joshua Tree National Park preserves some, but hardly all, of the finest stands of these odd, tree-sized plants.

The San Jacinto Mountains

Moving south from the San Bernardino Mountains and Joshua Tree National Park, we find the northwest-southeast-trending San Jacinto Mountains and their southerly extension, the Santa Rosa Mountains. These lofty ranges comprise the northern ramparts of what geologists call the Peninsular Ranges—so named because they extend, more or less continuously, south across the Mexican border and comprise the spine of the long, thin peninsula of Baja California.

As the highest peak in the entire Peninsular Ranges province, 10,800-foot San Jacinto Peak would outrank all other Southern California peaks were it not for the slightly higher San Gorgonio massif looming just 20 miles north. For sheer dramatic impact, however, San Jacinto wins hands down. Viewed from I-10 outside Palm Springs, the north and east escarpments of San Jacinto appear to rise nearly straight up from the desert floor—10,000 feet in 10 miles or less. Every plant community we have mentioned so far except Joshua tree woodland thrives at one level or another on the mountain.

San Jacinto's pine-clad western slopes shelter several resort communities (such as Idyllwild); otherwise nearly all of the mountain's upper elevations lie within national-forest wilderness or state wilderness areas.

The Colorado Desert

East of the northernmost Peninsular Ranges lie Palm Springs, the Coachella Valley, and the Salton Trough (Salton Sea). They are within the domain known as the Colorado Desert—California's low desert—so called because it stretches west from the lower Colorado River, which divides California from Arizona. A 1,000-square-mile chunk of the Colorado Desert lies within Anza-Borrego Desert State Park, by far the largest state park in California. Especially close and convenient for San Diegans, Anza-Borrego's vast acreage ranges from intricately dissected, desiccated terrain known as badlands to the pinyon-juniper and yellow-pine forests of the Peninsular Ranges.

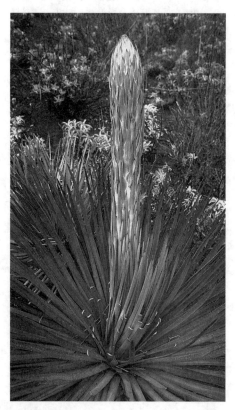

Lord's candle yucca ranges from the coast to the desert rim.

The Laguna, Cuyamaca, Palomar, and Santa Ana Mountains

East and north of San Diego, the Peninsular Ranges consist of a number of parallel ranges—primarily the Laguna, Cuyamaca, and Palomar Ranges—each attaining heights of a little more than 6,000 feet. Chaparral blankets the slopes of these mountains, while the typical yellow-pine assemblage of oak, pine, cedar, and fir dominates the higher elevations. Farther north and west, bordering the rapidly expanding urban zones of southwestern Riverside and southern Orange County, lie the Santa Ana Mountains. They are the northernmost coastal expressions of the Peninsular Ranges.

Suburban sprawl has crept into the foothills of these far-southern ranges, and in some cases threatens to degrade the

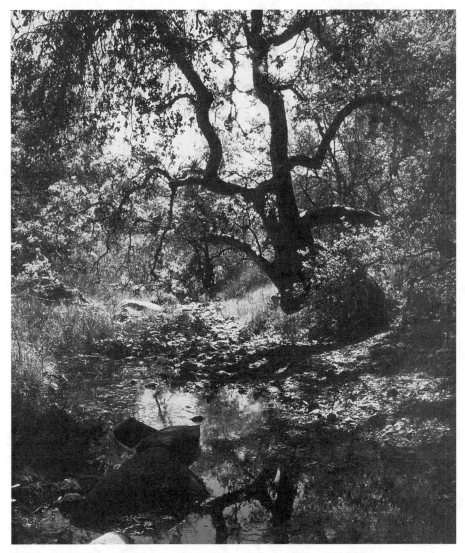

Oak woodland shelters Cole Creek, Santa Rosa Plateau Ecological Reserve (Hike 70).

higher elevations as well. Fortunately, large parts of this mountainous region lie within the jurisdiction of Cleveland National Forest and various state parks.

All the mountain ranges rimming San Diego have been hard-hit recently by both drought and catastrophic wildfire. The 300,000-acre Cedar Fire, which blazed an elongated path across central San Diego County in October 2003, burned through primarily chaparral and oak woodland, and secondarily through prime oak and coniferous forest, mostly in the Cuyamaca Mountains. The chaparral and oak woodlands of lower elevation, adapted to periodic fires, have largely recovered. The formerly lush Cuyamaca Mountains may never look quite the same, however, unless the climate shifts back to a wetter regime.

Health, Safety, and Courtesy

GOOD PREPARATION is always important for any kind of recreational pursuit. Hiking the Southern California backcountry is no exception. Although most of the Southland's natural environments are seldom hostile or dangerous to life and limb, there are some pitfalls to be aware of.

Preparation and Equipment

An obvious safety requirement is being in good health. Some degree of physical conditioning is always desirable, even for the trips in this book designated as easy or moderate. The more challenging trips require increasing amounts of stamina and technical expertise. Running, bicycling, swimming, aerobics, or any similar exercise that develops both your leg muscles and the aerobic capacity of your whole body are recommended as preparatory exercise.

For the longest hikes in this book, there is no really adequate way to prepare other than hiking itself. Start with easy- or moderate-length trips, and then work gradually toward extending both distance and time.

Several of the hiking trips in this book reach elevations of 7,000 feet or more—altitudes at which sea-level folks may notice a big difference in their rate of breathing and stamina. A few hours or a day spent at altitude before exercising will help almost anyone acclimate, but that's often impractical for day trips. Still, you might consider spending a night or two at a campground with some altitude before tackling the likes of 11,500-foot San Gorgonio Mountain. Altitude sickness strikes some victims at elevations as low as 8,000 feet. If you become dizzy or nauseated, or suffer from congested lungs or a severe headache, the antidote may be as simple as descending 1,000–2,000 feet.

Your choice of equipment and supplies on the longer hikes in this book can be critically important. The essentials you should carry with you at all times in the remote backcountry are the things that would allow you to survive, in a reasonably comfortable manner, one or two unscheduled nights out. It's important to note that no one ever plans these nights! No one plans to get lost, injured, stuck, or pinned down by the weather. Always do a "what if" analysis for a worst-case scenario, and plan accordingly. These essential items are your safety net; keep them with you on day hikes, and take them with you in a small day pack if you leave your backpack and camping equipment behind at a campsite.

Chief among the essential items is *warm clothing*. Inland Southern California is characterized by wide swings in day and night temperatures. In mountain valleys susceptible to cold-air drainage, for example, a midday temperature in the 70s or 80s is often followed by a subfreezing night. Carry light, inner layers of clothing consisting of polypropylene or wool (best for cool or cold weather) or cotton (adequate for warm or hot weather but very poor for cold and damp weather). Include a thicker insulating layer of synthetic fill, wool, or down to put on whenever you need it, especially when you are not moving around and generating heat. Add to these items a cap, gloves, and a waterproof or water-resistant shell (a large trash bag will do in a pinch)—and you'll be quite prepared for all but the most severe weather. In hot, sunny weather, sun-shielding clothing, including a sun hat and a light-colored, long-sleeve top, may also be essential.

Water and *food* are next in importance. Most streams and even some springs in the mountains have been shown to contain unacceptably high levels of bacteria or other contaminants. Even though most of the remote watersheds are probably pristine, it's wise to treat by filtering or chemical methods any water obtained outside of developed camp or picnic sites. Unless the day is very warm or your trip is a long one, it's usually easiest to carry (preferably in sturdy plastic bottles or a CamelBak) all the water you'll need. Don't underestimate your water needs: During a full day's hike in 80° temperatures you may require as much as a gallon of water. Know, too, that many springs and watercourses—even some shown as being permanent on topographic maps—may run dry at some point during the summer. Food is necessary to stave off the feeling of hunger and keep your energy stores up, but it is not nearly as critical as water is in emergency situations where you are in danger of dehydration.

Farther down the list but still essential are a *map* and *compass* (or a GPS unit and knowing how to use it), a *flashlight, fire-starting devices* (for example, waterproof matches, a lighter, or a candle), and a *first-aid kit*.

Items not always essential, but potentially very useful and convenient, are sunglasses, a pocketknife, a whistle (or other signaling device), sunscreen, and toilet paper. (*Note:* Sunglasses are an essential item for travel over snow.)

Every member of a hiking party should carry all these essential items because individuals or splinter groups may end up separating from the party

for one reason or another. If you plan to hike solo in the backcountry, being well-equipped is very important. If you hike alone, be sure to check in with a park ranger or leave your itinerary with a responsible person. That way, if you do get stuck, help will probably come to the right place—eventually.

Special Hazards

Other than the possibility of your getting lost or pinned down by a rare sudden storm, the most common hazards found in the Southland are steep, unstable terrain; icy terrain; spiny plants; rattlesnakes; mountain lions; ticks; and poison oak.

Falls

Exploring some trails—especially those of the San Gabriel Mountains—may involve traveling over structurally weak rock on steep slopes. The erosive effects of flowing water, of wedging by roots and by ice, and of brush fires tend to pulverize such rock even further. Slips on such terrain usually lead to sliding down a hillside some distance. If you explore cross-country, always be on the lookout for dangerous run-outs, such as cliffs, below you. The sidewalls of many canyons in the San Gabriels may look like fun places to practice rock-climbing moves, but this misconception has caused many deaths over the years.

Snow and Ice

Statistically, mishaps associated with snow and ice have caused the greatest number of fatalities in the San Gabriel and San Bernardino Mountains. This is not because our local mountains are inherently more dangerous than the Sierra Nevada, the Cascades, or other ranges. Rather, it is because the novelty of snow and easy access by way of snow-plowed highways attract inexperienced lowlanders, who never picture their backyard mountains as true wilderness areas. Icy chutes and slopes capable of avalanching

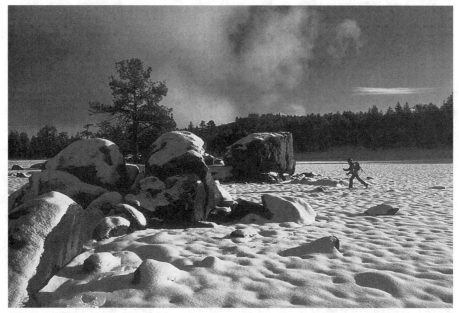

Winter at 6,000 feet in the Laguna Mountains

can easily trap such visitors unaware. Visitors can explore the gentler areas of the high country on snowshoes or skis, but the steeper slopes require technical skills and equipment such as an ice ax and crampons, just as other snow-covered mountain ranges do.

Puncturing Plants

Most desert hikers will sooner or later suffer punctures by thorns or spines. This is most likely to happen during close encounters with the cholla, or jumping, cactus, whose spine clusters readily break off and attach firmly to your skin, clothes, or boots. A comb will allow you to gently pull away the spine clusters, and tweezers or lightweight pliers will help you remove any individual embedded spines. Another problematic spiny plant is the agave, or century plant. It consists of a rosette of fleshy leaves, each tipped with a rigid thorn containing a mild toxin. A headlong fall into either an agave or one of the more vicious kinds of cacti could easily make you swear off desert travel

permanently. It's best to give these devilish plants as wide a berth as possible.

Rattlesnakes

Rattlesnakes are common everywhere in Southern California below an elevation of about 7,000 feet. Seldom seen in either cold or very hot weather, they favor temperatures in the 75°–90° range—spring and fall in the desert and coastal areas and summer in the mountains. Most rattlesnakes are as interested in avoiding contact with you as you are with them.

Watch carefully where you put your feet and especially your hands during the warmer months. In brushy or rocky areas where you cannot see as far, try to make your presence known. Tread with heavy footfalls, or bang a stick against rocks or bushes. Rattlesnakes will pick up the vibrations through their skin and will usually buzz (an unmistakable sound) before you get too close for comfort. Most bad encounters between rattlesnakes and hikers occur in April and May, when

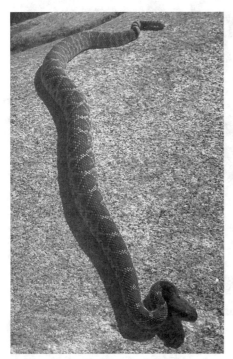

Red diamond rattlesnake

snakes are irritable and hungry after their long hibernation period.

Mountain Lions

Mountain-lion attacks, although statistically rare, have been increasing all over California in the past three decades. This trend may continue as the natural habitat for these carnivorous cats becomes more and more fragmented by suburban and rural development. Several attacks and many more incidents of threatening behavior by mountain lions toward humans have taken place in urban-edge park and national-forest lands, such as those covered in this book.

Here are some basic tips for dealing with this potential hazard:

- Hike with one or more companions.
- Keep children close at hand.
- Never run from a mountain lion. This may trigger an instinct to attack.
- Make yourself large: face the animal, maintain eye contact with it, shout, blow a whistle, and do not act fearful. Do anything you can to convince the animal that you are not its prey.

Ticks

Ticks can be the scourge of overgrown trails in the coastal foothills and lower mountain slopes, particularly during the first warm spells of the year, when they climb to the tips of shrub branches and lie in wait for warm-blooded hosts. If you can't avoid brushing against vegetation along the trail, be sure to check yourself for ticks frequently. Upon finding a host, a tick will usually crawl upward in search of a protected spot, where it will try to attach itself. If you are aware of the slightest irritation on your body, you'll usually intercept ticks long before they attempt to bite. Ticks would be of relatively minor concern here, except that tick-borne Lyme disease, which can have serious health effects, has been reported within Southern California.

Poison Oak

Poison oak grows profusely along many of the coastal and mountain canyons below 5,000 feet in elevation. It is often found on the banks of streamcourses in the form of a bush or vine, where it prefers semi-shady habitats. Quite often, it's seen beside or encroaching on well-used trails. Learn to recognize its distinctive three-leafed structure, and avoid touching it with skin or clothing. Since poison oak loses its leaves during the winter months (and sometimes during summer and fall drought), but still retains some of the toxic oil in its stems, it can be extra hazardous at that time because it is harder to identify and avoid. Mid-weight pants, like blue jeans, and a long-sleeve shirt will serve as a fair barrier against the toxic oil of the poison oak plant. Do, of course, remove these clothes as soon as the hike is over, and make sure they are washed carefully afterward.

Other Safety Concerns

Deer-hunting season in Southern California usually runs through the middle part

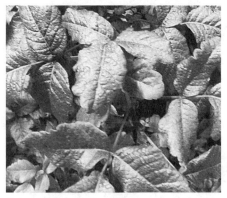

Poison oak leaves

of the autumn. Although conflicts between hunters and hikers are rare, you may want to confine your autumn explorations to state and county parks, as well as wilderness areas where hunting is prohibited.

There is always some risk in leaving a vehicle unattended at a trailhead. It may be worthwhile to disable your car's ignition or attach an antitheft device to your steering wheel. Never leave valuable property visible in an automobile, so as to be an invitation for a break-in. Report all theft and vandalism of personal or public property to the local county sheriff or the appropriate park or forest agency.

Permits and Camping

Some trails on national-forest lands (Angeles, San Bernardino, and Cleveland National Forests) are at present subject to the National Forest Adventure Pass program. This applies only to vehicles parked on national forest land and not to users who arrive on foot or by bicycle. Adventure passes are available at all national-forest offices, ranger stations, and fire stations. They are also sold through hundreds of vendors—typically sport shops throughout the region, gas stations and markets near the principal national-forest entry roads, and small businesses within national-forest borders. Adventure passes cost $5 per day

or $30 for a year. The adventure pass must be prominently displayed on your parked car—otherwise your car will likely be ticketed and fined.

If you plan to visit national-forest territory more than two or three times a year, it is time-efficient at the very least to purchase the $30 yearly pass instead of worrying about obtaining one each day you come up for a visit. Rules for the adventure pass program tend to change rapidly; in fact, the program may be rescinded in the future. Another option is the $80 Interagency Annual Pass, which also covers national parks and many other federal lands.

If you are planning an overnight trip of some type into the Southern California backcountry, be aware that camping in roadside campgrounds is not always a restful experience. Off-season camping (late fall through early spring) offers relief from crowds, but not from chilly nighttime weather. Most national forest campgrounds are less well supervised than those in state and county parks, which means that they sometimes attract a noisy crowd. In my experience, facilities with a campground host promise a quieter clientele and a better night's sleep.

The nice advantage of a developed campground is that you can always have a campfire there—unless the facility is closed. On trails where backpacking is allowed, fire regulations vary. Most jurisdictions prohibit campfires all or part of the year. Others permit fires, as long as you have the necessary free permit.

Some national forest areas allow remote, primitive-style camping: you are not always restricted to staying at a developed campground or designated trail camp. For sanitation reasons, you must locate your camp well away from the nearest source of water. And, of course, you must observe the fire regulations stated earlier. Always check with the US Forest Service to confirm these rules if you intend to do any remote camping.

Most federally managed wilderness areas around the state require special wilderness permits for entry. Many in Southern California have self-registering permits at trailheads; others require permits only for overnight visits. The San Gorgonio and San Jacinto Wildernesses are so popular that their managing agencies sometimes implement trailhead quotas.

Trail Courtesy

Whenever you travel the backcountry, you take on a burden of responsibility—keeping the wilderness as you found it. Aside from commonsense prohibitions against littering, vandalism, and inappropriate campfires, there are some less obvious guidelines every hiker should be aware of. We'll mention a few:

Never cut trail switchbacks. This practice breaks down the trail tread and hastens erosion. Try to improve designated trails by removing branches, rocks, or other debris. Springtime growth can quite rapidly obscure pathways in the chaparral country, and funding for trail maintenance is often scarce; try to do your part by joining a volunteer trail crew or by performing your own small maintenance tasks while walking the trails. Report any damage to trails or other facilities to the appropriate ranger office.

When backpacking, be a Leave No Trace camper. Leave your campsite as you found it—or leave it in an even more natural condition.

Collecting specimens of minerals, plants, animals, and historical objects without a special permit is prohibited in most jurisdictions. These regulations usually cover common things, such as pinecones, wildflowers, and lizards, too. Leave them for all visitors to enjoy. Limited collecting of items like pinecones may be allowed on some national forest lands—check with the local agency first.

We've covered most of the general regulations associated with Southern California's public lands, but you, as a visitor, are responsible for **knowing any additional rules as well.** Each hike described in this book includes a reference to the agency responsible for the area you'll be visiting. Phone numbers for those agencies appear in the back of this book. Internet research is often helpful, too. Using a search engine, enter key words for the park or area in question to find an abundance of information. The quality of this information, however, varies, and it is important to note the date of its posting and the source itself.

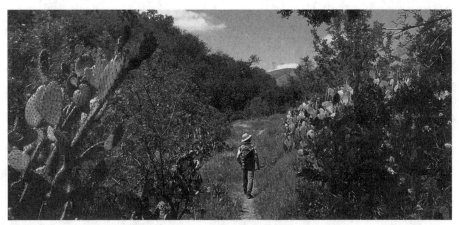

Water Canyon Trail, Chino Hills State Park

Using This Book

THERE ARE THREE PRINCIPAL WAYS to find hiking trips in this book that are suitable for you. First, you can check the overview map for all 101 hikes in this book, pages x–xi, and restrict your search to a specific geographic area. Second, you can scan the hike overview table (pages xii–xv) that appears after the overview map. Third, you can leaf through the book, browsing hike summaries, descriptions, and photos.

To get the most out of this guide, please take the time to carefully read, below, about the meaning of the capsulized information that appears before each hike description.

Sketch maps are provided for each hike. The boxed T (trailhead) symbol on each map denotes the start point of the hike it depicts, and it lists the GPS coordinates for the trailhead in decimal degrees. One-way (point-to-point) hikes have two T symbols—one for the beginning of the hike and one for end of the hike. For

nearly all hikes described in this book, the sketch map we provide is adequate for basic navigation. For a few hikes, the capsulized summary recommends a specific detailed topographic map by name.

Capsulized Summaries

Each hike begins with a capsulized summary that details its location, highlights, distance, elevation gain and loss, time required, optional or recommended maps, best times, managing agency, difficulty rating, and trail uses.

Location. The general location of the hike is stated: a well-known park, mountain range, or nearby city or town.

Highlights. One or two engaging features of the hike are mentioned.

Distance. An estimate of total distance is given. For hikes shorter than 6 miles, the distance is given to the nearest tenth of a mile. For hikes 6 miles and longer, their distance is rounded to the nearest

---

Map Legend

Freeway	**T** Trailhead
Highway	**P** Parking Area
Secondary Highway	**△** Campground
Minor Road	Ranger Station/Visitor Center
Unpaved Road	**A** Picnic Area
Trail/Hiking Route	**▲** Mountain
Cross Country Route	**■** Point of Interest
Drainage (canyon, creek)	●—● Gate
	Ϯ Oasis

whole number. Out-and-back trips show the sum of the distances of the out-and-back segments. This section also indicates what type of trip it is: out-and-back, one way, or loop.

Total Elevation Gain/Loss. These are estimates of the sum of all the vertical gain segments and the sum of all the vertical loss segments along the total length of the route (both ways for out-and-back trips). This is often considerably more than the net difference in elevation between the high and low points of the hike.

Hiking Time. This figure is for the average hiker, and includes only the time spent in motion. It *does not* include time spent for rest stops, lunch, and so on. Fast walkers can complete the routes in perhaps 30% less time, and slower hikers may take 50% longer. We assume the hiker is traveling with a light day pack. (*Important note:* The hiking time stated in this book is for *time-in-motion* only. Also, hikers carrying heavy packs could easily take nearly twice as long, especially if they are traveling under adverse weather conditions. Remember, too, that the progress made by a group as a whole is limited by the pace of its slowest member.)

Optional or Recommended Map(s). The topographic maps listed are nearly all U.S. Geological Survey 7.5-minute series topographic maps. Usually, these are the most complete and accurate maps of the physical features (if not always the cultural features and trails) of the area you'll be traveling in. These maps are typically stocked by backpacking, outdoor sports, and map shops around the Southland. Topographic maps available on CD or downloadable from the Internet are popular alternatives to hard-copy topographic maps.

Best Times. Because of the extreme heat, avoid the longer desert trips in this book during any period except the one recommended here. Trips elsewhere in Southern California are usually safe enough, but less rewarding, outside their best times.

Agency. These code letters refer to the agency or office that has jurisdiction over or manages the area being hiked (for example, CNF/TD means Cleveland National Forest, Trabuco District). Contact the agency for more information about a particular hike and its current regulations. Full names, phone numbers, and some addresses (of larger agencies) are listed in "Agencies and Information Sources" (page 267).

Difficulty. This subjective, overall rating takes into account the length of the hike and the nature of the terrain. The following are general definitions of the five categories:

Easy. Suitable for every member of the family.

Moderate. Suitable for all physically fit people.

Moderately strenuous. Long length, substantial elevation gain, and/or difficult terrain. Recommended for experienced hikers only.

Strenuous. A full day's hike (or a backpack trip) over a long and/or challenging route. Suitable only for experienced hikers in excellent physical condition.

Very strenuous. Long and rugged route in extremely remote area. Suitable only for experienced hikers or climbers in top physical condition. Only three hikes in this book—Down the East Fork (Hike 30), San Jacinto Peak: Hard Way (Hike 53), and Villager Peak (Hike 96)—get this rating.

Each higher level represents more or less a doubling of the difficulty.

Trail Use. This field mentions whether dogs are allowed, whether a given hike is appropriate for kids, and more.

Permit. This section is included only for trips that require permits, usually for overnight use.

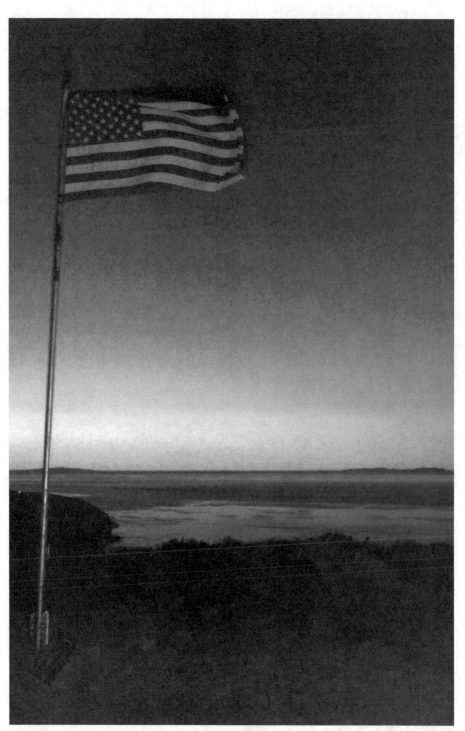

Sunrise on Mugu Peak (Hike 3)

HIKE 1

Paradise Falls

Location	Wildwood Park, City of Thousand Oaks
Highlights	Gem of a waterfall in a steep gorge
Distance	2.7 miles (loop)
Total Elevation Gain/Loss	400'/400'
Hiking Time	2 hours
Optional Map	USGS 7.5-minute *Newbury Park*
Best Times	All year
Agency	CRPD
Difficulty	Moderate
Trail Use	Dogs allowed, good for kids

Wildwood Park in Thousand Oaks is Ventura County's most scenic suburban park. The scenery here has been imprinted in the minds of many in the over-50 age group: The area was once an outdoor set for old Hollywood movies, as well as for television's *The Rifleman, Gunsmoke,* and *Wagon Train.* The short but steep hike—down and then up—described here takes you to Wildwood Park's scenic gem: the Arroyo Conejo gorge and Paradise Falls. The lovingly maintained park offers drinking fountains, picnic tables, interpretive signs, and shady rest spots along this fine loop.

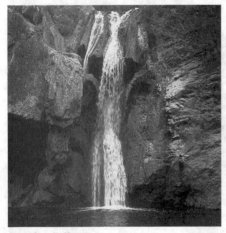

Paradise Falls

To Reach the Trailhead: From the 101 Freeway at Exit 45 in Thousand Oaks, take Lynn Road north 2.5 miles to Avenida de los Arboles. Turn left and follow Avenida de los Arboles 1 mile west. At this point traffic goes sharply right on Big Sky Drive; you make a U-turn and park on the right at Wildwood Park's principal trailhead, open 8 a.m.–5 p.m. Nearby curbside parking is also available.

Description: Three trails radiate from the Avenida de los Arboles trailhead. Two are wide and relatively bland dirt roads. The third (the one you want), the narrow and scenic Moonridge Trail, descends sharply from the east side of the parking area. This is the left side of the parking area as you drive in. Right away you come to a T-intersection amid oak woods. Turn right, remaining on the Moonridge Trail. The trail descends a sunny slope covered with aromatic sage-scrub vegetation and dappled with succulent live-forever plants that sprout white, comical-looking flower stalks. Beware of the prickly pear cactus flanking the trail. There's a brief passage across a shady ravine using wooden steps and a plank bridge. At 0.5 mile, you cross over a dirt road and continue on the narrow Moonridge Trail.

Ahead, the trail curls around a deep ravine, edging into the crumbly sedimentary rock. At 0.9 mile you join another dirt road and use it to descend toward a large wooden teepee structure on a knoll just below. Make a right at the teepee, further descending into the Arroyo Conejo gorge. As you descend, watch for the narrow side trail on the left that will take you straight down to Paradise Falls—a beautiful, 30-foot-high cascade that makes its presence known by sound before sight. The high water table in the canyon bottom ensures a nearly year-round flow of water. Watch for poison oak, especially on the far side of the creek.

After you've admired the falls, continue by climbing back up the slope in the direction you came, and take the fenced, cliff-hanging trail around the left (east) side of the falls. Beyond that fenced stretch, the narrow trail descends a little and sidles up alongside the creek, where large coast live oaks spread their shade. Soon, you continue on a path of dirt-road width. Stay with that path until you reach a major crossroads. It's worth a 0.1-mile detour straight ahead to walk through Indian Cave. Then, returning to the junction, cross the bridge. The small Wildwood Nature Center is just around the bend to the right, and your return route up along Indian Creek is to the left.

On the Indian Creek Trail, you pay your debt to gravity by ascending nearly 300 feet in about 0.7 mile. The beautifully tangled array of live oak and sycamore limbs along this trail keeps your mind off the climb. At one point, you can look down into a deep ravine where an inaccessible mini-waterfall and pool lie practically hidden. When you finally reach Avenida de los Arboles, turn left and then return a short distance to the trailhead parking lot.

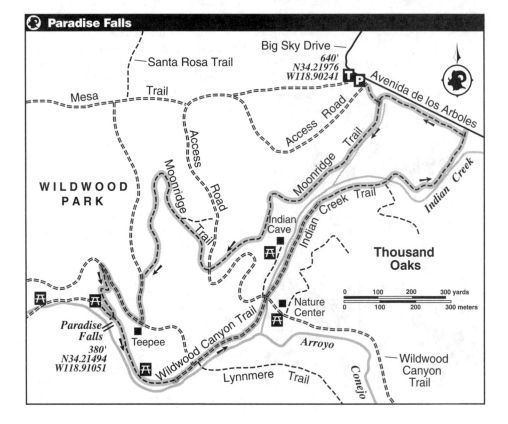

HIKE 2

Happy Camp Canyon

Location	Near Moorpark and Simi Valley
Highlights	Prime oak woodland and strange rock formations
Distance	11 miles (loop)
Total Elevation Gain/Loss	1,300'/1,300'
Hiking Time	5 hours
Optional Map	USGS 7.5-minute *Simi*
Best Times	October–June
Agency	SMMC
Difficulty	Moderately strenuous
Trail Use	Suitable for mountain bikes

Happy Camp Canyon nuzzles in a crease between the long, rounded ridge called Big Mountain, just north of Simi Valley, and Oak Ridge, a taller parallel ridge to the north. These ridges and plenty more, like the Santa Monica Mountains, are caterpillarlike, parallel segments of the Transverse Ranges, which stretch from Santa Barbara County in the west to San Bernardino County to the east.

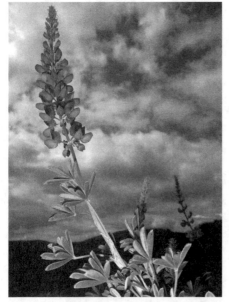

Lupine on Middle Range Fire Trail

Oil-bearing shales predominate in this region, evidenced by various oil wells and dirt roads built to access them scattered across the surrounding hillsides. On your ramble through the lower and middle parts of the canyon, keep an eye out for bright red stones, sometimes exhibiting a glassy texture, some right under your feet and others visible in outcrops. These rocks were formed by the slow combustion of organic material trapped in layers of shale.

Happy Camp Canyon itself remains quite pristine. Several groups of Chumash Indians called this place home in past centuries; later it became a part of an immense cattle ranch founded by a pioneer Simi Valley family. Purchased as a future state park in the late 1960s, it was traded to Ventura County for use as a regional park. Today, save for a few dirt roads and a smattering of artifacts from the days of cattle ranching, the 3,000-acre canyon park serves as prime natural habitat for native plants and animals and a restful retreat for hikers seeking to escape from the sights and sounds of city and suburban life. Beware that you may still run into cattle in the canyon. The October 2003 Simi Fire consumed most of the canyon's hillside sage-scrub and chaparral vegetation, and the scorched trees still show scars.

To Reach the Trailhead: To get to the Happy Camp Canyon's principal trailhead, follow the 118 Freeway west from Simi Valley or the 23 Freeway north from Thousand Oaks to the New Los Angeles Avenue exit. Go west 1 mile to Moorpark Avenue (signed Highway 23), turn right, and proceed 2.6 miles to where Highway 23 makes a sharp bend to the left. Keep going straight here, but then make an immediate right turn on Broadway. Proceed a short way to the east end of Broadway to a spacious dirt parking lot and trailhead.

Description: On foot, follow the trail that winds north and east along gentle, grassy slopes down onto the wide floor of Happy Camp Canyon. As you look down on a golf course at the canyon's mouth, note the terraced aspect of the landscape on both sides. These are fluvial (streamside) terraces, sedimentary deposits from earlier flows of Happy Camp Canyon's Creek.

Pass two minor side trails on the left (leading up to a maze of equestrian trails on the hill) and then another two on the right. At 1.0 mile you join the dirt Happy Camp Canyon Fire Road in the bottom of the canyon. Turn left, and 0.2 mile later you pass through a gate marking the start of the wilderness section of Happy Camp Canyon Park. At a fork just beyond, stay left (north) into the main canyon.

By 2.0 miles, the canyon floor has narrowed, and you've turned decidedly east and are strolling through beautiful

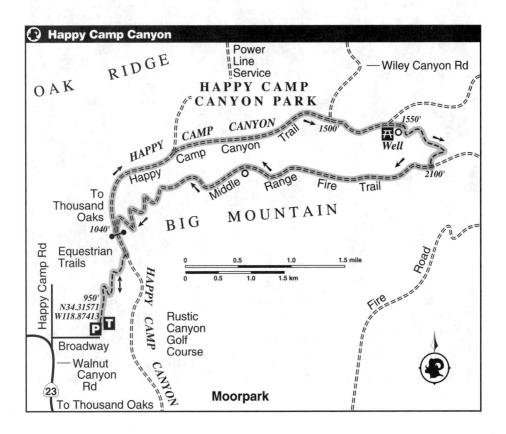

coast live-oak woods (plus native syca-more and walnut trees), which continue intermittently up the canyon in the next 3 miles. A little stream flows in the bottom of the canyon during and for some weeks or months after the winter rains. You're climbing at a gentle rate of about 200 feet per mile. You pass the ascending Wiley Canyon Road on the left at 4.1 miles, and at 4.7 miles you reach the site of an old well and pump. Large oak trees shade a cluster of picnic tables for a convenient lunch stop.

Continue following the graded dirt road about 300 yards past the well. The road ends, but a bulldozed track, eroded and very steep at first, curls 0.7 mile up the south slope of Happy Camp Canyon and then joins Middle Range Fire Trail on the crest of Big Mountain. If you are coming from the other direction, the easy-to-miss junction is marked by a cairn on a saddle. Use that ridge-running fire trail to return to lower Happy Camp Canyon at a point just above the gate marking the wilder-ness area boundary.

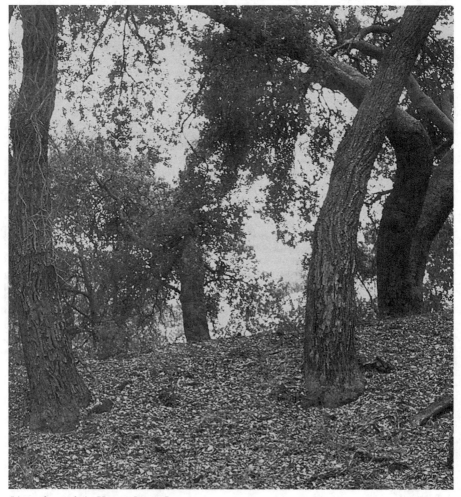

Live-oak woods in Happy Camp Canyon

HIKE 3

La Jolla Valley Loop

Location	Point Mugu State Park
Highlights	Spectacular ocean views and rare native vegetation
Distance	11 miles (loop)
Total Elevation Gain/Loss	1,950'/1,950'
Hiking Time	6 hours
Optional Maps	Trails Illustrated Santa Monica Mountains National Recreation Area, Point Mugu State Park map, or USGS 7.5-minute *Point Mugu*
Best Times	8 a.m.–sunset, October–June
Agency	PMSP
Difficulty	Moderately strenuous
Trail Use	Suitable for backpacking
Permit	Required for overnight use

Lazily curving up the rumpled slopes of the western Santa Monica Mountains, the Ray Miller Trail takes in sweeping views of the Point Mugu coastline and the distant Channel Islands. This is the westernmost link in the nearly completed Backbone Trail, which skims along the crest of the Santa Monicas for some 65 miles. The Ray Miller Trail offers a well-graded and scenic approach to the rounded ridge that divides the two largest canyons in Point Mugu State Park: La Jolla and Big Sycamore. The trail was named after California's first official State Park Campground Host, who served here from 1979 until his death in 1989.

The Ray Miller Trail is just the start of the big loop we're suggesting here: a comprehensive trek through the western quadrant of Point Mugu State Park. If this is too big a chunk to bite off for a single day, there are shortcuts, as our map suggests. You could also extend your trip by staying overnight at La Jolla Valley Walk-In Camp. For that, you must register with a park ranger across the highway at Thornhill Broome Beach Campground.

The May 2013 Springs Fire, driven by unseasonably high temperatures, strong winds, and dry conditions, swept from Thousand Oaks to the Pacific and damaged the state park. Check if the park is open before paying a visit, and stay on trail to protect regenerating vegetation.

To Reach the Trailhead: Point Mugu State Park lies some 32 miles west of Santa Monica via Pacific Coast Highway (Highway 1). Immediately west of the Thornhill Broome Beach Campground, turn north onto a poorly marked road, and follow it to the end for the Ray Miller Trailhead parking. If you haven't registered for overnight camping, pay your day-use fee at the parking area.

Description: Two trails diverge from the parking lot. The wide one going up along the dry canyon bottom ahead is the La Jolla Canyon Trail, your return route. To begin, take the narrower Ray Miller Trail to your right. It doggedly climbs 2.7 miles to a junction with the Overlook Trail, a wide fire road. This is the major ascent along the loop—better to get it over with at the beginning. Ever-widening views of the ocean and fine, springtime wildflower displays keep your mind off the effort.

Turn left when you reach the Overlook Trail, and wend your way around several bumps on the undulating ridge. Enjoy the terrific views of Boney Mountain's eroded volcanic core to the east and La Jolla Valley's grassy fields to the west. You arrive at a saddle (4.5 miles from the start), where five wide trails diverge. Take the trail to the left (west) that descends into the green- or flaxen-colored (depending on the season) La Jolla Valley.

The valley is managed by the state park as a natural preserve to protect the native bunchgrasses that flourish there. Because so much of California's coast ranges have been biologically disturbed by grazing for more than a century, opportunistic, non-native grasses have taken over just about everywhere. The authentic California tallgrass prairie in parts of La Jolla Valley is a notable exception.

The La Jolla Valley Walk-In Camp ahead has an outhouse and oak-shaded picnic tables. Bring your own water if you plan to camp; the faucets are not operational at the time of this writing. Just south of there, beside a trail leading directly back to the Ray Miller Trailhead, you'll find a tule-fringed pond, seasonally dry in some years. Look for chocolate lilies on the slopes around it.

From the camp, continue west in the direction of a military radar installation on Laguna Peak. Stay right where marked trails diverge to the left, circling the perimeter of the La Jolla Valley grassland and

rising sharply on the Chumash Trail to a saddle (7 miles) on the northwest shoulder of the Mugu Peak ridge. At that saddle you'll have a great view of the Pacific Ocean. The popping noises you may hear below are from a military shooting range, near the Pacific Coast Highway. Up the coast is the Point Mugu Naval Air Station.

Beyond the saddle, the Chumash Trail descends sharply to the Pacific Coast Highway. You veer left on the Mugu Peak Trail, and contour south and east around the south flank of Mugu Peak. (Alternatively, a use trail on the left just before the saddle shortcuts directly to the peak.) You arrive (8 miles) at another saddle just east of Mugu's 1,266-foot summit. Five minutes of climbing on a steep path puts you on top, where there's a dizzying view of the east-west-oriented coastline. You can look down upon The Great Sand Dune (coastal dunes) and the Pacific Coast Highway where it squeezes past some coastal bluffs. On warm days there's a desertlike feel to this rocky and sparsely vegetated mountain, oddly juxtaposed with the sights and sounds of the surf below.

Return to the saddle east of the peak, and continue descending to a junction in a wooded recess of La Jolla Canyon. Turn right, proceed east along a hillside, and then hook up with the La Jolla Canyon Trail, where you turn right.

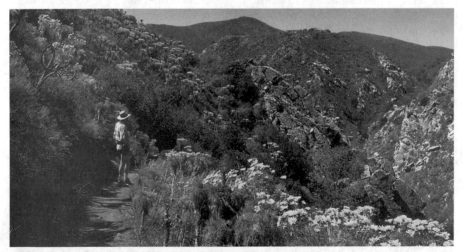

La Jolla Canyon Trail, with giant coreopsis in bloom

There's an exciting stretch through a rock-walled section of La Jolla Canyon, where giant coreopsis bloom in spring. Quite common in the Channel Islands, this plant is found only in scattered coastal locales from far western Los Angeles County to San Luis Obispo County. Some coreopsis plants have forked stems towering as high as 10 feet. The massed, yellow, daisylike flowers are an unforgettable sight in March and April.

Descending toward the canyon's mouth, you pass a little grove of native walnut trees and a small, seasonal waterfall. After a final descent, join a dirt road built to haul stone out of the area for the construction of the coast highway, and arrive a few minutes later at the trailhead.

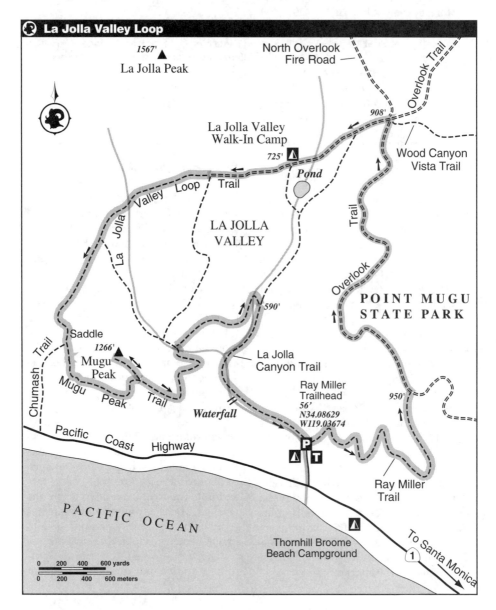

HIKE 4

Sandstone Peak

Location	Circle X Ranch (Santa Monica Mountains National Recreation Area)
Highlights	Most inclusive view in the Santa Monicas and volcanic rock formations
Distance	6 miles (loop)
Total Elevation Gain/Loss	1,400'/1,400'
Hiking Time	3½ hours
Optional Maps	Trails Illustrated Santa Monica Mountains National Recreation Area or USGS 7.5-minute *Triunfo Pass* and *Newbury Park*
Best Times	October–June
Agency	SMMNRA
Difficulty	Moderately strenuous
Trail Use	Dogs allowed

Sandstone Peak is the quintessential destination for peak baggers in the Santa Monica Mountains. The 3,111-foot summit can be efficiently climbed from the east via the Backbone Trail in a mere 1.5 miles, but the far more scenic way to go is the loop outlined below. Take a picnic lunch, and plan to make a half day of it. Try to come on a crystalline day in late fall or winter to get the best skyline views. Or, if it's wildflowers you most enjoy, come in April or May, when the native vegetation blooms most profusely at these middle elevations. In addition to blue-flowering stands of ceanothus, the early- to mid-spring floral bloom includes monkeyflower, nightshade, Chinese houses, wild peony, wild hyacinth, morning glory, and phacelia. Delicate, orangish Humboldt lilies unfold by June. Beware of poison oak growing alongside the trail.

Sandstone Peak lies within Circle X Ranch, formerly owned by the Boy Scouts of America and now a federally managed unit of the Santa Monica Mountains National Recreation Area. The National Park Service generously provides free trail maps at the trailhead.

To Reach the Trailhead: The Sandstone Peak Trailhead is located near the western end of the Santa Monica Mountains, a few miles (by crow's flight) south of Thousand Oaks. From the Pacific Coast Highway near mile marker 1 VEN 1.00, turn north onto Yerba Buena Rd. and proceed 6.4 miles.

Or from US 101 in Thousand Oaks, take CA 23 south for 7.2 miles. Turn right (west) on Mulholland Highway, then in 0.4 mile turn right again onto Little Sycamore Canyon, which soon becomes Yerba Buena Road and reaches the trailhead in 4.5 miles. On either approach, you face a white-knuckle drive on paved, but very narrow and curvy roads.

Description: Start hiking at the large parking lot on the north side of Yerba Buena Road, 1.1 miles east of the Circle X Ranch park office. Proceed on foot past a gate and up a fire road 0.3 mile to where the marked Mishe Mokwa Trail branches right. On it, right away you plunge into tough, scratchy chaparral vegetation.

The hand-tooled route is delightfully primitive, but it requires frequent maintenance so as to keep the chaparral from knitting together across the path. Both your hands and your feet will come into play over the next 40 or 50 minutes as you're forced to scramble a bit over rough-textured outcrops of volcanic rock. You make intimate acquaintance with mosses and ferns and several of the more attractive chaparral shrubs: toyon, holly-leaf cherry, manzanita, and red shanks (also known as ribbonwood), which is identified by its wispy foliage and perpetually peeling, rust-colored bark. You also pass several small bay trees. After about a half hour on the Mishe Mokwa Trail, keep an eye out for an amazing balanced rock that rests precariously on the opposite wall of the canyon that lies just below you.

By 1.7 miles from the start you will have worked your way around to the north flank of Sandstone Peak, where you suddenly come upon a picnic table shaded beneath glorious oaks beside Split Rock, a fractured volcanic boulder with a gap wide enough to walk through

(please do so to maintain the Scouts' tradition). An unmaintained trail on the right leads to Balanced Rock, but you continue on the vestiges of an old dirt road that crosses the canyon and turns west (upstream). You pass beneath some hefty volcanic outcrops, and at 3.1 miles come to a signed junction and turn left onto the Backbone Trail toward Sandstone Peak.

Pass some water tanks on the right and an unsigned service road up to the tanks. Shortly thereafter, a sign on the right indicates a side trail to Inspiration Point. It takes you about 50 yards to the top of a rock outcrop. The direction-finder there indicates local features as well as very distant points such as Mount San Antonio (Old Baldy), Santa Catalina Island, and San Clemente Island.

Press on with your ascent. At a point just past two closely spaced hairpin turns in the wide Backbone Trail, make your way up a slippery path to Sandstone Peak's windswept top. The plaque on the summit block honors W. Herbert Allen, a

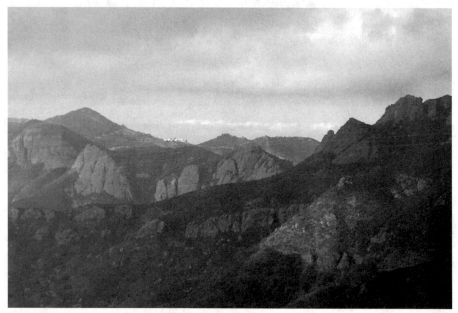

Boney Mountain

longtime benefactor of the Scouts and Circle X Ranch. To the Scouts this mountain is Mount Allen, although cartographers have, so far, not accepted that name. In any event, the peak's real name is misleading. It, along with Boney Mountain and most of the western crest of the Santa Monicas, consists of beige- and rust-colored volcanic rock, not unlike sandstone when seen from a distance.

On a clear day the view is truly amazing from here, with distant mountain ranges, the hazy L.A. Basin, and the island-dimpled surface of the ocean occupying all 360 degrees of the horizon. To complete the loop, return to the Backbone Trail and resume your travel eastward. Descend a twisting 1.5 miles to return to the trailhead.

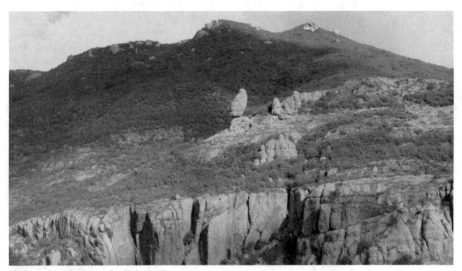

Balanced rock above the Dihedrals

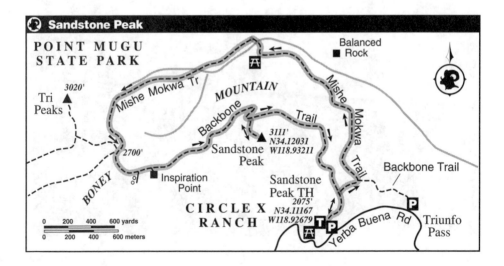

HIKE 5

The Grotto

Location	Circle X Ranch (Santa Monica Mountains National Recreation Area)
Highlights	Spooky rock formations and live oak groves
Distance	2.8 miles (out-and-back)
Total Elevation Gain/Loss	650'/650'
Hiking Time	2 hours
Optional Maps	Trails Illustrated Santa Monica Mountains National Recreation Area or USGS 7.5-minute *Triunfo Pass*
Best Times	All year
Agency	SMMNRA
Difficulty	Moderate
Trail Use	Dogs allowed, good for kids

The 1,655-acre Circle X Ranch, formerly run by the Boy Scouts of America but now administered by the National Park Service, is positively riddled with Tom Sawyer–esque hiking paths. Chief among those is the Grotto Trail, perfect for young or young-in-thought adventurers. This hike is almost entirely downhill on the way in and uphill on the way back. Plan accordingly and bring enough drinking water.

To Reach the Trailhead: The Circle X Ranch Ranger Station is located near the western end of the Santa Monica Mountains, a few miles (by crow's flight) south of Thousand Oaks. From the Pacific Coast Highway near mile marker 1 VEN 1.00, turn north onto Yerba Buena Road and proceed 5.4 miles.

Or from US 101 in Thousand Oaks, take CA 23 south for 7.2 miles. Turn right (west) on Mulholland Highway, then in 0.4 mile turn right again onto Little Sycamore Canyon, which soon becomes Yerba Buena Road and reaches the trailhead in 5.5 miles. On either approach, you face a white-knuckle drive on paved, but very narrow and curvy roads.

You may park at the ranger station or drive 0.1 mile down a dirt road behind the ranger station to signed day-use parking. The trailhead is 0.1 mile farther down at the bottom of the road beside the Circle X Ranch Group Campground (camping by reservation only).

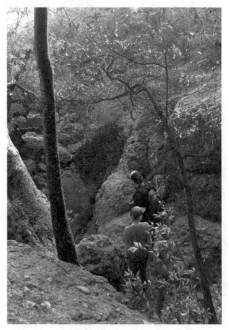

Rock-hopping in the Grotto

Description: Start hiking at the Circle X Ranch park office. Walk down to the group campground, where you find and follow the Grotto Trail heading south down along a shady, seasonal creek. Keep going downhill as you pass the Canyon View Trail intersecting on the left. Shortly afterward, you cross the creek at a point immediately above a 30-foot drop, which becomes a trickling waterfall in winter and spring. You then go uphill, gaining about 50 feet of elevation, and cross an open meadow offering fine views of both Boney Mountain above and a deep-cut gorge (the west fork of Arroyo Sequit) below. Maintain your descent, which becomes sharper as you get closer to the bottom of the gorge.

When you come upon an old roadbed at the bottom, stay left, cross the creek, and continue downstream on a narrowing trail along the shaded east bank. Curve left when you reach a grove of fantastically twisted live oaks at the confluence of two stream forks. On the edge of this grove, an overflow pipe coming out of a tank discharges tepid spring water. Continue another 200 yards down along the now-lively brook to the trail's abrupt end at The Grotto, a narrow, spooky constriction flanked by sheer volcanic-rock walls. If your sense of balance is good, you can clamber over gray rock ledges and massive boulders fallen from the canyon walls—just as thousands of Boy Scouts have done in the past. At one spot you can peer cautiously into a gloomy cavern, where you more easily hear than see the subterranean stream. Watermarks on the boulders above are evidence that this part of the gorge probably supports a two-tier stream in times of flood.

When you've had your fill of adventuring, return by the same route, uphill almost the whole way.

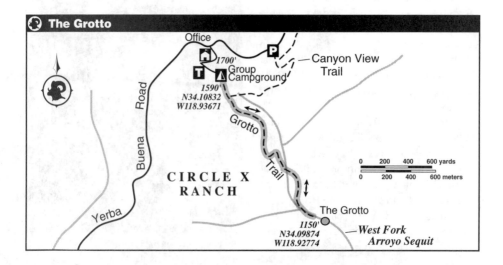

HIKE 6

Charmlee Wilderness Park

Location	Santa Monica Mountains
Highlights	Spring wildflowers and ocean views
Distance	2.8 miles (loop)
Total Elevation Gain/Loss	500'/500'
Hiking Time	1½ hours
Optional Maps	Trails Illustrated Santa Monica Mountains National Recreation Area or USGS 7.5-minute *Triunfo Pass*
Best Times	8 a.m.–sunset, all year
Agency	CW
Difficulty	Easy
Trail Use	Dogs allowed, good for kids

Charmlee Wilderness Park (also known as Charmlee Natural Area), 590 acres of meadow, oak woodland, sage scrub, and chaparral, was first opened to the public in 1981 as a unit of the Los Angeles County park system. Today the City of Malibu administers the park, which lies on that coastal city's western extremity. Never designed to accommodate a large number of visitors, Charmlee's parking lot is often full on the weekends. A spiderweb of trails totaling 8 miles covers the park, making it a great place to ramble with family and friends for wildflower spotting in spring and ocean watching on any clear day. The perimeter route described below is pieced together out of the maze of unevenly signed footpaths and old ranch roads in the park. Never fear if you find yourself straying from the route; aim downhill to get to the ocean views and uphill to return to the parking area.

To Reach the Trailhead: To reach Charmlee Wilderness Park from Santa Monica, drive 25 miles west on Pacific Coast Highway (Highway 1) to a point 0.5 mile west of mile marker 001 LA 59.0. Turn north on Encinal Canyon Road, and proceed 4 miles to the park's well-marked entrance.

Gates are open 8 a.m.–sunset daily. Pay the $4 parking fee at the iron ranger.

Description: From the parking lot, walk on pavement to the nature center (if it is open, pick up a guide for the interpretive signposts). Head uphill on a paved road, which soon becomes dirt and bends north up a slope. Make an acute left turn at the top by a gate, and then follow Potrero Rd. along the ridge road past a hilltop water tank. Boney Mountain, the eroded core of an old volcano, stands prominently on the crest of the Santa Monicas. Curve left at a junction, and head east to meet Charmichael Road. From here, consider a short detour left (south) to visit the foundation of an old ranch home in the oaks on a hilltop overlooking the meadow.

Resuming your walk, continue down Potrero Road to the edge of the park's large central meadow, where the road turns left and crosses the meadow. Continue all the way to a dry ridge topped by some old eucalyptus trees and a concrete-lined cistern, both relics of cattle-ranching days. From there descend to the southeast, making a broad switchback. Pass a connector trail on the left, then make a right onto a short spur leading to Ocean Vista, which delivers in a big way what its name suggests. In addition to miles of surf and sand seemingly at your feet, your eyes drink in perhaps a thousand square miles of wind-ruffled ocean. From here you can identify at least six Channel Islands if the ocean is free of haze. The small island to the west is Anacapa, with mountainous Santa Cruz Island looming behind. As your eyes roam left, you might glimpse the low ridge of San Nicholas Island far out to sea. It has become famous in children's literature as the Island of the Blue Dolphins, based on the true story of Juana Maria, a Nicoleño Indian girl, who survived there alone for 18 years after being stranded when her tribe fled. Closer in, Santa Barbara Island rises from the sea like a broken tooth. Continuing left, look for the low form of San Clemente Island, now a Navy firing

range, behind large Catalina Island. Continuing your panoramic sweep to the left, look for the Palos Verdes Hills, Santa Monica Bay, and Point Dume.

Circle north from Ocean Vista, passing the unsigned connector trail on the left. Watch for a charming oak-shaded glade on the right, where boulders tempt you to stop and sit a bit. Just beyond, pass the East Meadow Cutoff Trail on the left, and continue straight on the East Meadow Trail. At the next junction, stay straight onto the Botany Trail and follow it into the woods. The trail ends at a shady picnic area near the parking lot.

If it's a spring day and you've kept a tally of wildflowers spotted on the hike, you may be surprised to find your list includes as many as two dozen or more.

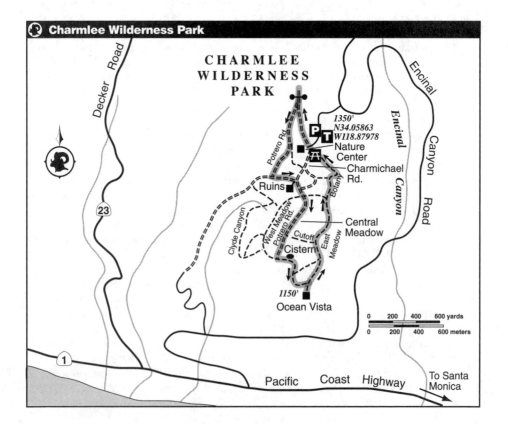

Zuma Canyon

Location	Santa Monica Mountains
Highlights	Spectacular, wild canyon trek and ocean views on the return
Distance	9 miles (loop)
Total Elevation Gain/Loss	1700'/1700'
Hiking Time	6 hours
Optional Maps	Trails Illustrated Santa Monica Mountains National Recreation Area or USGS 7.5-minute *Point Dume*
Best Times	8 a.m.–sunset, October–June
Agency	SMMNRA
Difficulty	Strenuous

Although it slices only 6 miles inland from the Pacific shoreline, Zuma Canyon harbors one of the deepest gorges in the Santa Monica Mountains. Easily on a par with nearby Malibu and Topanga Canyons in scenic wealth but much less known, Zuma Canyon holds the further distinction of never having suffered the invasion of a major road. Under cover of junglelike growths of willow, sycamore, oak, and bay, the canyon's small stream cascades over sculpted sandstone boulders and gathers in limpid pools adorned with ferns. These natural treasures yield their secrets begrudgingly, as they should, only to those willing to scramble over boulders, plow through sucking mud and cattails, and thrash through scratchy undergrowth.

On this challenging trek, you'll proceed straight up the canyon's scenic midsection, climb out of the canyon depths via a powerline service road, and loop back to your starting point on the ridge-running Zuma Ridge Trail (a fire road). The roads are shadeless, yet they offer great vistas of the canyon, the ocean, and the seemingly interminable east-west sweep of the Santa Monica Mountains.

Hiking the canyon bottom is least problematic in the fall season before the heavy rains set in. The stream may have shrunk to isolated pools by then, and you'll step mostly on dry rocks with good traction. Winter flooding can render the canyon impassable, but such episodes are rare and short-lived. During spring, the stream flows heartily and there's plenty of greenery and wildflowers; at the same time there's an increased threat of exposure to poison oak (which grows in fair abundance along the banks), and you're likely to surprise a rattlesnake. Summer days are usually too oppressively warm and humid for such a difficult hike. Whatever the season, take along plenty of water; the water in the canyon is not potable. Expect to get your feet wet, and bring sandals or a change of socks.

To Reach the Trailhead: A good starting place is the north end of Bonsall Drive, in the Point Dume area of Malibu. From the intersection of Kanan Dume Road and Pacific Coast Highway (Highway 1) at mile marker 001 LA 54.00, drive 0.9 mile west on the highway to Bonsall Drive, turn right, and continue 1 mile to where Bonsall Drive ends at a trailhead for the Zuma Canyon trail system.

Description: From the end of Bonsall Drive, walk north on the Zuma Canyon Trail following the canyon's winter-wet, summer-dry creek. Several trails branch off along either side, but stay on the mail trail up the canyon bottom. You pass statuesque sycamores, tall laurel sumac bushes, and scattered wildflowers in season. This is a promising area for spotting wildlife anytime—squirrels, rabbits, and coyotes are commonly seen, deer and bobcats less so.

After about a mile's walk along the creek or dry canyon bottom, the canyon walls close in tighter, oaks appear in greater numbers, and you notice a small grove of eucalyptus trees on a little terrace. The path abruptly ends at a pile of sandstone boulders, 1.3 miles from the start. During the dry months, surface water may get only this far down the canyon. Often, however, the water trickles or tumbles past here, disappearing at some point downstream into the porous substrate of the canyon floor.

Now you begin a nearly 2-mile stretch of boulder-hopping (and possibly wading), 2 or 3 hours' worth depending on the conditions. Other than a few rusting pieces of pipeline from an old dam and irrigation system, you may find that the canyon is completely litter-free; please keep it that way.

The great variety of rocks that have been washed down the stream or have fallen from the canyon walls says a lot about the geologic complexity of the Santa Monicas. You'll scramble over fine-grained siltstones and sandstones, conglomerates that look like poorly mixed aggregate concrete, and volcanic rocks of the sort that make up Saddle Rock (a local landmark near the head of Zuma Canyon) and the Goat Buttes of nearby Malibu Creek State Park. Some of the larger boulders attain the dimensions of mid-sized trucks, presenting an obstacle course that you must negotiate by moderate climbing with your hands and feet.

In another 1.3 miles, pass directly under a set of high-voltage transmission lines—so high they're hard to spot. These

lines, plus the graded road built to give access to the towers, represent the major incursion of civilization into Zuma Canyon. If you can ignore them, however, it's easy to imagine what all the large canyons in the Santa Monicas were like only a century ago.

When you finally reach the Zuma Edison Road, turn left and follow it 2 miles to the top of the west ridge. From there, turn left on the Zuma Ridge Trail (another dirt road) and follow its lazily curving, downhill course toward the coastal plain, enjoying clear-air vistas of the vast Pacific Ocean much of the way. On a fine day, you can see all the way from San Jacinto, Santiago Peak, and the Palos Verdes Hills to Catalina, San Clemente, Anacapa, and Santa Cruz Islands. This and many other utility service roads in the Santa Monicas are closed to unauthorized motorized vehicles and are popular among hikers and mountain bikers.

When you reach the bottom of the Zuma Ridge Trail in 2.6 miles, where

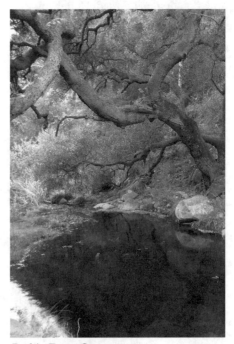

Pool in Zuma Canyon

Busch Drive and Cuthbert Road meet, take the path across the hillside to your left (east). You lose about 300 feet of elevation over 0.6 mile as you zigzag down to the bottom of the Zuma Canyon floodplain. Turn right when you reach the main Zuma Canyon Trail, and walk the final 0.2 mile over to where you began your hike.

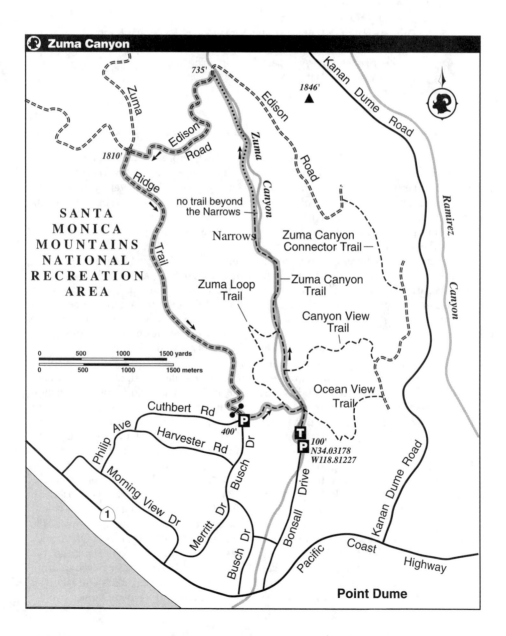

Zuma Canyon

735'

1846' ▲

Kanan Dume Road

Zuma

Edison Road

Edison Road

1810'

Zuma Canyon

Ridge

Ramirez Canyon

SANTA MONICA MOUNTAINS NATIONAL RECREATION AREA

no trail beyond the Narrows

Narrows

Zuma Canyon Connector Trail

Trail

Zuma Loop Trail

Zuma Canyon Trail

Canyon View Trail

| 0 | 500 | 1000 | 1500 yards |
| 0 | 500 | 1000 | 1500 meters |

Ocean View Trail

Cuthbert Rd

Philip Ave

Harvester Rd

400'

Busch Dr

Merritt Dr

Morning View Dr

1

Busch Dr

P

T P 100' N34.03178 W118.81227

Bonsall Drive

Kanan Dume Road

Pacific Coast Highway

Point Dume

HIKE 8

Point Dume to Paradise Cove

Location	Malibu coast
Highlights	Panoramic ocean vistas and superb intertidal exploration
Distance	2.1 miles (one way)
Total Elevation Gain/Loss	200'/200'
Hiking Time	1½ hours
Optional Maps	Trails Illustrated Santa Monica Mountains National Recreation Area or USGS 7.5-minute *Point Dume*
Best Times	All year (passable during low tide)
Agency	SMMNRA
Difficulty	Moderate
Trail Use	Good for kids

Like the armored bow of an icebreaker, flat-topped Point Dume juts into the Pacific about 20 miles west of Santa Monica. Just east of the point itself, an unbroken cliff wall shelters a secluded beach from the sights and sounds of the civilized world. Below the sometimes-narrow stretch of sand east of Point Dume, a strip of rocky coastline harbors tidepools and a mind-boggling array of plant and animal life.

A pleasant walk anytime the tide is low, this trip is doubly rewarding when the tide dips as low as negative 2 feet. Some of the tidepool inhabitants include: limpets, periwinkles, chitons, tube snails, sandcastle worms, sculpins, mussels, shore and hermit crabs, green and aggregating anemones, three kinds of barnacles, and two kinds of sea stars. Extremely low tides occur during the afternoon two or three times each month from October through March. During the summer, you'll have to get up early to catch the rare negative tides. Consult tide tables to find out exactly when.

To Reach the Trailhead: From the Pacific Coast Highway (Highway 1) on Malibu's west side, 0.4 mile west of mile marker 001 LA 54.5, turn south onto Westward Beach Road. Drive down Westward Beach Road to the road's end at Westward Beach (which is open daylight hours and charges a parking fee). Alternatively, you may park for free along the roadside before reaching the pay station, and then stroll 0.7 mile southeast along the beach to Point Dume.

Description: Starting out at Westward Beach, you have a choice between two routes: over the top of the point or around the end of the point at sea level. The shorter, much easier route (and the only practical alternative during all but extremely low tides) is the first one, the trail slanting left up the cliff. On top is an area popular for sighting gray whales during their southward migration in winter and a state historic monument. Point Dume, you'll learn, was christened by British naval commander George Vancouver, who sailed by in 1793.

As you stand on Point Dume's apex, note the marked contrast between the lighter sedimentary rock exposed on the cliff faces both east and west and the darker volcanic rock just below. This unusually tough mass of volcanic rock has thus far resisted the onslaught of the ocean swells. After you descend from the apex, some metal stairs will take you down to crescent-shaped Dume Cove.

The alternate route is for skilled climbers only (and definitely inappropriate for small children). During the very lowest tides, you round the point itself, making your way by hand-and-toe climbing in a couple of spots over huge, angular shards of volcanic rock along the base of the cliffs. The tidepools here and to the east along Dume Cove's shoreline have some of the best displays of intertidal marine life in Southern California. This visual feast will remain for others to enjoy if you refrain from taking or disturbing in any way the organisms that live there. (*Warning:* Exploring the lower intertidal zones can be hazardous. Be very cautious when traveling over slippery rocks, and always be aware of the incoming swells. Don't let a rogue wave catch you by surprise.)

The going is easy once you're on Dume Cove's ribbon of sand. Signs posted here warn against nude bathing and sunning. This was once a popular nude beach, much to the chagrin of some of those living in the cliffside mansions overlooking the area. You may see the *Zeus,* a sailboat shipwrecked at the cove, partially buried beneath the sands.

When you reach the northeast end of Dume Cove, swing left around a lesser point and continue another mile over a somewhat wider beach to Paradise Cove, site of an elegant beachside restaurant, private pier, and parking lot (the public is welcome for a hefty parking fee unless they spend at least $20 at the restaurant). If you've parked a bicycle or second car here, then your hike ends here. Otherwise you can return the way you came or wend your way along the residential streets of Point Dume to return to Westward Beach.

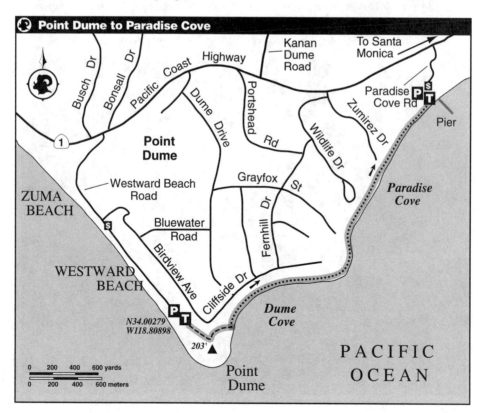

HIKE 9

Solstice Canyon Park

Location	Santa Monica Mountains (Malibu)
Highlights	Superb oak woodland and lessons in fire ecology
Distance	2.4 miles (out-and-back)
Total Elevation Gain/Loss	350'/350'
Hiking Time	1½ hours
Optional Maps	Trails Illustrated Santa Monica Mountains National Recreation Area or USGS 7.5-minute *Malibu Beach* and *Point Dume*
Best Times	All year
Agency	SMMNRA
Difficulty	Easy
Trail Use	Dogs allowed, good for kids

The easy-going but scenic Solstice Canyon Trail takes you through the grounds of the former Robert's Ranch—now Solstice Canyon Park, a site administered by the National Park Service. The canyon once hosted a private zoo where giraffes, camels, deer, and exotic birds roamed. At trail's end you come to Tropical Terrace, the site of an architecturally noted grand home that burned in a 1982 wildfire.

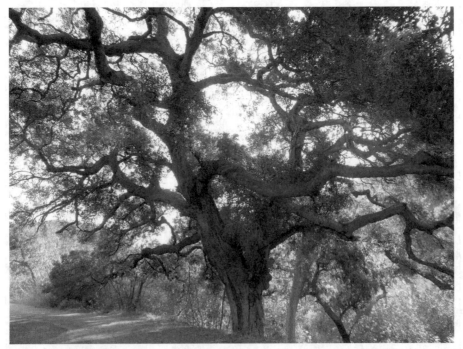

Live oak in Solstice Canyon

To Reach the Trailhead: From Highway 1 in Malibu 0.3 mile west of mile marker 001 LA 50.0, turn north onto Corral Canyon Road. In 0.2 mile, turn left into the park. There's overflow parking space for several cars at the entrance, and a more spacious lot 0.3 mile farther inside at the main trailhead. Parking is free. Carpooling is encouraged since parking space is limited. Posted park hours are 8 a.m.–sunset. The trail description begins from the inside parking lot.

Description: Starting at the main trailhead, pass through a gate and continue upstream alongside the canyon's melodious creek. The path is paved for much of the way. You travel through a fantastic woodland of alder, sycamore, bay, and live oak—the latter with trunks up to 18 feet in circumference. In 0.7 mile, you

pass an 1865 stone cottage on the right—thought to be the oldest existing stone building in Malibu.

At 1.2 miles, you arrive at the remains of Tropical Terrace. In a setting of palms and giant birds-of-paradise, curved flagstone steps sweep toward the roofless remains of what was for 26 years one of Malibu's grand homes. Beyond the house, crumbling stone steps and pathways lead to what used to be elaborately decorated rock grottoes, as well as a waterfall on Solstice Canyon's creek. Hidden among the Tropical Terrace ruins are the remains of a concrete bomb shelter. For all its perfectly natural setting, Tropical Terrace's destiny was that of a temporary paradise, wiped out by both fire and flood.

The steep and rugged Sostomo Trail continues up the canyon, eventually joining the Deer Valley Loop for those who

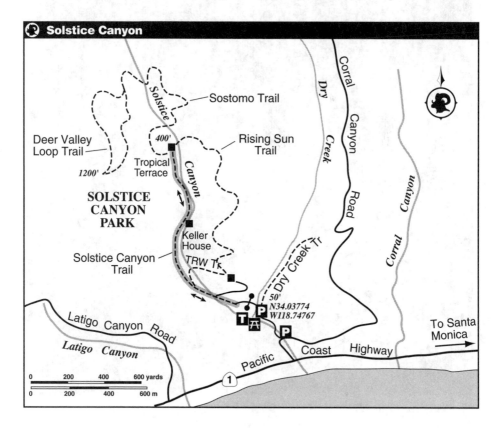

want a longer trip. A beautiful but strenuous option for a loop hike is to return via the Rising Sun Trail, which adds 500 feet of climbing onto the canyon wall but offers fantastic coastline views stretching from the Palos Verdes Peninsula to Point Dume. Otherwise, you can turn around at Tropical Terrace and start an easy, gentle descent back to the trailhead.

Back at the trailhead parking lot you may want to check out the Dry Creek Trail, which goes northeast up an oak-shaded ravine for about 0.6 mile before entering private property. An outrageously cantilevered "Darth Vader" house overlooks the ravine as well as a 150-foot-high precipice that infrequently becomes a spectacular waterfall.

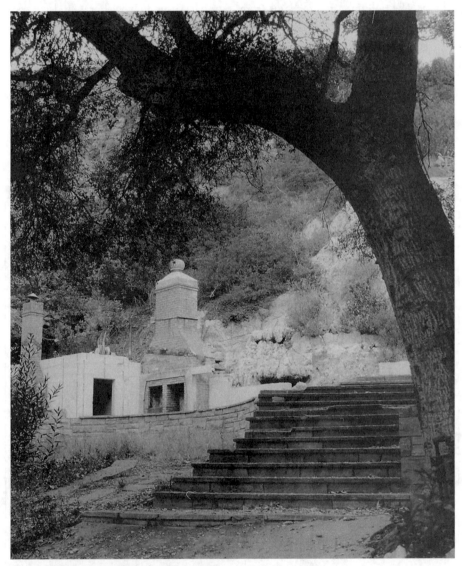

Tropical Terrace ruins in Solstice Canyon

HIKE 10

Temescal Canyon

Location	Santa Monica Mountains (Pacific Palisades)
Highlights	Pseudoaerial coastline views and shady riparian and oak woodland
Distance	2.8 miles (loop)
Total Elevation Gain/Loss	850'/850'
Hiking Time	1½ hours
Optional Maps	Trails Illustrated Santa Monica Mountains National Recreation Area or USGS 7.5-minute *Topanga*
Best Times	All year
Agency	SMMNRA
Difficulty	Moderate
Trail Use	Good for kids

Spring lingers long on the coastal slopes of the Santa Monica Mountains, which are frequently bathed from May until July in the sopping-wet breath of the marine layer. This is quintessential coastal sage-scrub and chaparral country, a particular habitat that is fast succumbing to urban development all over Southern California. All through spring and early summer, you can enjoy the scents of sage and wildflowers on the trails of Temescal Canyon, part of the Santa Monica Mountains National Recreation Area and Topanga State Park. With an early start on a foggy morning, you may find yourself punching right through the mist as you ascend into the bright, sunny world above.

To Reach the Trailhead: Begin at Temescal Gateway Park, just north of the intersection of Sunset Boulevard and Temescal Canyon Road in Pacific Palisades, 1 mile north of Pacific Coast Highway by way of Temescal Canyon Road. Park for a fee inside the park from sunrise to sunset. Pets are allowed on the short paths in Temescal Gateway Park, but they are prohibited on the outlying trails ahead, which enter Topanga State Park.

Description: This hike traverses the Temescal loop clockwise, climbing the scrubby west wall of Temescal Canyon on the way up and then making a nice, easy descent down through the canyon. To do

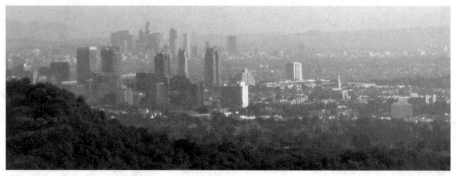

City views from Temescal Ridge

this, head north up the road past several buildings that comprise the former Presbyterian conference grounds. Stay left onto a dirt path and climb to a signed junction where you can pick up the Temescal Ridge Trail on the left. The narrow trail immediately starts a vigorous ascent up the scrubby canyon slope to the west. After several twists and turns, the trail gains a moderately ascending crest and sticks to it. Pause often so you can turn around and look at the ever-widening view of the coastline curving from Santa Monica Bay to Malibu.

Ahead, two short trails (the Leacock and Bienveneda Trails) strike off to the left toward the end of Bienveneda Avenue. Ignore those paths and continue a junction (1.3 miles from the start) with the Temescal Canyon Trail on the right. At this juncture you have the option of making a side trip north 0.4 mile to a wind-carved, sandstone outcrop known as Skull Rock. To stay on the loop route, turn right and follow the Temescal Canyon Trail into the shady bottom of Temescal Canyon.

At the bottom you cross Temescal Canyon's creek on a footbridge. Above and below that bridge are small, trickling waterfalls and shallow, limpid pools. You can poke around the creek a bit for a look at its typical denizens—water striders and newts. When you've finished sightseeing, continue down the canyon trail back to the conference buildings, a mile away. That final stretch follows the canyon bottom and then contours along a slope behind the buildings. Lots of live oak, sycamore, willow, and bay trees, their woodsy scents commingling on the ocean breeze, highlight your return.

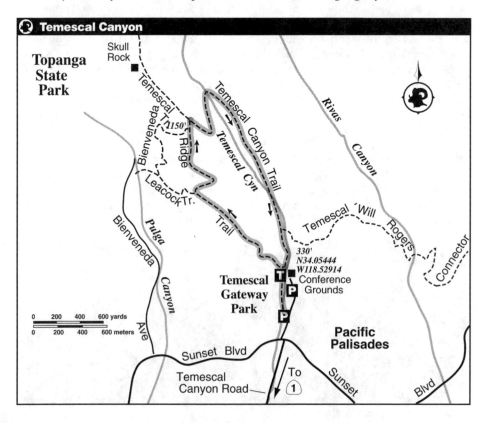

HIKE 11

Will Rogers Park

Location	Santa Monica Mountains (Pacific Palisades)
Highlights	City, ocean, and mountain views in a single stance
Distance	2.0 miles (loop)
Total Elevation Gain/Loss	350'/350'
Hiking Time	1 hour
Optional Maps	Trails Illustrated Santa Monica Mountains National Recreation Area or USGS 7.5-minute *Topanga*
Best Times	All year
Agency	WRSHP
Difficulty	Easy
Trail Use	Suitable for mountain biking, dogs allowed, good for kids

Drive up a short mile from the speedway known as Sunset Boulevard toward Will Rogers State Historic Park, and you'll instantly leave the rat race behind. Especially on weekdays or early on weekend mornings, this quiet spot is perfect for getting some exercise and taking advantage of multimillion-dollar views of Santa Monica, West L.A., and downtown L.A.

Newspaperman, radio commentator, movie star, and pop-philosopher Will Rogers purchased this 182-acre property in 1922 and lived with his family here from 1928 until his death in 1935. Historic only by Southern California standards, his 31-room mansion is nevertheless interesting to tour. Your main goal, however, is to reach Inspiration Point, a flat-topped bump on a ridge overlooking the entire spread.

To Reach the Trailhead: Drive 1.5 miles east on Sunset Boulevard from the commercial district of Pacific Palisades (Sunset Boulevard and Temescal Canyon Road) to reach the Will Rogers Park entrance road. Or take Sunset Boulevard 4 miles west from I-405 to reach the same entrance. The park is open daily, except certain holidays, 8 a.m.–sunset and charges a parking fee.

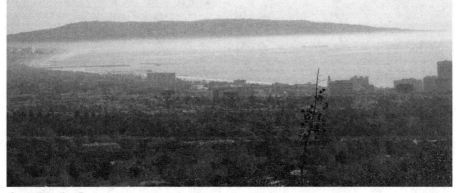

Santa Monica Bay

Description: You may want to obtain a copy of the detailed hikers' map, available at the gift shop in a wing of the home. Printed on the map is one of Will's memorable (if not apropos) aphorisms, "If your time is worth anything, travel by air. If not, you might just as well walk." To reach Inspiration Point, follow the main, wide, riding and hiking trail that makes a 2-mile loop, starting at the north end of the big lawn adjoining the Rogers home. Or use any of several shorter, more direct paths (mountain bikes and leashed pets are only allowed on the main, looping trail).

Relaxing on the benches at the top on a clear day, you can admire true-as-advertised, inspiring vistas stretching east to the front range of the San Gabriel Mountains and southeast to the Santa Ana Mountains. South past the swelling Palos Verdes Peninsula you can sometimes spot Santa Catalina Island, rising in ethereal majesty from the shining surface of the sea.

Will Rogers Park serves as the east terminus of the Backbone Trail, which skims some 65 miles along the crest of the Santa Monica Mountains. Its west end lies in Point Mugu State Park (described in Hike 3).

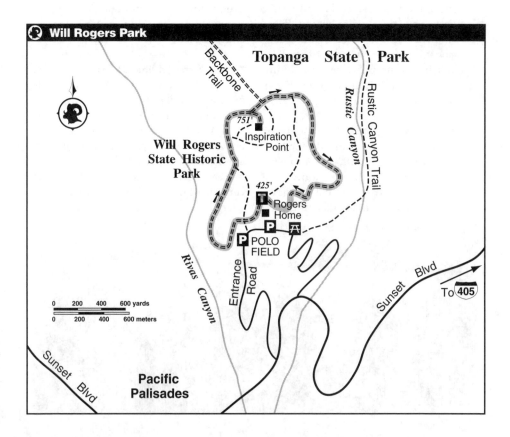

HIKE 12

Malaga Cove to Bluff Cove

Location	Palos Verdes Peninsula
Highlights	Boulder-hopping beneath sea cliffs and past small tidepools
Distance	2.0 miles (loop)
Total Elevation Gain/Loss	200'/200'
Hiking Time	2 hours
Optional Map	USGS 7.5-minute *Redondo Beach*
Best Times	All year
Agency	PVESP
Difficulty	Moderate
Trail Use	Good for kids

When the tide is not too high, curious hikers can thread their way along a narrow strip of rocks between the ocean and the sea cliffs at the northern end of the Palos Verdes Peninsula. Watch for sea life in small tidepools and debris from an old shipwreck. While young children may love this trip, folks uncomfortable hopping along slippery rocks will prefer exploring elsewhere.

To Reach the Trailhead: From the 110 Freeway, exit west on the Pacific Coast Highway (Highway 1). In 0.6 mile, turn left on Normandie. Then in 0.5 mile, veer right onto Palos Verdes Drive North.

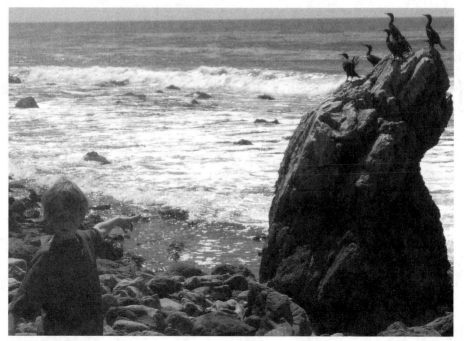

Near Bluff Cove

Follow this scenic winding road for 6.7 miles, then keep left onto Palos Verdes Drive West. In 0.2 mile, turn right onto Via Almar. In 0.5 mile, turn right again onto Via Arroyo, and in 0.1 mile, turn right yet again onto Paseo del Mar, where you will find a large parking area.

Description: Walk to the east end of the parking area, where you will see a trail just beyond a gazebo overlooking the Pacific. Follow the trail down to Malaga Cove. This hike leads left (southwest) along the rocks beneath the sea cliffs. If the tide looks too high or the surf is excessive, consider diverting right instead and taking a stroll along Torrance Beach.

Otherwise, pick a path over the sedimentary rocks. Surfers flock to the cove to test their skills on the waves. Look carefully for small sea anemones, snails, and hermit crabs in the tidepools. In 0.3

mile, watch and sniff for a natural mineral spring emerging from the rocks near the ocean's edge. Continuing along the rocks, watch for rusted metal debris from an unknown wreck. The famous 1961 wreck of the *Dominator* freighter is located south on the peninsula near Rocky Point.

After a slow mile of picking your way through the rocks, reach Flat Rock Point, another popular spot to view tidepools. Bluff Cove lies on the far side of the point. Your goal is to reach Paseo del Mar above. An extremely steep and potentially hazardous trail leads straight up from Flat Rock Point. A safer choice is to continue along the cove to find a graded path on the left. In either event, once you reach Paseo del Mar, turn left and walk a half mile back to your vehicle, enjoying the elaborately landscaped mansions along the way.

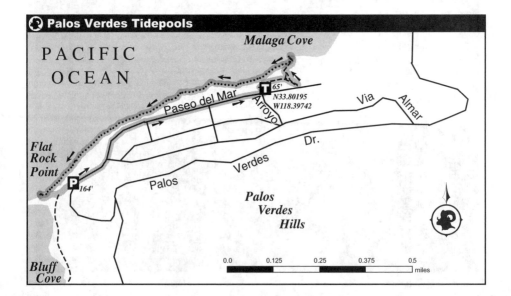

HIKE 13

Cheeseboro and Palo Comado Canyons

Location	Simi Hills (east of Thousand Oaks)
Highlights	Classic green or golden California grassland dotted with oaks
Distance	10 miles (loop)
Total Elevation Gain/Loss	1,200'/1,200'
Hiking Time	5 hours
Optional Maps	Trails Illustrated Santa Monica Mountains National Recreation Area or USGS 7.5-minute *Calabasas*
Best Times	October–June
Agency	SMMNRA
Difficulty	Moderately strenuous
Trail Use	Suitable for mountain biking, dogs allowed

The Cheeseboro and Palo Comado Canyons park site, a unit of the Santa Monica Mountains National Recreation Area, serves as an important wildlife corridor between the interior Transverse Ranges in the north and the Santa Monica Mountains to the south. Self-propelled travelers by the thousands have discovered the place, but there's plenty of room for visitors to spread out. The long, leisurely loop route described here visits the two canyons, both surprisingly serene and pristine despite extensive suburban development in the surrounding region. Deer, bobcats, coyotes, rabbits, owls, and various birds of prey can be spotted in both canyons, especially in the early morning.

Without question, the period between the emergence of tender green grass (December or January) and the shift from green to gold (April or May) is the very best time to visit Cheeseboro and Palo Comado Canyons. July through September brings midday temperatures in the 90s, making this area unpleasant for all but perhaps mountain bikers, who may

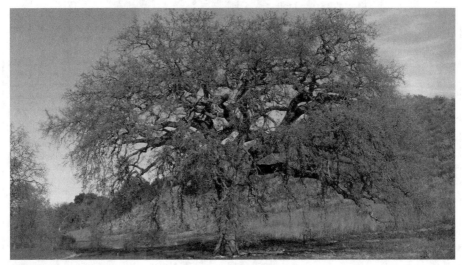

Valley oak

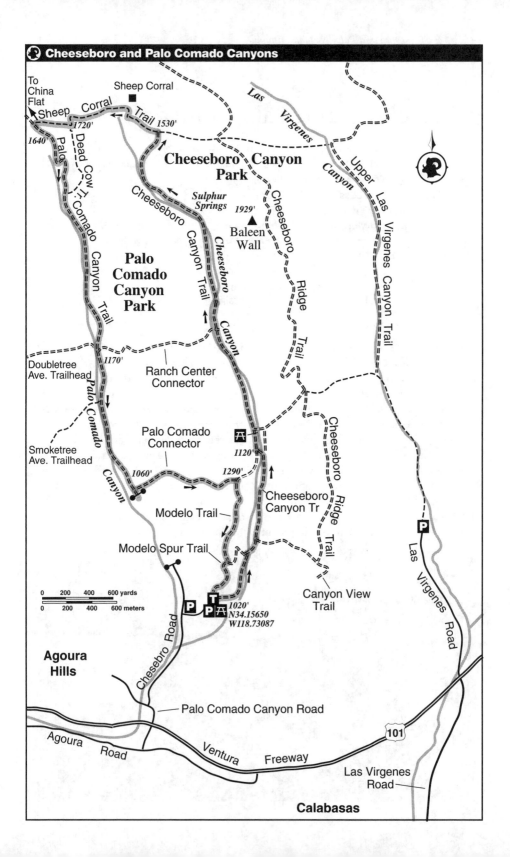

enjoy the benefit of evaporative cooling if they move fast enough.

To Reach the Trailhead: From US 101 at Exit 35 in Agoura Hills, take the Cheesebro (sic) Road exit, go north about 200 yards on what is signed Palo Comado Canyon Road, then turn right on Cheesebro Road. Drive 0.7 mile north to the main entrance to the Cheeseboro and Palo Comado Canyons site, on the right. Gates to the trailhead parking lot swing open at 8 a.m.—often earlier on weekends, when volunteers sometimes staff a National Park Service information booth here. A fenced trail into Cheeseboro Canyon bypasses the parking area, and hikers, bikers, and equestrians use it even when the gates are shut. Be aware that soggy trail conditions may close the park.

Description: From the trailhead parking lot, follow the wide Cheeseboro Canyon Trail, which goes briefly east and then bends north up along the wide, nearly flat canyon floor. Stay on the broad main path; disregard narrow trails branching off either side. Two kinds of oak trees dominate the Cheeseboro landscape: evergreen coast live oaks cluster along the canyon bottoms, and deciduous valley oaks, widely spaced, strike statuesque poses in the meadows and on the hillsides. It looks like typical California cattle-grazing land, and indeed it was for a period of about 150 years. Now that the cattle have been removed, oak seedlings are taking root in increasing numbers, and native spring wildflowers are returning to the hillsides, creating splashes of color across the grassy hillsides.

At 1.6 miles on Cheeseboro Canyon Trail, near the Palo Comado Connector joining from the west, you come upon a pleasant trailside picnic area. Stay on the main, wide trail going north through the canyon bottom. At 3.0 miles you pass Sulphur Springs. Let your nose be your guide for locating the springs. There's not much to see—mere seeps if they are flowing at all.

As you continue, the oaks clustering along the canyon bottom thin out, and you can gaze upward, to your right, at the whitish sedimentary outcrop known as the Baleen Wall. The trail narrows and becomes rocky in places. At 4.1 miles, reach a T-junction at Shepherds Flat. Pause here for a picnic, perhaps, before resuming your trip.

From the corral continue west on the narrow Sheep Corral Trail through the brush. This is a segment of the Juan Bautista de Anza National Historic Trail, a 1,200-mile trail commemorating the Spanish captain's famed 1775 expedition leading 240 people across the desert to found San Francisco. You pass over a saddle and briefly descend to meet the graded-dirt Palo Comado Canyon Trail (5.2 miles). Turn left now, and commence a short mile of crooked descent on the wide dirt road. You look down on a lovely tapestry of canyon-bottom woods and slopes adorned with dense patches of chaparral and sandstone outcrops. Soon you are amid those woods, which are mostly live oaks and sycamores. The going is easy for another 2 miles as you proceed almost imperceptibly downhill along the canyon bottom.

At 8.2 miles, there's a forced left turn out of the canyon (off-limits private land lies ahead) and onto the Palo Comado Connector. You meander uphill and across two minor canyons for 1.0 mile to a rounded ridge, where you meet the Modelo Trail on the right. It and the Modelo Spur Trail are the most expeditious route back to the trailhead.

HIKE 14

Placerita Canyon

Location	Santa Clarita
Highlights	Wooded ravines, waterfall, and historically interesting features
Distance	5.0 miles (out-and-back)
Total Elevation Gain/Loss	700'/700'
Hiking Time	2½ hours
Optional Maps	USGS 7.5-minute *Mint Canyon* and *San Fernando*
Best Times	October–June
Agency	PCP
Difficulty	Moderate
Trail Use	Dogs allowed, good for kids

Barely 10 minutes' drive from northern San Fernando Valley and the sprawling suburban city of Santa Clarita, Placerita Canyon Park nestles comfortably at the foot of one of the more verdant slopes of the San Gabriel Mountains. A very civilized nature center housing exhibits on local history, pre-history, geology, plants, and wildlife complements the park's wild backcountry sector (the subject of this hike).

Placerita Canyon's fascinating history is highlighted by the discovery of gold there in 1842. That event, which touched off California's first (and relatively trivial) gold rush, predated by six years John Marshall's famous discovery of gold at Sutter's Mill in Northern California. By the 1950s, Placerita Canyon had become one of the more popular generic Western site locations used by Hollywood's moviemakers and early television producers. First the state and then county eventually acquired the canyon as parkland.

To Reach the Trailhead: Take Exit 3 for Placerita Canyon from Antelope Valley Freeway (Highway 14) at Newhall, and drive east 1.5 miles to reach the park's main gate, which is open from sunrise to sunset. Nearby lie the nature center

and a paved path leading under Placerita Canyon Road to the Oak of the Golden Dream, the exact site (according to legend) where in 1842 a herdsman pulling up wild onions for his after-siesta meal discovered gold.

Description: This trip begins at the signed Main Trailhead near the Nature Center and parking lot. Go straight ahead on the Canyon Trail, which soon veers left. Pass an unsigned junction on the right leading to a water tank, and continue east up Placerita Canyon.

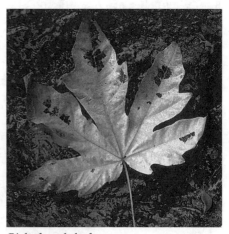

Bigleaf maple leaf

The canyon's melodious creek flows decently about half the year (winter and spring), caressing the ears with white noise that echoes off the canyon walls. During the fall, when the creek may be bone-dry, you make your own noise instead by crunching through the crispy leaf litter of sycamore and live oak. Down by the grassy banks are wild blackberry vines, lots of willows, and occasionally cottonwood and alder trees.

Soaring canyon walls ahead tell the story of thousands of years of natural erosion, as well as the destructive effects of hydraulic mining, which involved aiming high-pressure water hoses at hillsides to loosen and wash away ores. Used extensively in Northern California during the big Gold Rush, hydraulicking was finally banned in 1884 after catastrophic damages to waterways and farms downstream. At Placerita Canyon, several hundred thousand dollars' worth of gold were ultimately recovered, but at considerable cost, effort, and general messiness.

Cross and recross the creek. In 1.85 miles, you reach the scant remains of some early-20th-century cottages hand-built by settler Frank Walker, his wife, and some of their 12 children. The area is now used as a group campground, and it has drinking water.

Our way lies ahead, along the Waterfall Trail, which leads into Los Pinetos Canyon. Don't confuse this trail with the Los Pinetos Trail on the right. The Waterfall Trail momentarily slants upward along the canyon's steep west wall, and then drops onto the canyon's sunny floodplain. Presently you bear right into a narrow ravine (Los Pinetos Canyon), avoiding a wider tributary bending left (east).

Continue past and sometimes over water-polished, metamorphic rock. Live oaks and bigcone Douglas-firs cling to the slopes above, and a few bigleaf maples grace the canyon bottom. Beware of the poison oak that abounds along the trail and near the waterfall, especially in the winter when its bare twigs are difficult to recognize. About 0.2 mile after the first fork in the canyon, there's a second fork.

Go right and continue 50 yards to a small waterfall and a sublime little grotto, cool and dark except when the sun passes almost straight overhead. As you listen to water dashing or dribbling down the chute, enjoy the serenity of this private place and contemplate that it lies only 3 miles—but a world away—from the creeping boundary of the L.A. metropolis. Return the way you came.

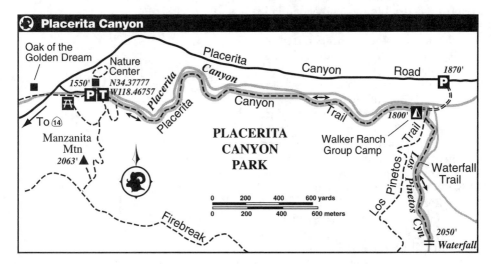

HIKE 15

Mount Lee

Location	Griffith Park
Highlights	Hollywood sign
Distance	3.2 miles (out-and-back)
Total Elevation Gain/Loss	750'/750'
Hiking Time	1½ hours
Optional Map	USGS 7.5-minute *Burbank*
Best Times	All year
Agency	GP
Difficulty	Moderate
Trail Use	Suitable for mountain biking, dogs allowed, good for kids

Mount Lee is recognizable around the world for the iconic Hollywood sign. This trip draws a steady stream of hikers to see the sign up close. Located at the western end of Griffith Park, Mount Lee also provides a stupendous view of Los Angeles and out to the Pacific Ocean. Don't mix up this summit with nearby Mount Hollywood, which is not the site of the eponymous sign.

To Reach the Trailhead: From the westbound 101 Freeway, take Exit 8C for Gower St. Before the ramp reaches Gower St., turn right onto Beachwood Dr. Follow Beachwood Dr. 1.9 miles north to its end in the Hollywood Hills just outside Sunset Ranch Stables. Park in the dirt hikers lot; if this parking lot is full, head a quarter mile south to look for streetside parking.

Description: The broad Hollyridge Trail climbs briefly south to a saddle with an excellent view of the Hollywood sign. It makes a hairpin turn and continues north to a junction with Mulholland Highway (here, an unpaved road) in 0.5 mile.

Turn hard left and follow it 0.3 mile, then turn right onto the Mount Lee Service Road (paved but closed to traffic). Continue 0.9 mile to the road's end immediately above the sign. The sheer slope is fenced off to discourage vandalism.

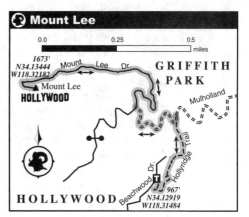

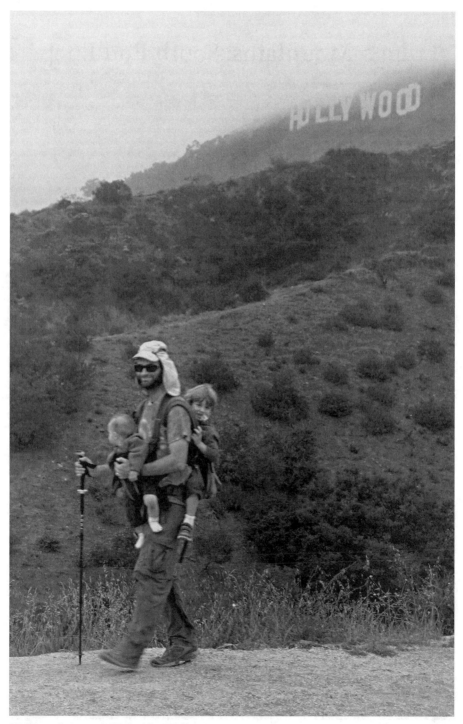

Hollywood sign over Hollyridge Trail

HIKE 16

Verdugo Mountains: South End Loop

Location	Glendale
Highlights	Incomparable city and regional views
Distance	6 miles (loop)
Total Elevation Gain/Loss	1,500'/1,500'
Hiking Time	3½ hours
Optional Maps	USGS 7.5-min *Pasadena, Burbank*
Best Times	November–May
Agency	GPR
Difficulty	Moderately strenuous
Trail Use	Suitable for mountain biking, dogs allowed

The Verdugo Mountains stand as a remarkable island of undeveloped land—a haven for wildlife such as deer and coyotes—completely encircled by an urbanized domain. Public access to the network of trails and fire roads on the mountain is by foot, horse, or mountain bike—great news if you're looking for a quick escape from the ubiquitous automobile and the pressures of city life.

Along the south crest of the Verdugos, your gaze takes in the San Gabriel Mountains, much of the L.A. megalopolis, and even the ocean on occasion. Do this trip late in the day if you want to

enjoy both a spectacular sunset and a blaze of lights after twilight fades. At best, try this on any cloud-free, smog-free day that falls within two weeks on either side of the winter solstice (December 21). During that period, the sun sets on the flat ocean horizon behind Santa Monica Bay, at around 5 p.m. At other times of year, the sun's sinking path is likely to intersect the coastal mountains. The seemingly strange fact of the sun setting over land most of the year is a consequence of the east-west orientation of California's coastline in the first miles up-coast from Los Angeles.

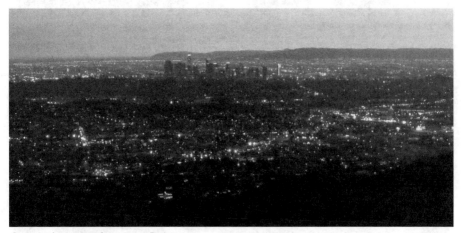

Sunset views over downtown L.A.

To Reach the Trailhead: From I-210 in Glendale, exit south on La Crescenta Avenue. In 1 mile, turn right onto Oakmont View Drive. In 0.2 mile, turn left (south) onto Country Club Drive. In 0.7 mile, turn right onto Beaudry Boulevard, and proceed 0.4 mile to the trailhead where the road veers right. Park on the street.

Description: From Beaudry Boulevard, walk up a paved segment of fire road, bypass a vehicle gate, and continue on dirt past a debris basin to where the fire road splits (0.3 mile). Choose for your way the shadier right branch, Beaudry North Fire Road. You'll return to this junction by way of the left branch, the Beaudry South

Fire Road, which has better views. About halfway up the north road you come to a trickling spring and a water tank nestled in a shady ravine, a good place for a breather.

When you reach the summit ridge (2.3 miles), turn sharply left on Verdugo Fire Road, and continue climbing another 0.4 mile toward a cluster of brightly painted radio towers atop a 2,656-foot bump, the highest point along this hike. From the towers, continue south along the ridge 0.6 mile to a road junction at 2,420 feet. The right branch descends to Sunshine Drive in Glendale; take the left branch, and return along an east ridge to the split just above the debris basin.

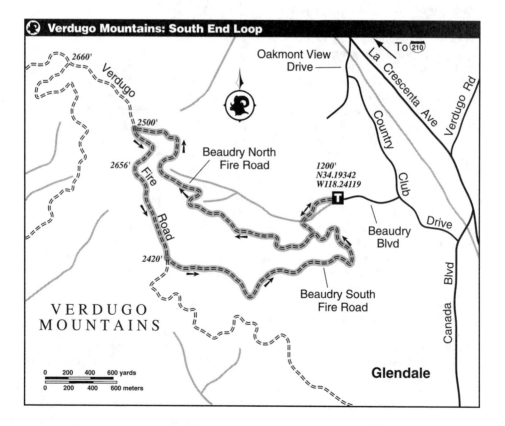

Mount Wilson

Location	San Gabriel Mountains above Pasadena
Highlights	Prominent summit, historic trail, and great views
Distance	15 miles (out-and-back)
Total Elevation Gain/Loss	4,800'/4,800'
Hiking Time	9 hours
Optional Maps	Tom Harrison Maps Angeles Front Country or USGS 7.5-minute *Mt. Wilson*
Best Times	October–May
Agency	ANF/LARD
Difficulty	Strenuous
Trail Use	Dogs allowed

Mount Wilson (5,710 feet) is the most prominent peak in the San Gabriel Front Range overlooking Pasadena. The mountain was named for Benjamin David Wilson, who, in 1864, improved an old American Indian footpath into the first modern trail into the San Gabriels. Although his logging venture failed, the trail became popular in the 1880s for the newly emerging sport of recreational hiking. In the area's great hiking era (1895–1938), hundreds would disembark from the red Pacific Electric trollies in Sierra Madre each Saturday, intent on a weekend at the mountain resorts.

Before the turn of the century, a massive telescope was hauled up the trail piece by piece, and Mount Wilson soon became home to the world's leading observatory of the era. Light pollution in the L.A. Basin now limits its capabilities. Eventually, the Mount Wilson Toll Road from Henninger Flats became the preferred route for vehicle traffic to the summit, and Frank Benedict set the automotive speed record of 22 minutes in 1922.

Mount Wilson has more trails than any other peak in the San Gabriel Mountains. This hike follows Benjamin Wilson's original route. Although it is described as an out-and-back, you could arrange a car

or bicycle shuttle to do it as a one-way trip either up or down, or you could link to the Winter Creek Trail, Sturtevant Trail, or old Mount Wilson Toll Road to find an alternative descent (with a shuttle).

The lower portion of the trail sometimes closes during periods of extreme fire danger. Check with the US Forest Service to avoid disappointment. The road to the summit is generally open 10 a.m.–5 p.m., April 1–November 30, weather permitting. Guided tours of the Mount Wilson Observatory generally run on weekends at 1 p.m. when the road is open.

To Reach the Trailhead: From I-210 in Arcadia, exit north on Baldwin Ave. In 1.5 miles, turn right on Mira Monte Ave. The trailhead is on the left in two blocks.

If you wish to station a vehicle at the summit, return to I-210 and follow it west to the Angeles Crest Highway (CA 2), which leads 13.5 miles north and east up to Red Box Station. Turn right on Mount Wilson Road and proceed 4 miles to the Skyline Park parking area at the end of the road. The drive between trailheads takes about 50 minutes.

Description: The signed route, initially a road, detours left onto a trail around

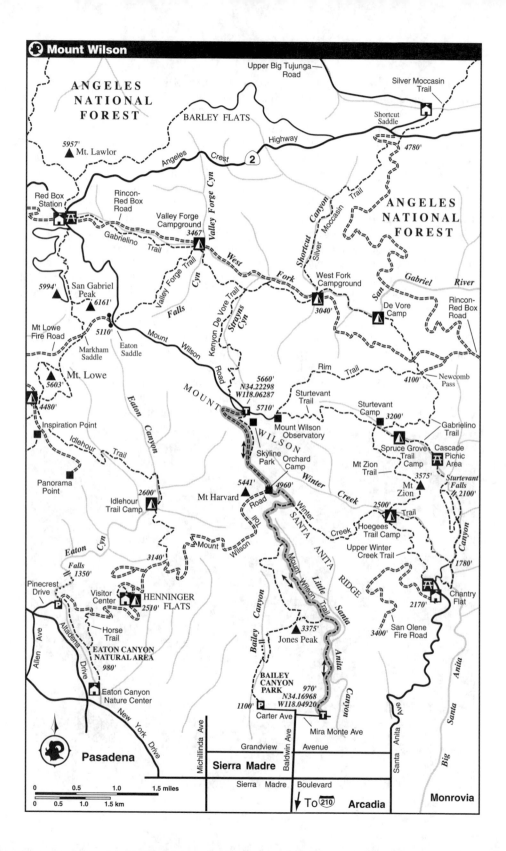

ANGELES
NATIONAL
FOREST

BARLEY FLATS

Upper Big Tujunga Road

Silver Moccasin Trail

Shortcut Saddle

Highway

5957' ▲ Mt. Lawlor

Angeles Crest

(2)

4780'

Red Box Station

Rincon-Red Box Road

Valley Forge Campground *3467'*

Valley Forge Cyn

ANGELES
NATIONAL
FOREST

Gabrielino Trail

Valley Forge Trail

West Fork

West Fork Campground *3040'*

Shortcut Canyon

Silver Moccasin Trail

San Gabriel River

5994'

San Gabriel Peak ▲ *6161'*

Falls

Kenyon De Vore Trail

Shanns Cyn

De Vore Camp

Rincon-Red Box Road

Mt Lowe Fire Road

5110'

Markham Saddle

Eaton Saddle

Mount Wilson Road

Rim Trail

4100'

Newcomb Pass

▲ Mt. Lowe
5603'

MOUNT

5660'
N34.22298
W118.06287
5710'

Sturtevant Trail

Sturtevant Camp *3200'*

Gabrielino Trail

4480'

Eaton Canyon

WILSON

Mount Wilson Observatory

Spruce Grove Trail Camp

Cascade Picnic Area

Inspiration Point

Idlehour Trail

Skyline Park

Orchard Camp

Mt Zion Trail

3575'

Mt Zion ▲

Sturtevant Falls *2100'*

Panorama Point

2600'

Idlehour Trail Camp

5441'
Mt Harvard

4960'

Winter Creek

2500'

Hoegees Trail Camp

Trail

1780'

Eaton Cyn

Falls *1350'*

3140'

Mount Wilson Toll Road

Winter Creek Trail

SANTA ANITA RIDGE

Upper Winter Creek Trail

Santa Anita Canyon

Chantry Flat

Pinecrest Drive

Visitor Center

HENNINGER FLATS *2510'*

Mount Wilson Toll Road

Bailey Canyon

Mount Wilson Trail

Little Santa Anita Canyon

2170'

San Olene Fire Road

3400'

Allen Ave

Altadena Drive

Horse Trail

EATON CANYON NATURAL AREA *980'*

3375'
Jones Peak

BAILEY CANYON PARK
970'
N34.16968
W118.04920

1100'

Eaton Canyon Nature Center

New York Drive

Carter Ave

Mira Monte Ave

Santa Anita Ave

Big Santa Anita

Pasadena

Michillinda Ave

Grandview

Baldwin Ave

Avenue

Sierra Madre

Sierra Madre Boulevard

To (210) Arcadia

Monrovia

0   0.5   1.0   1.5 miles
0   0.5   1.0   1.5 km

private property, rejoins the road in a quarter mile, and soon narrows to a trail again. Only the dedicated work of many volunteers keeps this trail on the steep wall of Little Santa Anita Canyon from collapsing.

At 1.6 miles, pass a branch to the canyon bottom (First Water), then make a steep climb through the chaparral. Eventually, the grade relaxes in a grove of oaks. In another 1.1 miles, watch for a trail on the left leading up to the ridge by Jones Peak. In another 0.9 mile, reach the shady streamside ruins of Orchard Camp. In its heyday of 1911, 40,000 hikers and equestrians signed the camp register, but now only foundations remain. Wilson originally established a construction camp at this spot and called it Halfway House because it marks the midpoint of the route. Here you can find the last dependable water of the trip. The huge canyon oak here is one of the largest and

oldest in the San Gabriels, estimated to be 1,500 years old.

The Mount Wilson Trail now kicks off an earnest climb with a set of switchbacks, eventually reaching a ridgeline in 1.6 miles where it meets the Winter Creek Trail on the right. Your path turns left up the ridge. In 0.6 mile, meet the dirt roadbed of the Mount Wilson Toll Road just east of Mount Harvard. Follow this road north for 0.5 mile to a point north of Mount Harvard where you can veer right onto trail again. The trail climbs directly 0.8 mile to Mount Wilson's flat summit.

The domes here are part of the Mount Wilson Observatory. The radio antennas to the northwest include most of the major television stations of Los Angeles, along with much of the basin's emergency communications network. Their location was of concern to firefighters in the 2009 Station Fire, which threatened the structures on the mountaintop.

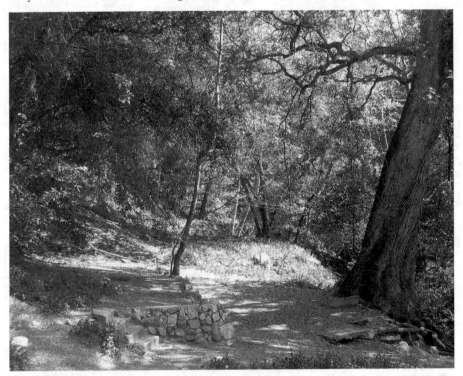

Orchard Camp

HIKE 18

Down the Arroyo Seco

Location	San Gabriel Mountains above Pasadena
Highlights	Sylvan glens and a sparkling stream
Distance	10 miles (one way)
Total Elevation Gain/Loss	450'/2,600'
Hiking Time	5 hours
Optional Maps	Tom Harrison Maps Angeles Front Country or USGS 7.5-minute *Condor Peak* and *Pasadena*
Best Times	October–June
Agency	ANF/LARD
Difficulty	Moderately strenuous
Trail Use	Suitable for backpacking

The Spanish colonists who christened Arroyo Seco ("dry creek") evidently observed only its lower end—a hot, boulder-strewn wash emptying into the Los Angeles River. Upstream, inside the confines of the San Gabriels, Arroyo Seco is a scenic treasure—all the more astounding when you consider that its exquisite sylvan glens and sparkling brook lie just 12–15 miles from L.A.'s city center. If you haven't yet been freed from the notion that Los Angeles is nothing but a seething megalopolis, a walk down the canyon of the Arroyo Seco will convince you otherwise.

The 2009 Station Fire ravaged much of the canyon. Most of the western San Gabriel Mountains, including the middle of this trail, remains closed as the vegetation recuperates. Although most of the burned trails have been removed from this edition of this guidebook, Arroyo Seco is such a special place that it remains in the book. Contact the Los Angeles River Ranger District office of the Angeles National Forest at 626-574-5200, and check if the trail has been reopened before you consider going.

Although the fire killed many of the splendid trees in the canyon, many others remain standing, and wildflowers flourish after fire. A quick census one spring day before the fire (in a dry year, no less) yielded the following blooming plants: golden yarrow, prickly phlox, western wallflower, Indian pink, live-forever, wild pea, deerweed, bush lupine, Spanish broom, baby blue eyes, yerba santa, phacelia, chia, black sage, bush poppy, California buckwheat, shooting star, western clematis, Indian paintbrush, sticky monkeyflower, scarlet bugler, and purple nightshade. Beware of the extensive stands of poison oak that impinge upon the trail, and watch for poodle dog bush below the Brown Canyon debris dam.

Some kind of car-shuttle or drop-off-and-pick-up transportation arrangement is obviously required for this long one-way trip.

To Reach the Switzer Picnic Area Trailhead: Switzer Picnic Area is one of the most popular destinations in the San Gabriel Mountains. Plan to arrive early—the gates normally swing open at 8 a.m. By 10 a.m. on weekends the picnic area's adjacent parking lot is usually filled to capacity. Overflow and off-hours parking is available at the well-marked entrance to the picnic area, at mile marker 34.2 on Angeles Crest Highway (CA 2), 10 miles from I-210 at La Cañada. If you park at this entrance, you must hike down a narrow paved road to the picnic area, adding 0.4 mile and 250 feet of elevation loss to your one-way trip. Any car left at or near this upper trailhead must display a National Forest Adventure Pass.

To Reach the Pasadena Trailhead: Exit I-210 at Arroyo Boulevard and Windsor Avenue, and drive north on Windsor Avenue for 0.8 mile to the intersection of Windsor Avenue and Ventura Street. Free parking is available here, at the trailhead for the Gabrielino Trail.

Description: You'll be traveling the westernmost leg of the Gabrielino Trail, one of four routes in Angeles National Forest specially designated as National Recreation Trails. The trip is a testament to the San Gabriel Mountains' awesome powers to wipe itself clean of humankind's imprint through fire, flood, and avalanche. In the early 1900s, many tourist camps and cabins were erected along the canyon. Virtually all the structures were either destroyed by flooding in 1938 or removed through condemnation proceedings (based on water and flood-control needs) in the 1920s through the 1940s. Many of these sites were converted to picnic sites and trail camps, but the Station Fire largely obliterated much of what remained.

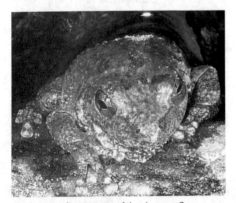
Endangered arroyo toad in Arroyo Seco

Note: Carry whatever drinking water you'll need for the duration of the trip; there may be piped water at one or another of the rest stops along the way, but don't count on it.

For the easier, downhill direction suggested here, you start hiking from the west end of Switzer Picnic Area on the Gabrielino Trail. Make your way across the bridge and along a road past outlying picnic tables, and then down along the alder-shaded stream. Soon nothing but the clear-flowing stream and rustling leaves disturb the silence. Remnants of an old paved road will occasionally appear underfoot. In a couple of spots you ford the stream by boulder-hopping—easy except after heavy rain.

One mile down the canyon you come upon the foundation remnants of Switzer's Camp—now occupied by a trail campground. Established in 1884, the camp became the San Gabriels' premier wilderness resort in the early 1900s, patronized by Hollywood celebrities and anyone who had the gumption to hike or ride a burro up the tortuous Arroyo Seco Trail from Pasadena. After the construction of Angeles Crest Highway in the early 1930s and a severe flood in the 1938, the resort lost its appeal. It was finally razed in the late 1950s.

The main trail crosses to the west side of the creek at Switzer's Camp. Don't be lured onto one of the use trails continuing down the east side to some crumbling cliffs above Switzer Falls; a sign warns that an unfathomable 118 accidental falls occurred there between 1975 and 1977!

Walk down to a fork in the trail 0.2 mile beyond the trail camp. You will probably hear, if not clearly see, the 50-foot cascade known as Switzer Falls, to the east. Your way continues on the right fork (Gabrielino Trail), which now begins a mile-long traverse through burned chaparral. This stretch avoids a narrow, twisting trench called Royal Gorge,

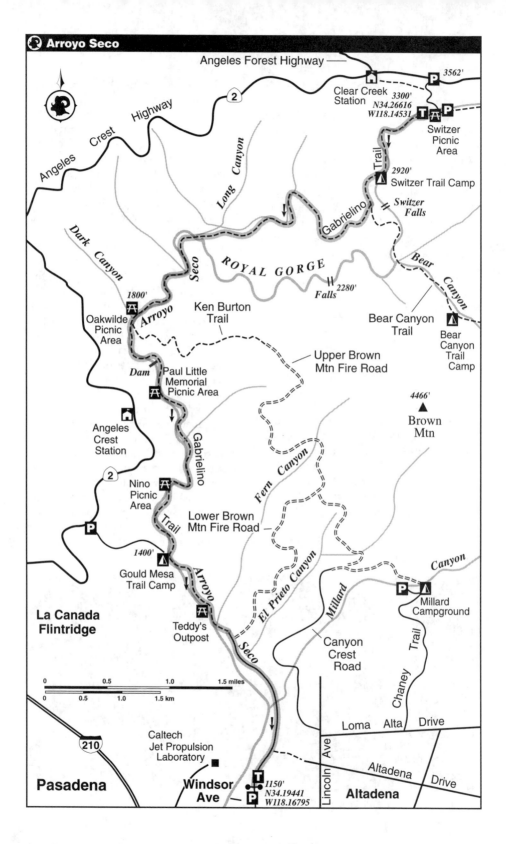

Angeles Forest Highway

2

Angeles Crest Highway

Long Canyon

Dark Canyon

Seco Arroyo

1800'
Oakwilde Picnic Area

Ken Burton Trail

ROYAL GORGE

Falls 2280'

Clear Creek Station
3300'
N34.26616
W118.14531

3562'

T A P
Switzer Picnic Area

2920'
Switzer Trail Camp

Gabrielino Trail

Switzer Falls

Bear Canyon

Bear Canyon Trail

Bear Canyon Trail Camp

Upper Brown Mtn Fire Road

4466'
Brown Mtn

Dam
Paul Little Memorial Picnic Area

Angeles Crest Station

2

Nino Picnic Area

Gabrielino

Lower Brown Mtn Fire Road

Fern Canyon

P

1400'
Gould Mesa Trail Camp

Trail

Arroyo

Teddy's Outpost

El Prieto Canyon

Millard

Canyon

P
Millard Campground

Chaney Trail

La Canada Flintridge

Canyon Crest Road

0   0.5   1.0   1.5 miles
0   0.5   1.0   1.5 km

Loma Alta Drive

Lincoln Ave

210

Caltech Jet Propulsion Laboratory

Seco Arroyo

Altadena Drive

Pasadena

Windsor Ave

T
P
1150'
N34.19441
W118.16795

Altadena

through which Arroyo Seco tumbles and sometimes abruptly drops.

At 2.3 miles (from the start) the trail joins a shady tributary of Long Canyon, and later Long Canyon itself, replete with a trickling stream. The trail mostly clings to a narrow ledge cut at great effort into the east wall of the canyon. The canyon bottom largely survived the Station Fire. Alongside the trail you'll discover at least five kinds of ferns, plus mosses, miner's lettuce, poison oak, and Humboldt lilies (in bloom during early summer).

At 3.4 miles, the waters of Long Canyon swish down through a sculpted grotto to join Arroyo Seco. The trail descends to Arroyo Seco canyon's narrow floor and vanishes. The portions once cut into the east wall have mostly collapsed or become overgrown, and the trail on the floor has been washed away. Pick the best route down the canyon, crossing the creek many times over the next few miles. In the springtime, expect to get your feet wet. The fire killed most of the gorgeous oaks, maples, and alders that once filled the canyon. Look for a tributary on the right at 4.5 miles where Camp Oak Wilde stood from 1911 until its destruction by flood in 1938. The Oakwilde Picnic Area was rebuilt in the same place, but the Station Fire wiped it out.

The canyon widens a bit. At 5.5 miles, the large Brown Canyon Debris Dam abruptly blocks your way. Built in the 1940s to reduce the flow of detritus into Pasadena, it has completely filled up and no longer serves its purpose, but it remains as a scar on the canyon that will take nature many more years to demolish. Look for a faint trail bypassing the dam high on the east wall of the canyon. Backtrack 0.2 mile and look for an obscure cairn marking the start of the trail, which climbs sharply and then descends steeply to reach the canyon bottom at a sign for the Paul Little Memorial Picnic Area.

The hardest work is over, and a decent path takes you down the remainder of the gently sloping canyon. The trail gradually improves into a road and crosses several bridges in varying states of repair. At 7.5 miles, pass the Gould Mesa Campground, named for Will Gould, a homesteader who lived here in the 1890s. Reaching the south end of the burn area, watch for a gauging station on the right and some US Forest Service residences on the left. Since the last segment of the trail is paved, you are likely to run into cyclists, joggers, parents pushing strollers, and even skateboarders. Pass the imposing complex of Caltech's Jet Propulsion Laboratory on the right, and eventually emerge at the Arroyo Boulevard Trailhead.

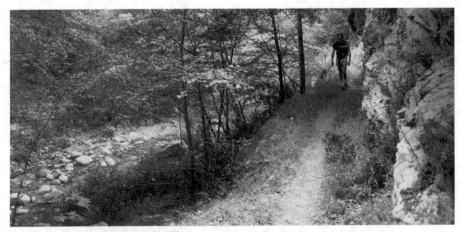

The Gabrielino Trail above Oakwilde

HIKE 19

Mount Lowe

Location	San Gabriel Mountains, above Pasadena
Highlights	Mountain, city, and ocean views
Distance	3.2 miles (out-and-back)
Total Elevation Gain/Loss	500'/500'
Hiking Time	1½ hours
Optional Maps	Tom Harrison Maps Angeles Front Country or USGS 7.5-minute *Mount Wilson*
Best Times	All year
Agency	ANF/LARD
Difficulty	Moderate
Trail Use	Dogs allowed, good for kids

Late in the year, when the smog lightens, but temperatures still hover within a moderate register, come up to Mount Lowe to toast the setting sun. You can sit on an old bench, pour some champagne, and watch Old Sol sink into Santa Monica Bay.

To Reach the Trailhead: To reach the starting point from I-210 at La Cañada, drive up Angeles Crest Highway (CA 2) for 14 miles to Red Box Divide, and turn right on Mount Wilson Road. Proceed 2.4 miles to a large roadside parking area at unmarked Eaton Saddle.

Description: Walk past the gate on the west side, and proceed up the dirt road (Mount Lowe Fire Road) that carves its way under the precipitous south face of San Gabriel Peak. The dramatic peak ahead to the west is Mount Markham. As you approach a short tunnel (0.3 mile) dating from 1942, look for the remnants of a former cliff-hanging trail to the left of the tunnel's east entrance.

At Markham Saddle (0.5 mile), reach the edge of the burn area from the vast 2009 Station Fire. Beware of fire-following poodle dog bush, which grows close to the trail and causes a severe rash. Don't continue on the road. Instead, find the

unmarked Mount Lowe Trail on the left (south). On it, you contour southwest above the fire road for 0.6 mile, and then cross a saddle between Lowe and Markham and start climbing south across the east flank of Mount Lowe.

In 0.2 mile, make a sharp right turn at a sign for Mount Lowe. Proceed 0.2

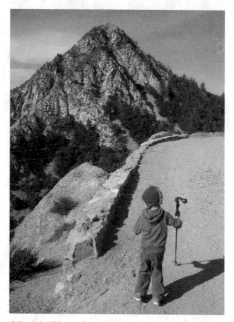

Mt. Markham from the Mt. Lowe Fire Road

mile uphill, then go left on a short spur trail to Mount Lowe's summit, where a small grove of live oaks miraculously survived the fire. Mount Lowe was the proposed upper terminus for Professor Thaddeus Lowe's famed scenic railway (see Hike 20). Funding ran out, however, and tracks were never laid higher than Ye Alpine Tavern, 1,200 feet below. During the railway's heyday in the early 1900s, thousands disembarked at the tavern

and tramped Mount Lowe's east- and west-side trails for world-class views of the basin and the surrounding mountains. Some reminders of that era remain on the summit of Mount Lowe and along some of the trails: volunteers have repainted, relettered, and returned to their proper places some of the many sighting tubes that helped the early tourists familiarize themselves with the surrounding geography.

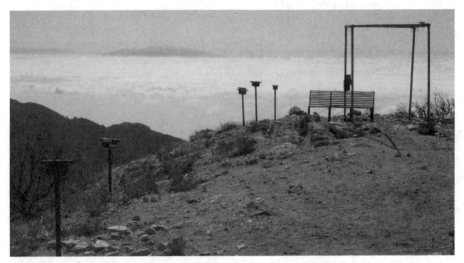

Mount Lowe Summit

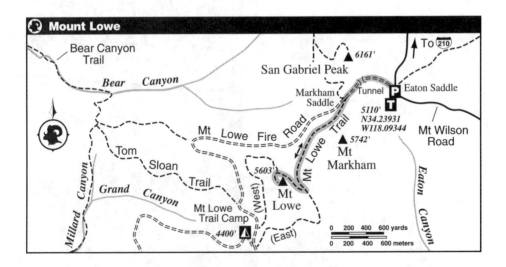

HIKE 20

Mount Lowe Railway

Location	San Gabriel Mountains, above Pasadena
Highlights	Grand vistas and historically interesting
Distance	11 miles (loop)
Total Elevation Gain/Loss	2,800'/2,800'
Hiking Time	6 hours
Optional Maps	Tom Harrison Maps Angeles Front Country or USGS 7.5-minute *Mount Wilson* and *Pasadena*
Best Times	October–May
Agency	ANF/LARD
Difficulty	Moderately strenuous
Trail Use	Suitable for backpacking, dogs allowed

An engineering marvel when it was built in the 1890s, the Mount Lowe Railway has lived a checkered past full of both glory and destruction. Before its final abandonment in the mid-1930s, the line carried more than 3 million passengers—virtually all of them tourists. Unheard of by millions of Southland newcomers today, the railway was for many years the most popular outdoor attraction in Southern California.

Today hikers are taking a new interest in the old roadbed; the Rails-to-Trails Conservancy (which promotes the conversion of abandoned rail corridors into recreation trails) ranked the Mount Lowe Railway as one of the nation's 12 most scenic and historically significant recycled rail lines.

The line consisted of three stages, of which almost nothing remains today. Passengers rode a trolley from Altadena into lower Rubio Canyon and then boarded a steeply inclined cable railway that took them 1,300 feet higher to Echo Mountain, where two hotels, a number of small tourist attractions, and an observatory stood. At Echo Mountain, nonacrophobic passengers hopped onto the third phase, a mountain trolley that climbed another 1,200 vertical feet along airy slopes to the

end of the line—Ye Alpine Tavern (later Mount Lowe Tavern, on whose ruins stands today's Mount Lowe Trail Camp). The US Forest Service and volunteers have put together a self-guiding trail, featuring 10 markers fashioned from railroad rails, along the route of the mountain trolley.

To Reach the Trailhead: The Sam Merrill Trailhead lies on the grounds of the long-demolished Cobb Estate, at the intersection of Lake Avenue and Loma Alta Drive in Altadena. Take the Lake Avenue exit from I-210 in Pasadena, and drive 3.6 miles north to where Lake Avenue turns left (west) and becomes Loma Alta Drive. Park on the street (no National Forest Adventure Pass needed).

Description: Walk east past the stone pillars at the Cobb Estate entrance, and continue 150 yards on a narrow, blacktop driveway. The driveway bends left, but you keep walking straight (east). Soon you come to a water fountain on the rim of Las Flores Canyon and a sign indicating the start of the Sam Merrill Trail. This trail goes left over the top of a small debris dam and begins a switchbacking ascent of Las Flores Canyon's precipitous east wall, while another trail (the Altadena Crest equestrian trail) veers to the right, down the canyon.

Inspired by the fabulous views (assuming you're doing this early on one of L.A.'s clear winter days), the 2.5 miles of steady ascent on the Sam Merrill Trail may seem to go rather quickly. Turn right at the top of the trail, and walk south over to Echo Mountain, which is more like the shoulder of a ridge. There you'll find a historical plaque and some picnic tables near a grove of incense-cedars and bigleaf maples. Poke around and you'll find many foundation ruins and piles of concrete rubble. An old bullwheel and cables for the incline railway were thoughtfully left behind after the US Forest Service cleared away what remained of the buildings here in the 1950s and '60s. After visiting Echo Mountain, go north on the signed Echo Mountain Trail, where you walk over railroad ties still embedded in the ground.

The rail bed is now marked with a series of interpretive signs highlighted on the following pages. Numbers in parentheses refer to hiking mileage starting from Echo Mountain.

Station 1 (0.0), Echo Mountain. This area was known as the White City during its brief heyday in the late 1890s, but most of its tourist facilities were destroyed by fire or windstorms in the first decade of the 1900s. The mountain remained a transfer point for passengers until the mid-1930s.

Station 2 (0.5), View of Circular Bridge. You can't see it from here, but passengers at this point first noticed the 400-foot-diameter circular bridge (Station 6) jutting from the slope above. As you walk on, you'll notice the many concrete footings that supported trestles bridging the side ravines of Las Flores Canyon.

Station 3 (0.8), Cape of Good Hope. You're now at the junction of the Echo Mountain Trail and Sunset Ridge Fire Road where the route crosses from Las Flores to Millard Canyon. The tracks swung in a 200-degree arc around the rocky promontory just west, Cape of Good Hope. (Walk around the Cape, if you like,

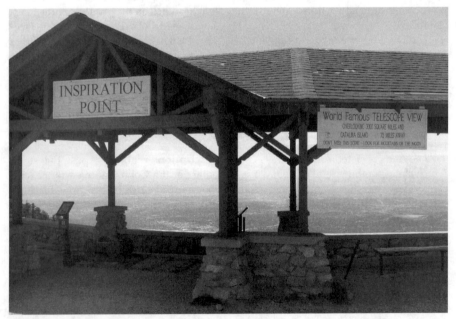

Inspiration Point

to get a feel for the experience.) North of this dizzying passage, riders were treated to the longest stretch of straight track— only 225 feet long. The entire original line from Echo Mountain to Ye Alpine Tavern had 127 curves and 114 straight sections. The Cape of Good Hope also marks the edge of the vast burn area from the 2009 Station Fire. (*Note:* Plenty of mountain bikers use this section of the old railroad grade. They mostly arrive by way of the Sunset Ridge Fire Road.)

Station 4 (1.0), Dawn Station and Devil's Slide. Gold-bearing ore, packed up by mules from Dawn Mine in the bottom of Millard Canyon, was loaded onto

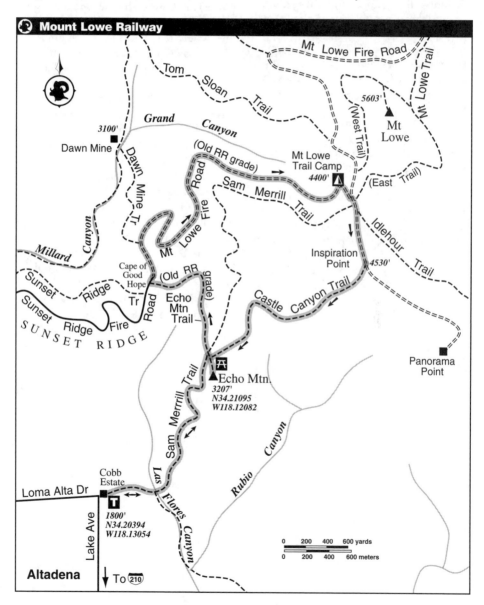

the train here. Ahead lay a treacherous stretch of crumbling granite, the Devil's Slide, which was eventually bridged by a trestle. (The current fire road has been shored up with much new concrete, and cement-lined spillways seem to do a good job of carrying away flood debris.)

Station 5 (1.2), Horseshoe Curve. Just beyond this station, Horseshoe Curve enabled the railway to gain elevation above Millard Canyon. The grade just beyond Horseshoe Curve was 7%, the steepest on the mountain segment of the line.

Station 6 (1.6), Circular Bridge. An engineering accomplishment of world-wide fame, the Circular Bridge carried startled passengers into midair over the upper walls of Las Flores Canyon. Look for the concrete supports of this bridge down along the chaparral-covered slopes to the right.

Station 7 (2.0), Horseshoe Curve Overview. Passengers here looked down on Horseshoe Curve and could also see all three levels of steep, twisting track climbing the east wall of Millard Canyon.

Station 8 (2.4), Granite Gate. A narrow slot carefully blasted out of solid granite on a sheer north-facing slope, Granite Gate took eight months to cut. Look for the electric wire support dangling from the rock above.

Station 9 (3.4), Ye Alpine Tavern. The tavern, which later became a fancy hotel, was located at Crystal Springs, the source that still provides water (which now requires purification) for backpackers staying overnight at today's Mount Lowe Trail Camp. The railway never got farther than here, although it was hoped they would one day reach the summit of Mount Lowe, 1,200 feet higher. The Station Fire thankfully spared this splendid forest of oak and bigcone Douglas-fir here.

Station 10 (3.9), Inspiration Point. From Ye Alpine Tavern, tourists could saunter over to Inspiration Point along part of the never-finished rail extension to Mount Lowe. Sighting tubes (still in place there) helped visitors locate places of interest below.

Inspiration Point is the last station on the self-guiding trail. The fastest and easiest way to return is by way of the Castle Canyon Trail, which descends directly below Inspiration Point. After 2 miles you arrive back on the old railway grade just north of Echo Mountain. Retrace your steps on the Sam Merrill Trail.

HIKE 21

Eaton Canyon

Location	Altadena (Pasadena)
Highlights	Lessons in fire ecology and a waterfall
Distance	3.4 miles (out-and-back)
Total Elevation Gain/Loss	400'/400'
Hiking Time	1½ hours
Optional Maps	Tom Harrison Maps Angeles Front Country or USGS 7.5-minute *Mount Wilson*
Best Times	All year
Agency	ECNA
Difficulty	Moderate
Trail Use	Dogs allowed, good for kids

Eaton Canyon Natural Area is a well-known gem at the foot of the San Gabriel Mountains. On a pleasant spring weekend, hundreds of people gather at the busy trailhead for a stroll. The canyon burned to ash in the 1993 Altadena Fire, but it has completely recovered. The rebuilt Nature Center is full of knowledgeable volunteers who will share their passion for the outdoors with you.

Upstream from the 190-acre park, where the waters of Eaton Canyon have carved a raw groove in the San Gabriel Mountains, you'll discover Eaton Canyon Falls. Impressive only during the wetter half of the year, the falls possesses, as John Muir once put it, "a low sweet voice, singing like a bird." The falls are well worth visiting, especially in the aftermath of a larger winter storm, if only to witness the power of large (by Southern California standards) volumes of falling water.

To Reach the Trailhead: From I-210 at Exit 29A, take Sierra Madre Boulevard north. In 0.3 mile, turn left on Orange Grove Boulevard. In 0.2 mile, turn right on Altadena Drive. Proceed 1.3 miles to Eaton Canyon Natural Area on the right. If the parking lot is full, follow signs to the overflow area.

(If you prefer, you can shorten the walk to the falls by starting from the lower gate of Mount Wilson Toll Road on Pinecrest Drive in Altadena. Be sure to observe any signs about parking restrictions in that neighborhood.)

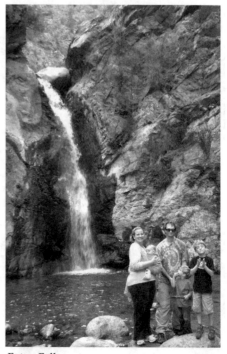

Eaton Falls

Description: The Eaton Canyon Trail splits near the trailhead. Both branches run in parallel and rejoin before crossing to the east side of the canyon; the west branch has a picnic area. Pass many splits along the way, but stay on the wide dirt track. After crossing the canyon's cobbled bottom, the trail sticks to an elevated stream terrace, passing some beautiful live-oak woods.

At 1.1 miles you rise to meet the Mount Wilson Toll Road bridge over Eaton Canyon. Just before the bridge, veer left onto a narrower track at a sign for Eaton Canyon Falls. The rough path leads up the canyon, crossing the creek eight times. Expect plenty of boulder-hopping, and you may get your feet wet if the stream is lively. (This is not a place to be when the creek is flooding.) Except for a line of alders along part of the stream and some live oaks on benches just above the reach of floods, the canyon bottom and the precipitous walls are desolate and desertlike. After a half mile of canyon-bottom travel, you come to the falls, where the water slides and then free-falls for a total of about 35 feet down a narrow chute in the bedrock.

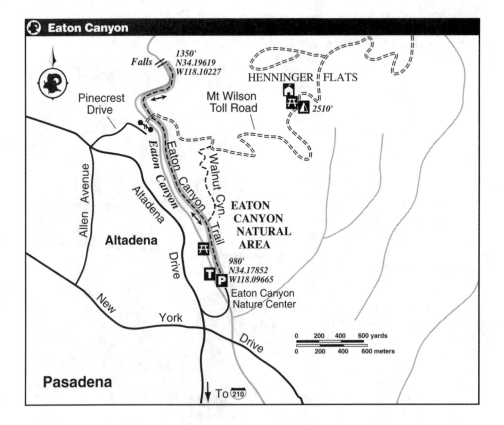

HIKE 22

Santa Anita Canyon Loop

Location	San Gabriel Mountains, above Arcadia
Highlights	Sparkling streams and botanically and historically interesting
Distance	9 miles (loop)
Total Elevation Gain/Loss	2,300'/2,300'
Hiking Time	5 hours
Optional Maps	Tom Harrison Maps Angeles Front Country or USGS 7.5-minute *Mount Wilson*
Best Times	October–June
Agency	ANF/LARD
Difficulty	Moderately strenuous
Trail Use	Suitable for backpacking, dogs allowed

In the lush, shady recesses of Santa Anita Canyon and its tributary, Winter Creek, you can easily lose all sight and sense of the hundreds of square miles of dense metropolis and the millions of people that lie just over the ridge to the south. With easy access from the San Gabriel Valley by city street and mountain road, you can be strolling along a fern-lined path less than a half hour after leaving the freeway traffic behind.

To Reach the Trailhead: From I-210 in Arcadia, follow Santa Anita Avenue north. Continue to the edge of the city, pass a sturdy gate (open 6 a.m.–8 p.m.), and ascend along a curling and precipitous ribbon of asphalt to your destination

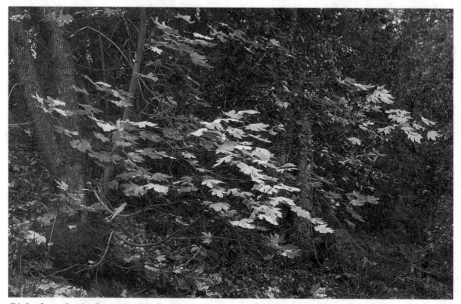

Bigleaf maples in Santa Anita Canyon

at the end of the road: Chantry Flat. Spacious, but often inadequate parking lots (National Forest Adventure Pass required), a picnic ground, and a mom-and-pop concession stand are here.

Chantry Flat also features an old-fashioned freight business—the last pack station operating year-round in California. Almost every day, horses, mules, and burros carry supplies and building materials from the station down into canyon bottom, where an anachronistic cabin community has survived since the early 1900s.

Description: In this scenic loop trip from Chantry Flat, you'll climb by way of the Gabrielino Trail to historic Sturtevant Camp, and return by way of the Mount Zion and Upper Winter Creek Trails. Do it in a day, or take your time on an overnight backpacking trip, with a stay at Spruce Grove Trail Camp. The camp is popular, so plan to get there early to secure a spot on the weekend—or go on a weekday. Be sure you can recognize poison oak because it grows beside many parts of the trail.

From the south edge of the lower parking lot at Chantry Flat, hike the first, paved segment of the Gabrielino Trail down to the confluence of Winter Creek and Santa Anita Canyon at 0.6 mile. Pavement ends at a metal bridge spanning Winter Creek. Pass the restrooms and continue up alder-lined Santa Anita Canyon on a wide roadbed following the left bank. Edging alongside a number of small cabins, the deteriorating road soon assumes the proportions of a foot trail.

At 1.4 miles, amid a beautiful oak woodland, you come to a four-way junction of trails. The right branch goes up-canyon to the base of 50-foot-high Sturtevant Falls, a worthy 0.6-mile round-trip detour during the wet season. The middle and left branches join again a mile upstream. The left, upper trail is recommended for horses. Take the middle (lower) trail—the more scenic and exciting alternative—unless you fear heights. The

lower trail slices across a sheer wall above the falls and continues through a veritable fairyland of miniature cascades and crystalline pools with giant chain ferns.

A half mile past the reconvergence of the upper and lower trails and at 2.8 miles from the trailhead, you come upon Cascade Picnic Area, which has tables and restrooms and is named for a smooth chute in the stream bottom just below. Press on past a hulking crib dam (flood-check dam) to reach Spruce Grove Trail Camp, at 3.5 miles, named for the bigcone Douglas-fir (bigcone spruce) trees that attain truly inspiring proportions on the surrounding hillsides.

Reach a junction in 0.2 mile, and turn left onto the signed Sturtevant Trail. After only 0.1 mile, Sturtevant Camp comes into view. This is both the oldest (1893) and the only remaining resort in the Santa Anita drainage. Run by the Methodist Church as a retreat (but available to other groups by reservation), the camp remains accessible only by foot trail. All supplies are packed in from Chantry Flat on the backs of pack animals, not unlike a century ago.

Before reaching the camp, cross above another crib dam to the opposite side of the creek from the camp, continue another 0.1 mile, and look for the Mount Zion Trail on the left at 3.9 miles. This restored version of the original trail to Sturtevant Camp (reconstructed in the late 1970s and early '80s) winds delightfully upward across a ravine and then along timber-shaded, north-facing slopes.

When the trail crests at a notch just northwest of Mount Zion, take the short side path up through manzanita and scrub oak to the summit at 5.0 miles, which has a broad if somewhat unremarkable view of surrounding ridges and a small slice of the San Gabriel Valley. You can see the telescope on Mount Wilson to the northwest.

Return to the main trail, and begin a long, switchback descent down the dry, north canyon wall of Winter Creek—a sweaty affair if the day is sunny and warm. At the foot of this stretch you reach the cool canyon bottom and a T-intersection with the Winter Creek Trail at 6.4 miles, just above Hoegee's Trail Camp. Turn right, going upstream momentarily, follow the trail across the creek, and climb to the next trail junction in 0.2 mile. Bear left on the Upper Winter Creek Trail, which briefly climbs and then gradually descends for 2.3 miles through the cool woods overlooking Winter Creek. Upon reaching the paved service road, follow it down 0.3 mile past a water tank and the picnic grounds to reach the signed Winter Creek Trailhead at the upper Chantry Flat parking area.

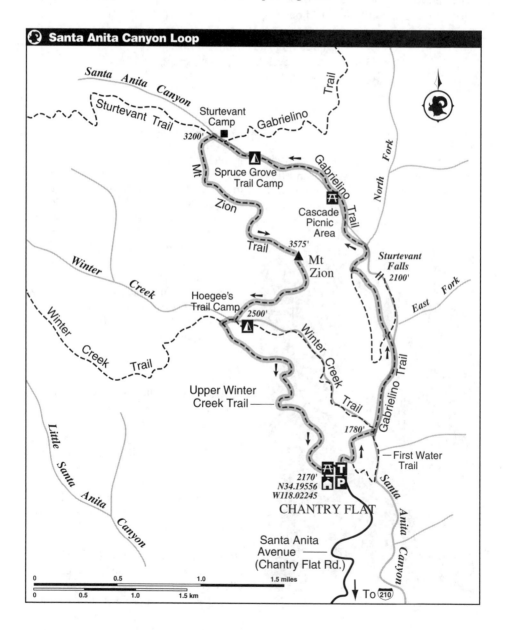

HIKE 23

Cooper Canyon Falls

Location	Central San Gabriel Mountains
Highlight	Beautiful, hidden waterfall
Distance	3.2 miles (out-and-back)
Total Elevation Gain/Loss	800'/800'
Hiking Time	1½ hours
Optional Maps	Tom Harrison Maps Angeles High Country or USGS 7.5-minute *Waterman Mtn.*
Best Times	April–November, especially spring
Agency	ANF/SCMRD
Difficulty	Moderate
Trail Use	Dogs allowed, good for kids

Cooper Canyon Falls roars with the melting snows of early spring and then settles down to a quiet whisper by June or July. You can cool off in the spray of the 25-foot cascade, or at least sit on a

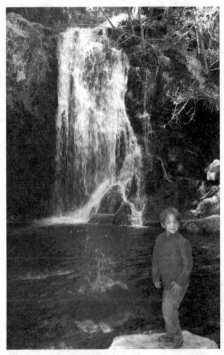

Cooper Canyon Falls

water-smoothed log and soak your feet in the chilly, alder-shaded pool just below the base of the falls. In the right season (April or May most years) these falls are one of the best unheralded attractions of the San Gabriel Mountains. The area has very little water by early in fall, but the chilly ravines offer outstanding displays of autumn color.

The Burkhart Trail takes you quickly to the falls, downhill all the way, and then uphill all the way back. The forest traversed by the trail is dense enough to give you plenty of cool shade for most of the unrelenting climb back up.

To Reach the Trailhead: From I-210 in La Cañada, drive 34 miles up Angeles Crest Highway (CA 2) to the Buckhorn Campground entrance road at mile marker 2 LA 58.25. Drive all the way through the campground to the far (northeast) end, where a short stub of dirt road leads to the Burkhart Trailhead. You must display a National Forest Adventure Pass in your car to park here.

Description: The Burkhart Trail takes off down the west wall of an unnamed, usually wet canyon garnished by two waterfalls. The first, a little gem of a cascade dropping 10 feet into a rock grotto, is easy to reach by descending from the trailside. The second, some 30 feet high, is dangerous to approach from above, but you can reach it from below by scrambling up the canyon bottom from Cooper Canyon.

At 1.2 miles, the trail bends east to follow Cooper Canyon's south bank. Continue another 0.3 mile, down past the junction with the Pacific Crest Trail that doubles back to follow the north bank upstream. Look or listen for water plunging over the rocky declivity to the left. A rough pathway leads down off the trail to the alder-fringed pool below. The bottom of the path is steep and slippery and might have a rope that you can use to steady yourself—inspect it before trusting it.

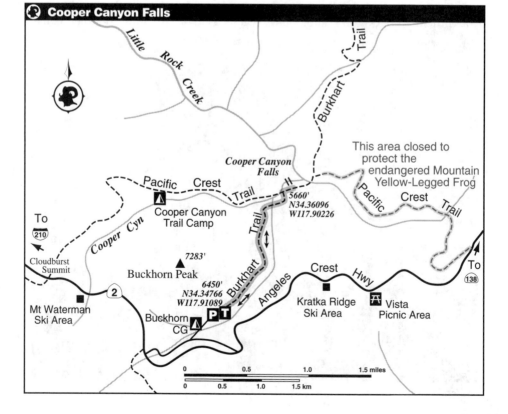

Cooper Canyon Falls

This area closed to protect the endangered Mountain Yellow-Legged Frog

HIKE 24

Mount Waterman Trail

Location	Central San Gabriel Mountains
Highlights	Vistas of yawning canyons, possible bighorn sheep sightings
Distance	8 miles (one way)
Total Elevation Gain/Loss	1,400'/2,250'
Hiking Time	4½ hours
Optional Maps	Tom Harrison Maps Angeles High Country or USGS 7.5-minute *Waterman Mtn.*
Best Times	May–November
Agency	ANF/SGRD
Difficulty	Moderately strenuous
Trail Use	Suitable for backpacking, dogs allowed

The Mount Waterman Trail traverse across the north rim of San Gabriel Wilderness provides almost constant views of statuesque pines, yawning chasms, and distant, hazy ridges. You start near the entrance to Buckhorn Campground, and you end up half-circling broad-shouldered Waterman Mountain by the time you arrive at Three Points, 5 miles away by car. Snow can linger on the easternmost mile of the trail until May, but it tends to disappear much earlier on the

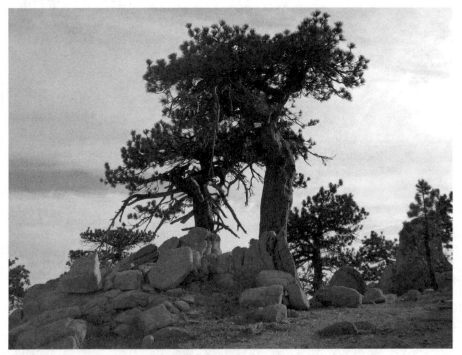

Waterman Mountain

remaining (mostly south-facing) parts of the trail. This is one of the most popular high-country summer hikes—one heartily recommend for all but the warmest days.

To Reach the Trailhead: To reach the Three Points Trailhead from I-210 in La Cañada, drive 29 miles up Angeles Crest Highway (CA 2) to an unmarked turnout on the left near mile marker 2 LA 52.66, where you will leave a getaway vehicle. The Pacific Crest Trail crosses the highway just beyond, but the small signs are easy to miss while driving. If you reach the Sulphur Springs and Santa Clara Divide Road, you've gone 0.1 mile too far. To reach the Mount Waterman Trailhead, continue 5 miles up to a large turnout on the left at mile marker 2 LA 58.02 across the road from the signed trailhead. Cars

parked at either trailhead must display a National Forest Adventure Pass.

If you would prefer to use a bicycle for your shuttle, it is more enjoyable to do the hike in reverse, leaving your bike at the Mount Waterman Trailhead so that your return is mostly downhill. This approach adds 850 feet of elevation gain to the trip.

Description: From the Buckhorn end, follow the well-graded Mount Waterman Trail—not the old roadbed paralleling the trail at first—along a shady slope. Soon, cross another dirt service road. After 1.0 mile of easy ascent through gorgeous mixed-conifer forest, you come to a saddle overlooking Bear Creek. The trail turns west, follows a viewful ridge, and then ascends on six long switchbacks to a trail junction at 2.1 miles. The trail on your right to Waterman Mountain's flat summit

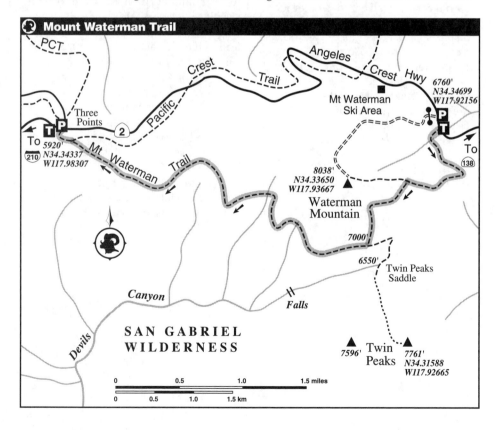

is a worthy side trip that adds 0.8 mile and 400 feet of climbing one way. The main trip stays left and contours west about 0.5 mile, then it zigzags south down to a second junction at 3.0 miles. Twin Peaks Saddle, a spacious spot suitable for camping, lies below to the left. If you're day-hiking this stretch, then stay right (west).

The remaining 5 miles take you gradually downhill (steeper at the very end) along a generally south-facing slope. You wind in and out of broad ravines, either shaded by huge incense-cedars and vanilla-scented Jeffrey pines or exposed to the warm sunshine on chaparral-covered slopes. The older cedar trees are gnarled veterans of past fires. Portions of this area burned again in the massive 2009 Station Fire, and the last 2 miles of the trail were nearly incinerated. Beware of poodle dog bush growing along the trail in the fresh burn area, especially at lower elevations. This rather attractive, leafy green shrub displays showy blue or purple flowers from June through August. Touching poodle dog bush causes unfortunate victims a nasty delayed rash, including itching and blisters. The bush sprouts after fire has cleared the ground, and it may persist for up to a decade after a fire. Then its seeds remain dormant in the soil until the next fire.

The rugged topography of San Gabriel Wilderness below conceals herds of Nelson bighorn sheep. This area and another to the east, Sheep Mountain Wilderness, were classified as statutory wilderness areas in part to preserve the habitat of these magnificent animals. The last 2 miles of the trip joins the Pacific Crest Trail, which leads down to your vehicle at the Angeles Crest Highway near Three Points.

An excellent way to extend and embellish this hike is to visit the summits of Waterman Mountain and Twin Peaks. Waterman Mountain is an easy 1.6-mile round-trip that adds 400 feet of climbing from the trail junction. Shortly before you reach the summit, watch for an unmarked junction; stay left on the main path that leads up to the summit.

A bit more involved, visiting Twin Peaks adds 4 miles and 1,800 feet of climbing. Take the trail that switchbacks down to Twin Peaks Saddle. A good climber's trail continues south, circling a bump to reach another minor saddle. It then steeply switchbacks up the north face of the peak. Upon reaching the ridgeline, it leads left to the taller and more accessible east summit of Twin Peaks. There, on rock outcrops just below the summit, you will have a dizzying view of the canyons below. Quite often you can look out over a low-lying blanket of smog in the L.A. Basin and see Santa Catalina Island floating out at sea beyond the hazy dome of Palos Verdes. The Santa Ana Mountains, Palomar Mountain, the Santa Rosa Mountains, San Jacinto Peak, and Old Baldy arc around the horizon from south to east.

HIKE 25

Devil's Punchbowl

Location	San Gabriel Mountains, north slope
Highlight	Spectacular geological formations
Distance	1.4 miles (loop)
Total Elevation Gain/Loss	300'/300'
Hiking Time	½ hour
Optional Maps	Tom Harrison Maps Angeles High Country or USGS 7.5-minute *Valyermo*
Best Times	Sunrise–sunset, all year
Agency	DPNA
Difficulty	Easy
Trail Use	Dogs allowed, good for kids

Tens of millions of years in the making, Devil's Punchbowl is without a doubt Los Angeles County's most spectacular geological showplace. Looking down into this 300-foot-deep chasm, you immediately sense the enormity of the forces that produced the tilted and tangled collection of beige sandstone slabs.

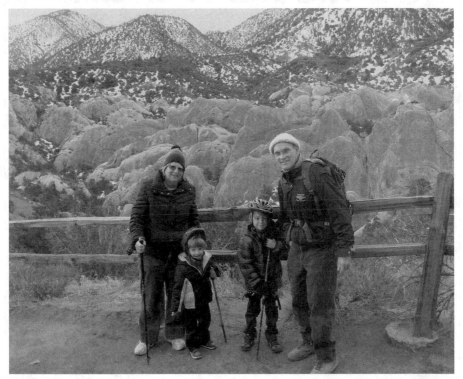

Devil's Punchbowl

The Punchbowl is caught between two active faults—the main San Andreas Fault and an offshoot, the Punchbowl Fault—along which old sedimentary formations have been pushed upward and crumpled downward, as well as transported horizontally. Weathering and erosion have put the final touches on the scene, roughing out the bowl-shaped gorge of Punchbowl Canyon and carving, in a host of unique ways, the rocks exposed at the surface.

Devil's Punchbowl Natural Area lies in the pinyon-juniper transition zone between the Mojave Desert and the richly forested slopes of the higher San Gabriels. The park features a superb nature center, a couple of short nature walks (including the loop trail described here), and the Punchbowl Trail—a part of the High Desert National Recreation Trail. South

of the punchbowl are long-distance trails leading through Angeles National Forest to the high country along Angeles Crest Highway.

To Reach the Trailhead: To reach Devil's Punchbowl from most parts of L.A., exit Antelope Valley Freeway (Highway 14) at Pearblossom Highway (Highway 138), and follow it east through the town of Littlerock to Pearblossom. At Pearblossom, turn right (south) on Longview Road (County Road N6), and follow signs for the park, 8 miles ahead. The park is open seven days a week from sunrise to sunset, with no admission charge.

Description: The 1-mile Loop Trail is a perfect introduction to the Punchbowl area. It begins just behind the nature center, zigzags down off the rim to touch the

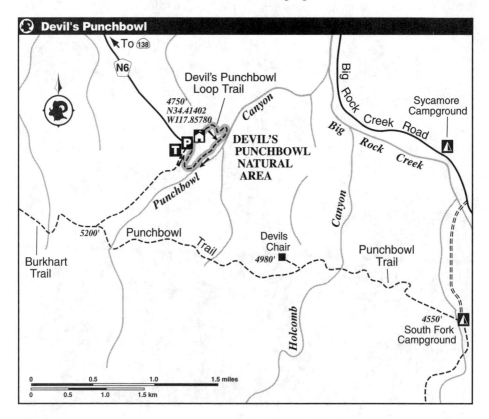

seasonal creek in Punchbowl Canyon, and then climbs back out of the canyon opposite some of the tallest upright rock formations in the park. Near the start of the trail is a side path, the 0.3-mile Pinon Pathway, a self-guiding nature trail that loops through the pinyon-juniper forest along the Punchbowl rim.

During winter, occasional snowfalls dust the Punchbowl and leave a lingering, thicker mantle of white on the pine-dotted slopes above it. At these times the Loop Trail can become muddy and slippery and is, therefore, unsuitable for small children.

Peripatetic walkers may wish to undertake the 6.4-mile round-trip trek via the Punchbowl Trail to the Devil's Chair, which perches on the upper rim of the canyon complex that generally encompasses the Punchbowl. From the parking area, head southwest up a broad path or 0.8 mile to a junction with a trail variously called the Burkhart Trail, the Devil's Chair Trail, the Punchbowl Trail, or the High Desert National Recreation Trail. The Pacific Crest Trail detours through here as well to avoid the endangered mountain yellow-legged frogs near Williamson Rock.

Turn left (east) and proceed 2.5 miles, crossing Punchbowl Creek, climbing, and then undulating. Turn left at a signed junction leading to the Devil's Chair. At the fenced viewpoint there, you can peer over what looks like frozen chaos—a vast assemblage of sandstone chunks and slabs tipped at odd angles, bent, seemingly pulled apart here, compressed there. There's a reason for this chaos: Devil's Chair sits astride the crush zone of the Punchbowl Fault.

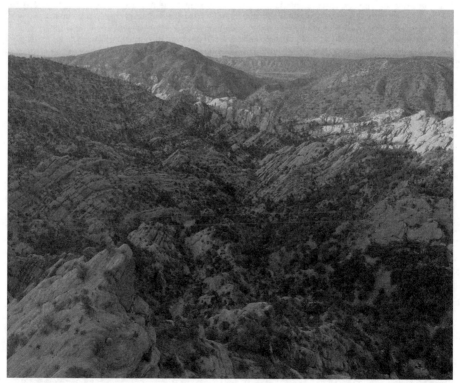

View from Devil's Chair

HIKE 26

Mount Williamson

Location	San Gabriel Mountains
Highlights	Views
Distance	4.4 miles (out-and-back)
Total Elevation Gain/Loss	1,600'/1,600'
Hiking Time	2½ hours
Optional Maps	Tom Harrison Maps Angeles High Country or USGS 7.5-minute *Crystal Lake*
Best Times	May–November
Agency	ANF/SCMRD
Difficulty	Moderate
Trail Use	Suitable for backpacking, dogs allowed

Mount Williamson is not as tall as its brethren on the opposite side of the Angeles Crest Highway, but it is nevertheless one of the most prominent and noteworthy because of its commanding position overlooking the Mojave Desert. This popular hike via the Pacific Crest Trail offers excellent views from the trail and summit.

The Pacific Crest Trail is closed at Eagles Roost, 4 miles west of Islip Saddle, to protect the endangered mountain yellow-legged frog. You may see detour signs directing PCT hikers down the South Fork Trail, but the detour does not impact this hike.

To Reach the Trailhead: The trail begins at Islip Saddle on the Angeles Crest Highway (CA 2) at mile marker 02 LA 64.17. Display a National Forest Adventure Pass.

Description: Two trails depart from the north side of the parking lot. This trip takes the one on the left, the official Pacific Crest Trail, which climbs steeply. Don't get lured onto the South Fork Trail,

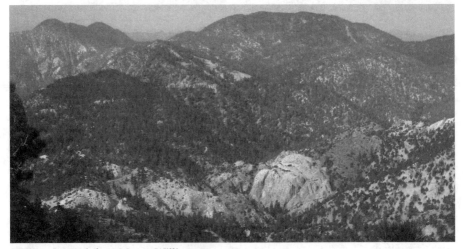

Williamson Rock from Mount Williamson

which may be marked as the PCT detour route. The trail climbs through a conifer forest, heading to a small saddle and then continuing to wind upward to a point on the south ridge of Mount Williamson, 1.6 miles from the start.

Veer right on an unmaintained but heavily used climber's trail leading up the ridge to Mount Williamson. The huge formation to the west above Little Rock Creek is Williamson Rock, which was a major Southern California sport-climbing destination before it was closed to protect the frogs. Pass a false summit on the right, and in 0.6 mile, reach Mount Williamson's slightly higher true summit. A third summit just beyond is about the same height.

From here, you can clearly identify the linear rifts formed by the San Andreas and Punchbowl Faults. On a particularly clear day, you can look across tens of thousands of square miles of desert to see the Southern Sierra Nevada and Telescope Peak above Death Valley. For those so inclined, there is adequate space to pitch a tent and enjoy exceptional stargazing. Looking north, you may see the metallic glint of wreckage on the northeast ridge of Pallett Mountain. A C119 Flying Boxcar from March Air Force Base crashed in 1966, killing all four crew and scattering aluminum on both sides of the ridge. The 1.5-mile ridge walk to inspect the site is fairly strenuous.

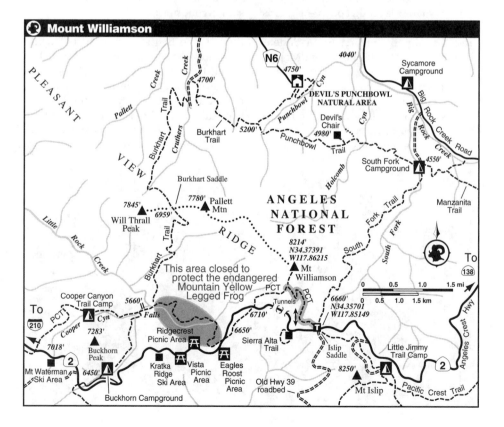

HIKE 27

Mount Baden-Powell Traverse

Location	Eastern San Gabriel Mountains
Highlights	Subalpine habitat, panoramic views, and possible bighorn sheep sightings
Distance	9 miles (one way)
Total Elevation Gain/Loss	2,400'/3,700'
Hiking Time	5 hours
Optional Map	Tom Harrison Maps Angeles High Country or USGS 7.5-minute *Crystal Lake*
Best Times	May–November
Agency	ANF/SGRD
Difficulty	Moderately strenuous
Trail Use	Suitable for backpacking, dogs allowed

Massive Mount Baden-Powell stands head and shoulders above the foggy or smoggy marine layer that often enshrouds the lowlands of the Los Angeles Basin and the Inland Empire. From Baden-Powell's flattish top, the brown Mojave Desert floor stretches interminably inland toward some hazy vanishing point. The disembodied summit ridges of mountain ranges as far west as Ventura County and as far south as San Diego County seem to float over opaque blankets of haze. Santa

Catalina, and sometimes other Channel Islands, are visible on an average early-summer morning.

Named in honor of Lord Baden-Powell, the British Army officer who started the Boy Scout movement in 1907, Baden-Powell soars higher (9,399') than any other mountain in the San Gabriel mountain range—except for the Mount San Antonio (Old Baldy) complex to the east. Many thousands of hikers troop to Baden-Powell's summit yearly, most of

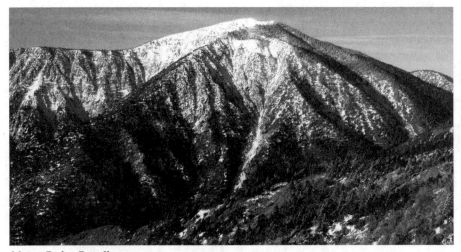

Mount Baden-Powell

them by way of the trail from Vincent Gap on Angeles Crest Highway. Baden-Powell's summit is the last major milestone on the 52-mile trek from Chantry Flat to Vincent Gap known as the Silver Moccasin Trail. The 5-day-long Silver Moccasin backpack is a rite-of-passage for L.A.-area Scouts.

If you want to climb Mount Baden-Powell without having to retrace your steps, you can try a one-way hike, described here, from Dawson Saddle to Vincent Gap. The effort is only bit more than what's involved in the usual round-trip from Vincent Gap, and you'll visit two other peaks as well. All three peaks offer their own unique and panoramic perspective of the rugged Sheep Mountain Wilderness to the south. As the name suggests, this wilderness protects the habitat of the Nelson bighorn sheep,

which number several hundred in the San Gabriel Mountains. Early-morning sightings of the bighorn are not unusual on and near Mount Baden-Powell.

At a moderate pace, including a few short breaks and a stop for lunch, the 9-mile hike should take you about 6 hours. Snow accumulations can blanket the area until June. Thereafter, little or no water can be found on the route, so carry plenty of it. The start and end points of the hike are 5 miles apart by way of Angeles Crest Highway, so you should plan to bring either two cars for a car shuttle, or one car plus a bicycle (to be left near the end point for use in retrieving the car from the start point after the hike is over). Those planning a bicycle shuttle may prefer to do this hike in reverse so they can coast down the road on the bike.

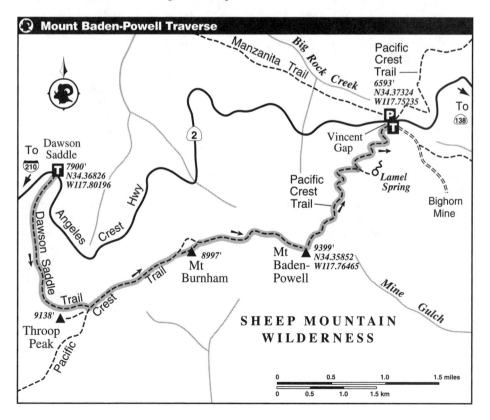

Baden-Powell is also a popular winter ascent because Caltrans usually plows the road to Vincent Gap. The icy climb demands crampons, an ice axe, and suitable experience. Most winter climbers return the way they came.

To Reach the Trailhead: From I-210 in La Cañada, drive 50 miles east on Angeles Crest Highway (CA 2) to reach the Vincent Gap Trailhead at mile marker 02 LA 74.75. Alternatively, you can approach this same trailhead from the east by way of I-15, Highway 138, and Angeles Crest Highway through Wrightwood. Vincent Gap is 10 miles west of Wrightwood via Angeles Crest Highway.

Your hike ends at Vincent Gap, but it begins about 5 miles west of Vincent Gap at a point just east of Dawson Saddle at mile marker 02 LA 69.6. There's room for parking along Angeles Crest Highway there, across from where the trail starts. To park at either trailhead, you must display a National Forest Adventure Pass. If you prefer to arrange a bicycle shuttle between the trailheads, do the hike in reverse so you can enjoy the steep downhill bike ride along the highway.

Description: Beginning at the highway just east of Dawson Saddle, the Dawson Saddle Trail immediately switchbacks uphill (south) through pines and firs to gain the top of a long, gradually ascending ridge that culminates at Throop Peak. Building this trail, which was completed in 1982, required an impressive 3,540 hours of volunteer labor by Boy Scouts. Note that another unsigned steeper trail starts at Dawson Saddle and joins the main trail in 0.25 mile. About halfway up the trail, lodgepole pines dominate the forest, but keen eyes will spot a few limber pines, which are relatively rare in Southern California. Look closely at the needles: Lodgepole-pine needles come in bundles of two, while limber pines have bundles of five. Where the trail veers east off the ridge to bypass Throop Peak, step off the trail to find a sheltered campsite on a flat part of the ridge that could accommodate a large Scout troop.

After 1.8 miles you join the Pacific Crest Trail. From this junction, the first side trip takes you southwest on the PCT for 200 yards and then off-trail in the same direction another 300 yards to Throop Peak. This summit and the other two you'll reach later has a hikers' register.

Return to the Dawson Saddle Trail junction, and continue northeast on the PCT, which follows the main, semi-shaded ridgeline. You descend to a saddle and then ascend to Mount Burnham's north flank, from where switchbacks take you over to its east shoulder. Double back (go west) if you want to take the easy side trip to the summit.

After bagging Burnham, continue east, climbing another breathless 400 feet, to reach the next trail junction. Just above it is Mount Baden-Powell's summit and an impressive monument constructed by the Boy Scouts. Weather-beaten lodgepole and limber pines dot the summit area.

Return to the junction and take the main, heavily traveled trail that descends Baden-Powell's northeast ridge. After 40 switchbacks and 3.8 miles of steady descent, you reach the end, the large Vincent Gap parking area on Angeles Crest Highway. About halfway down this trail, from the corner of the 25th switchback, a side trail leads about 200 yards east to a dribbling pipe at Lamel Spring, the only dependable source of water along the route.

HIKE 28

Lewis Falls

Location	San Gabriel Mountains, above Azusa
Highlights	Beautiful stream and cascades
Distance	0.8 mile (out-and-back)
Total Elevation Gain/Loss	300'/300'
Hiking Time	1 hour
Optional Maps	Tom Harrison Maps Angeles High Country or USGS 7.5-minute *Crystal Lake*
Best Times	All year
Agency	ANF/SGRD
Difficulty	Easy
Trail Use	Dogs allowed, good for kids

At the precipice called Lewis Falls, Soldier Creek shoots (or merely dribbles if it's not the rainy season or has been a dry year) some 50 feet down a two-tiered rock face. The volume of water splattering on rocks and sand below is seldom dramatic, but the cool spray and the sounds of falling water are refreshing. The hike to the base of the falls is short, a manageable adventure (with some assistance) for small children.

To Reach the Trailhead: Lewis Falls is located off CA 39, the road from Azusa into San Gabriel Canyon and Crystal Lake Recreation Area. Use the roadside mileage markers to identify the starting point, a small, shaded turnout on the right at mile 34.8, where Soldier Creek tumbles through a culvert under the highway. Don't forget to display a National Forest Adventure Pass on your car.

Description: From the highway turnout, make your way up a well-beaten trail on the east side of the creek, under shade-giving oaks, laurels, and bigcone Douglas-firs. Many summer cabins once lined the creek, but only a few remain. Nearly the entire Crystal Lake basin was burned in the 2002 Curve Fire, and you can still see the scars of the fire in singed tree trunks,

downed trees, and cabin foundations. In 0.3 mile, the main trail peters out. Scramble the last 0.1 mile along the banks of the creek, hopping along rocks and over logs.

Most of the year Soldier Creek is a tame brook that the average adult can easily jump. But a major storm or a rapid

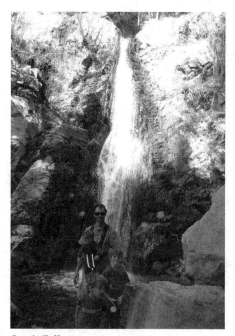

Lewis Falls

thaw in the snowpack above could produce runoff deep and swift enough to be hazardous—especially for kids.

Just above Lewis Falls, but inaccessible by the route just described, is a beautiful stretch of Soldier Creek featuring a half dozen small cascades. This secret hideaway is also a short walk away from CA 39. To go that way, drive to mile 36.8 on CA 39, from where a wide, gated dirt road goes east. Park so as not to block the gate, and on foot follow the dirt road 0.5 mile east to its end. Find a narrow trail on the left, contouring through the brush. It leads 300 yards, sometimes precariously, across a steep slope to the cascades.

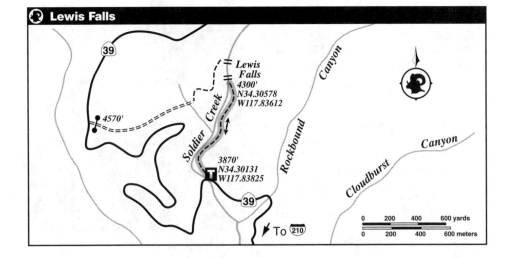

HIKE 29

Mount Islip

Location	Crystal Lake Recreation Area
Highlight	Ocean to desert views
Distance	8 miles (loop)
Total Elevation Gain/Loss	2,400'/2,400'
Hiking Time	4 hours
Optional Maps	Tom Harrison Maps Angeles High Country or USGS 7.5-minute *Crystal Lake*
Best Times	May–November
Agency	ANF/SGRD
Difficulty	Moderately strenuous
Trail Use	Suitable for backpacking, dogs allowed

The south approach of Mount Islip, one of the significant high points in the San Gabriel Mountains, feels a bit like real mountain climbing, despite its rather straightforward ascent by way of marked trails. You begin amid spreading oaks and tall conifers in Crystal Lake basin, rise through progressively smaller and sparser timber, and finally reach the nearly bald and often windblown summit. On clear days it offers a comprehensive view, both north over the Mojave Desert and south over the metropolis.

For the slight effort of an extra half mile on the way up or down, you can spend the night at Little Jimmy Campground, one of the nicest trail camps in the San Gabriels. The 2002 Curve Fire swept nearly the entire Crystal Lake basin, burning to the ground much of the low-growing vegetation and singeing or destroying most of the trees. The forest will take decades to return to its former stature.

To Reach the Trailhead: From I-210 in Azusa, drive north on Azusa Avenue, which becomes San Gabriel Canyon Road (CA 39) as it passes flood-control basins at the mouth of San Gabriel Canyon. Continue 24 miles north through the canyon to the Crystal Lake Recreation Area

turnoff. Drive a half mile past the Crystal Lake Visitor Center to the main hikers' parking lot, and don't forget to display a National Forest Adventure Pass on your parked car.

Description: Start hiking on the marked Windy Gap Trail. On the way to Windy Gap, you cross the Mount Hawkins Truck Trail twice (at the first crossing the road is paved and at the second it's dirt) and then tackle the steep, upper slopes of the cirquelike rim overlooking Crystal Lake basin. Windy Gap is the lowest spot on the north side of that rim.

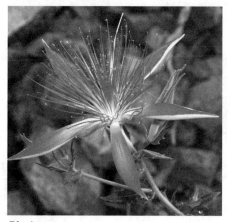

Blazing star

At Windy Gap and 2.5 miles into your hike, you meet the Pacific Crest Trail, which joins from the right (east). Continue briefly north on the PCT to the next junction. Going left takes you more directly to the summit of Mount Islip, while going right leads you to Little Jimmy Campground and a more roundabout ascent of the mountain. In either case, you'll end up on the trail that follows the sunny east ridge of Mount Islip to its summit. (*Note:* Hard snow or ice can linger on the steep, north-facing slopes north of Windy Gap until sometime in May. You can avoid that stretch if need be by going straight up the east shoulder of Mount Islip from

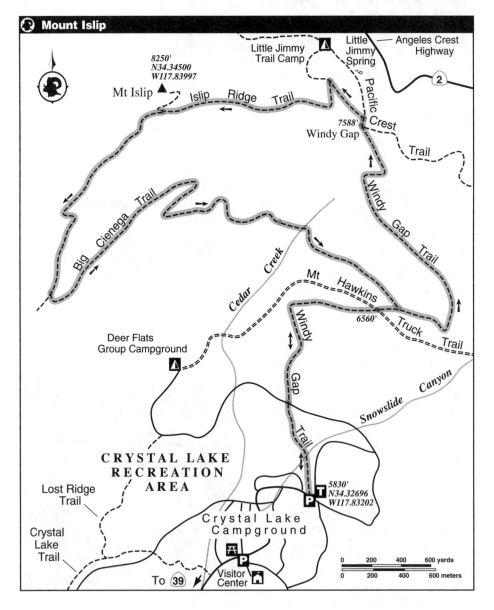

Windy Gap; that route becomes snow-free earlier in the season.)

On the summit at 3.5 miles you'll discover the shell of an old stone cabin and footings of a fire lookout tower that stood on Islip from 1927 until 1937, when the lookout was moved to a better site to the southeast, South Mount Hawkins. That structure was completely destroyed in the 2002 Curve Fire.

On your return, for the sake of variety, you can follow the Islip Ridge and Big Cienega Trails. Two switchbacks below the summit of Mount Islip, turn right on the Islip Ridge Trail, which goes down Islip's south ridge. A planned extension of that trail will go south and east all the way to Crystal Lake. You, however, travel just 1.0 mile down Islip Ridge Trail and then veer east on Big Cienega Trail. After another 2.0 miles of gradual descent along wooded south-facing slopes, you join the Windy Gap Trail just north of the upper crossing of Mount Hawkins Truck Trail. Turn right and return to the hikers' parking lot.

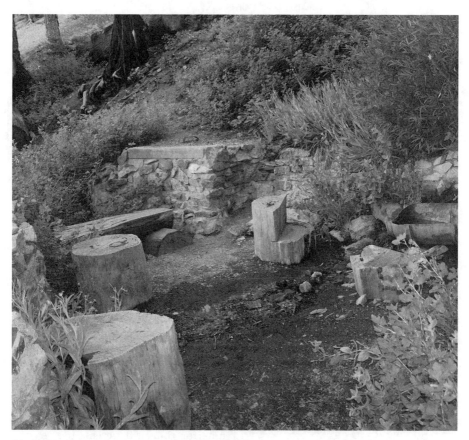

Little Jimmy Spring

HIKE 30

Down the East Fork

Location	San Gabriel River, San Gabriel Mountains
Highlights	An epic trek along a cascading stream and nearly a vertical mile of descent
Distance	16 miles (one way)
Total Elevation Gain/Loss	200'/4,800'
Hiking Time	11 hours
Recommended Maps	Tom Harrison Maps Angeles High Country or USGS 7.5-minute *Crystal Lake, Mount San Antonio,* and *Glendora*
Best Times	May–November
Agency	ANF/SGRD
Difficulty	Strenuous
Trail Use	Suitable for backpacking, dogs allowed
Permit	Self-issued permit required only if you are starting from the East Fork Trailhead

Born from snow-fed rivulets, the many tributaries of the East Fork San Gabriel River gather together to form one of the liveliest and most remote streams in the San Gabriel Mountains. At The Narrows of

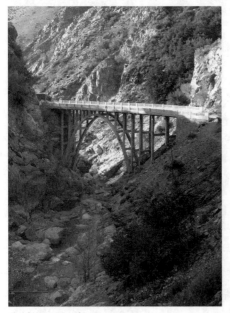

Bridge to Nowhere

the East Fork, the water squeezes through the deepest gorge in Southern California. From the bottom of The Narrows, the east wall soars about 5,200 feet to Iron Mountain, and the west wall rises about 4,000 feet to the South Mount Hawkins divide.

On this grand journey down the upper East Fork, you'll descend nearly a mile in elevation, travel from high-country pines and firs to sun-scorched chaparral, and cross three important geologic faults: the Punchbowl, Vincent Thrust, and San Gabriel Faults. During the course of a single day you could experience a temperature increase of as much as 60°F.

You can do this hike in one incredibly long day with an early start, or you can camp overnight on one of the shaded streamside terraces near the midpoint of the trek. The better camping sites include former trail camps at Fish and Iron Forks and the lower part of The Narrows.

The upper part of the canyon receives few visitors and remains pristine, while the lower portion is heavily traveled by day hikers and "prospectors" panning for gold in the creek. If everyone hauls out a bit of the detritus left behind by thoughtless users, the canyon will become more attractive.

This route passes through the Sheep Mountain Wilderness. Presently, a wilderness permit is only required if you start this trip from the south at the East Fork Trailhead, and they're available at a self-service trailhead kiosk at the parking area.

Navigation on the trip is easy throughout—you simply head down-canyon the whole way. Consult a detailed map often if you want to confirm exactly where you are. Heavy runoff after a storm or major snowmelt can create hazardous stream crossings, which is one of the reasons why this trip is only recommended from late spring through fall. Contact the Angeles National Forest rangers for current conditions. The other reason is that snow may block access to the upper trailhead at Vincent Gap, although CA 2 is usually plowed to Vincent Gap. Check dot.ca.gov for road conditions; if the highway is listed as "closed 5 miles west of Big Pines," it is open to Vincent Gap.

It's practical to have someone drop you off at the starting point, Vincent Gap, and later pick you up at the hike's end, East Fork Station. That being said, it is important to note that the amount of time required to complete the trip can vary greatly due to problems with adverse weather or swift-flowing water, excessive bushwhacking along the banks of the upper river, how heavy a pack you are carrying, and the hiking ability of your party's slowest member. This is not a trip for hikers without plenty of successful experience in off-trail wilderness travel. Allow some flexibility in your planned arrival time at the end.

Cars parked at either the start or the end point will need a National Forest Adventure Pass.

To Reach the Trailhead (Vincent Gap): From I-210 in La Cañada, drive 50 miles east on the Angeles Crest Highway (CA 2) to reach the Vincent Gap Trailhead (mile 74.8 according to the roadside mile markers). Alternatively, you can approach this same trailhead from the east by way of I-15, CA 138, and Angeles Crest Highway through Wrightwood. Vincent Gap is 10 miles west of Wrightwood via Angeles Crest Highway.

To Reach the Trailhead (East Fork Station): From I-210 in Azusa, drive north on Azusa Avenue and San Gabriel Canyon Road (CA 39) for 11 miles to East Fork Road. Continue up East Fork Road 6 miles to its gated terminus at the East Fork Trailhead.

Description: From the parking area on the south side of Vincent Gap, walk down the gated road to the southeast. At a wilderness kiosk in 0.2 mile, a footpath veers left, into Sheep Mountain Wilderness. Take it; the road itself continues toward the Bighorn Mine, an inholding of privately owned land inside the wilderness boundary.

Intermittently shaded by bigcone Douglas-firs, white firs, Jeffrey pines, and live oaks, the path descends along the south slope of Vincent Gulch. The gulch itself follows the Punchbowl Fault, a splinter of the San Andreas. At 0.7 mile, on a flat ridge spur, look for an indistinct path on the right that leads about 100 yards, passing a tangle of downed trees, to an old cabin believed to have been the home of Charles Vincent. Vincent led the life of a hermit, prospector, and big-game hunter in the Baden-Powell and Old Baldy area from 1870 until his death in 1926.

After a few switchbacks, the primitive trail crosses Vincent Gulch (usually dry at this point, but wet a short distance below) at 1.6 miles. Thereafter it stays on or above the east bank. Pass a tributary on the left in 0.4 mile, and then a second one in another 0.5 mile. An unsigned trail leads to some fine campsites in the second tributary, but you should be careful to stay right and drop onto the floor of the main drainage.

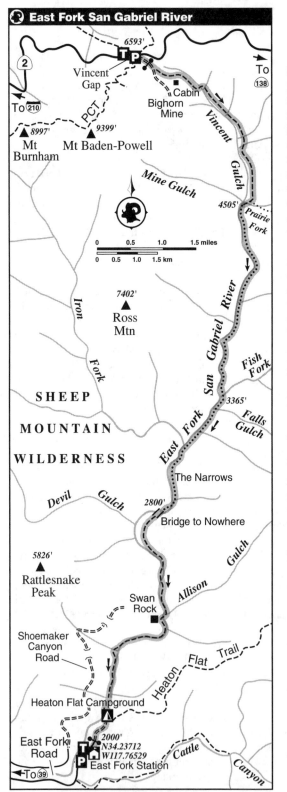

The trail soon becomes indistinct, and you must pick your own path down the rocky floor of Vincent Gulch. In 0.6 mile, watch for the wreck of a Schweizer sailplane. In February 1974, the plane was caught in a severe downdraft on the flank of Mount Baden-Powell and became trapped in the canyon. The occupants walked away with minor injuries, but the plane was unsalvageable.

A large sign marks the confluence of Prairie Fork, a wide drainage coming in from the east at 4.2 miles from the start. A trail once led up this canyon to Cabin Flat, but it was obliterated by the 1997 Beiderbach Fire and is now heavily overgrown with poison oak and stinging nettles. You veer right (west) down a gravelly wash, good for setting up a camp.

Shortly after, at the Mine Gulch confluence, you bend left (south) into the wide bed of the upper East Fork. For several miles to come, there is essentially no trail. It may take several hours to traverse this stretch, depending on your group's energy and motivation. To help you gauge your progress, you can often see Iron Mountain, the major summit to the south.

Proceed down the rock-strewn floodplain, crossing the creek (and battling alder thickets) several times over the next mile. The canyon becomes narrow for a while, and you must wade or hop from one slippery rock to another. Fish Fork, on the left at 7.9 miles from the start, is the first large stream south of Prairie Fork. One of the best campsites along the canyon can be found here.

If you have time for an intriguing side trip, Fish Fork canyon is well worth exploring. Chock-full of alder and bay, narrow with soaring walls, its clear stream tumbling over boulders, the canyon boasts one of the wildest and most beautiful settings in the San Gabriels. About 1.6 miles upstream lies a formidable impasse: There, the waters of Fish Fork drop 12 feet into an emerald-green pool set amid sheer rock walls. A bigger waterfall, inaccessible by means of this approach, lies farther upstream.

In another 0.3 mile, you may observe a thin column of water dropping over the cliff at the mouth of Falls Gulch on the left. In another mile, you enter The Narrows. A rough trail, worn in by hikers, traverses this 1-mile-plus section of fast-moving water. You'll pass swimmable (if chilly) pools cupped in the granite and schist bedrock and cross the stream when necessary. Listen and watch for water ouzels (dippers) by the edges of the pools. Old mining trails once threaded the canyon walls here and to the north, but they are all virtually obliterated now.

At the lower portals of The Narrows at 10.7 miles, you come upon the enigmatically named Bridge to Nowhere. During the 1930s, road-builders managed to push a highway up along the East Fork stream to just this far. The arched, concrete bridge, similar in style to those built along Angeles Crest Highway, was to be a key link in a route that would carry traffic between the San Gabriel Valley and the desert near Wrightwood. Fate intervened. A great flood in 1938 thoroughly demolished most of the road, leaving the bridge stranded. Another, later attempt to construct a road through the East Fork gorge also resulted in failure. High on the canyon's west rim lies Shoemaker Canyon Road, a "road to nowhere."

Below the bridge, on remnants of the old road washed out in 1938, you'll run into more and more hikers, anglers, and other travelers out for the day. The east side of the canyon generally has a decent trail, but that occasionally becomes harder to find when you are forced over to the west side. At 12.7 miles, Swan Rock, an outcrop of metamorphic rock branded with the light-colored imprint of a swan, comes into view on the right. At 15.0 miles you come upon Heaton Flat Campground. From there a final, easy 0.5-mile stroll takes you to the East Fork Station and trailhead at the end of East Fork Road.

HIKE 31

Fish Canyon Falls

Location	Foothills of the San Gabriel Mountains behind Duarte
Highlight	Arguably the most beautiful waterfall in Angeles National Forest
Distance	3.8 miles (out-and-back)
Total Elevation Gain/Loss	600'/600'
Hiking Time	2 hours
Optional Maps	Tom Harrison Maps Angeles High Country or USGS 7.5-minute *Azusa*
Best Times	Select spring weekends when the Vulcan shuttle operates
Agency	ANF/SGRD
Difficulty	Moderate
Trail Use	Dogs allowed, good for kids
Permit	Access allowed only on select spring Saturdays

Time-traveling visitors from a century ago would have a hard time recognizing Fish Canyon today. Long gone are the dozens of vacation cabins lining the canyon and the dance hall at the canyon's mouth. Today, the lower canyon is being chewed apart on an astounding scale by rock quarrying operations. These operations, however, extend only as far into the canyon as the Angeles National Forest boundary. Beyond lies perennially green Fish Canyon, its sparkling stream, and its magnificent, multitiered waterfall.

It is difficult to be definitive about how to hike into the upper canyon and visit the falls because the means of access have changed frequently over the past decades. During the 1980s and most of the '90s, public access to the canyon was made difficult or impossible by operations at the Vulcan Materials quarry. The access issue was at least temporarily resolved in 1998, when the city of Duarte opened a new trail bypassing the quarry on the canyon's steep, west wall. Unfortunately, the devilish climb and descent on this trail (if accomplished twice during the round-trip) occupies almost three-fourths of the time and

energy expended on the entire hike to the falls. The round-trip to and from the falls via this route totals 9 miles with elevation gains and losses of 3,100 feet. To make things worse, the lower part of the bypass trail quickly fell into disrepair due to its unfavorable route across perpetually sliding, steep slopes. It is still passable, though some consider it to be excessively dangerous.

For a time, hikers were given permission to pass through quarry property on Sundays, when mining operations were suspended. Lately, Vulcan Materials has started providing a shuttle through the quarry on select spring Saturdays, which allows hikers to avoid the brutally steep, rough bypass route. See azusarock.com /fishcreek/calendar.html for details.

To Reach the Trailhead: From I-210, exit north on Irwindale Avenue in Irwindale. In 0.2 mile, turn left (west) on Foothill Boulevard, which becomes Huntington Drive. In 0.7 mile, turn right on Encanto Parkway. Follow it 1.4 miles northeast as it turns into Fish Canyon Road. The quarry entrance is at the end of the road, and the bypass trail starts on the left.

Description: The Vulcan shuttle will take you the first half mile up the canyon through a literal no-man's land of raw earth and gargantuan machinery flanked by dynamite-blasted cliffs. After the shuttle drops you off, you enter a delightful, alder-lined riparian zone with the Fish Canyon stream alongside you and a trail to follow up the canyon. Around the first bend, the trail climbs to a bench on the left, and you instantly forget the ugliness of the quarry.

The remainder of the route features a gentle ascent, superb scenery, and many historical reminders. Notice the old cabin foundations, rock and mortar walls, and rusty household equipment. Check out the botanical evidence: nonnative ivy, vinca, trees-of-heaven, agaves, and ornamental yuccas. Plenty of native vegetation thrives here, too. Live oaks, bigleaf maples, and bay laurels cling tenaciously to the canyon's precipitous walls, helping to hold together the structurally precarious miscellany of smashed-up granitic and metamorphic rock. Be alert for poison oak.

After about 1.5 miles on the west bank, the trail crosses to the east bank—a foot- and leg-wetting exercise when the water's running high. A final 0.3-mile stretch leads to a point on the canyonside offering a fine but not intimately close view of Fish Canyon Falls. The water tumbles nearly 100 feet down a cliff with four separate tiers, slides through riparian vegetation a short way, and makes a final, small leap into a crystalline pool just below the trail. Expect to have plenty of company at the pool.

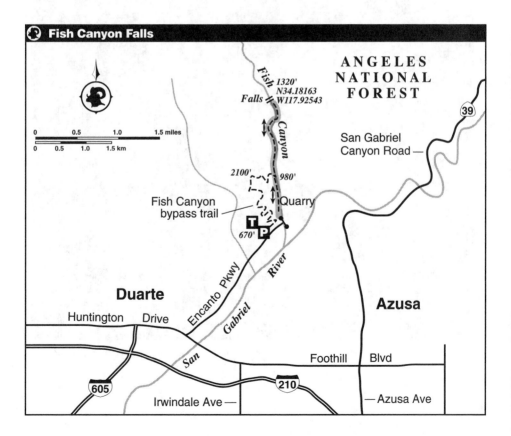

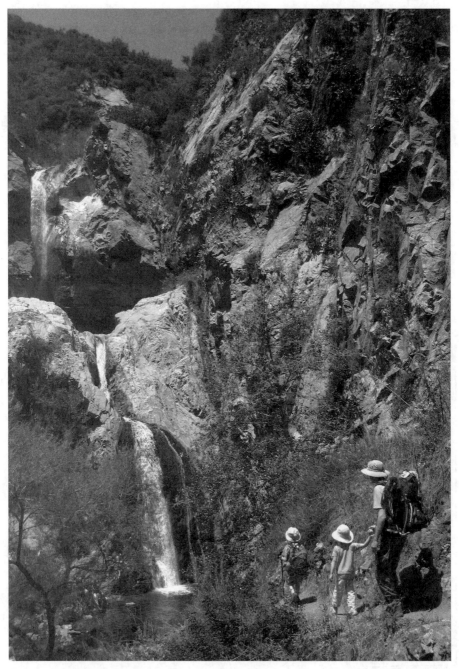

Fish Canyon Falls

HIKE 32

Old Baldy

Location	Eastern San Gabriel Mountains
Highlights	Panoramic views along the Devils Backbone and atop L.A. County's highest point
Distance	6 miles (out-and-back)
Total Elevation Gain/Loss	2,300'/2,300'
Hiking Time	3½ hours
Optional Maps	Tom Harrison Maps Angeles High Country or USGS 7.5-minute *Mount San Antonio, Telegraph Peak*
Best Times	May–November
Agency	ANF/SGRD
Difficulty	Moderately strenuous
Trail Use	Suitable for backpacking, dogs allowed

No Southland hiker's repertoire of experiences is complete without at least one ascent of Mount San Antonio, or Old Baldy. The east approach is the least taxing of the several routes to the summit, but it's by no means a picnic. You start at 7,800 feet, with virtually no altitude acclimatization, and climb expeditiously to higher than 10,000 feet. Given the easy access, it's beguilingly easy to come unprepared for high winds or bad weather, which, although fairly rare, may come up suddenly. Ice, if present, can be a serious hazard as well.

To Reach the Trailhead: By mechanical means (a car) you can get to the upper terminus of Mount Baldy Road in less than a half hour from the valley flatlands below. To do this, exit I-210 at Mills Avenue in Claremont, and follow Mills north toward the mountains. After 1.8 miles Mills veers right and becomes Mount Baldy Road. Continue 12 miles to the end of the road, where you enter the parking lot for the Mount Baldy Ski Lift.

By further mechanical means (the ski lift), you ascend effortlessly to an elevation of 7,800 feet at Mount Baldy Notch, where you begin the hike. Although the

ski lift caters mostly to skiers (daily during the winter season), it remains open during the summer season on weekends (9 a.m.–4:45 p.m.) for the benefit of sightseers and hikers. If it's a weekday or you don't like being dangled over an abyss, you can always walk up the ski-lift-maintenance road starting from Manker Flats. That option adds 3.6 miles and an elevation change of about 1,600 feet both on the way up and on the way down. A lodge at the upper terminus of the lift offers food and beverages.

Description: From Mount Baldy Notch, technically the spot about 200 yards northeast of the top of the ski lift, take the first maintenance road to the northwest that climbs moderately and then more steeply through groves of Jeffrey pine and incense-cedar. After a couple of bends, you come to the road's end at 1.3 miles and the beginning of the trail along the Devil's Backbone ridge.

The stretch ahead, once a hair-raiser, lost most of its terror when the Civilian Conservation Corps constructed a wider and safer trail, complete with guardrails, in 1935–36. The guardrails are gone now, but there's plenty of room to maneuver, unless there are strong winds or ice on the trail. Devil's Backbone offers grand vistas of both the Lytle Creek drainage on the north and east and San Antonio Canyon on the south.

The backbone section ends at about 2.0 miles as you start traversing the broad south flank of Mount Harwood. Scattered lodgepole pines now predominate. At 2.6 miles you arrive at the saddle between Harwood and Old Baldy, where backpackers sometimes set up camp (no water, no facilities here). Continue climbing up the rocky ridge to the west, past stunted, battered conifers barely surviving yearly onslaughts by cold winter

winds. You reach the summit after a total of 3.2 miles.

On the rocky summit, barren of trees, you'll find a rock-walled enclosure. Most days you can easily make out the other two members of the triad of Southern California giants—San Gorgonio Mountain and San Jacinto Peak—about 50 miles east and southeast, respectively. On days of crystalline clarity, the Old Baldy panorama includes 90 degrees of ocean horizon, a 120-degree slice of the tawny desert floor, and the far-off ramparts of the southern Sierra Nevada and the Panamint Range, as much as 160 miles away.

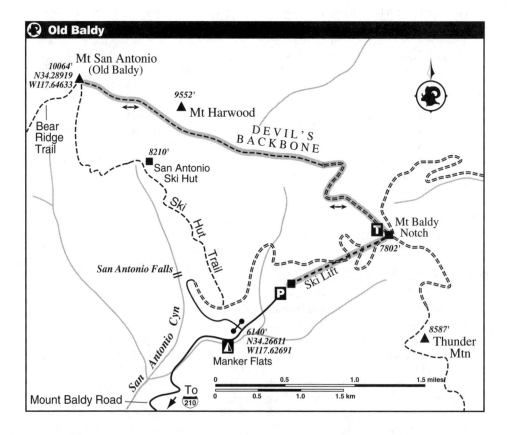

HIKE 33

Cucamonga Peak

Location	Eastern San Gabriel Mountains
Highlights	Alder-shaded stream and stupendous valley views during clear weather
Distance	12 miles (out-and-back)
Total Elevation Gain/Loss	4,300'/4,300'
Hiking Time	7 hours
Optional Maps	Tom Harrison Maps Angeles High Country or USGS 7.5-minute *Mt. Baldy* and *Cucamonga Peak*
Best Times	May–November
Agency	ANF/SGRD
Difficulty	Strenuous
Trail Use	Dogs allowed, suitable for backpacking
Permit	Cucamonga Wilderness permit required

Cucamonga Peak's south and east slopes feature some of the most dramatic relief in the San Gabriel range. At 8,859 feet, the peak stands sentinel-like only 4 miles from the edge of the broad inland valley region known as the Inland Empire. Go all the way to the top for the view, but don't be too disappointed if you see only haze and smog. So much beautiful high country can be seen along the way that reaching the top is just icing on the cake.

Most of the hike lies within Cucamonga Wilderness, which requires a permit for both day and overnight use. Near Cucamonga's summit you'll tackle a steep, north-facing gully that can retain snow into May. Be sure to discuss with a ranger the possible hazards of snow and ice if it's early or late in the year.

To Reach the Trailhead: Exit I-210 at Mills Avenue in Claremont, and follow Mills north toward the mountains. After 1.8 miles Mills veers right and becomes Mount Baldy Road. An 8-mile climb up through San Antonio Canyon on Mount Baldy Road takes you to the small village of Mount Baldy, and a national-forest ranger station on the left where you can pick up the needed wilderness permit.

Continue 1.5 miles past the village to a short spur road on the right, signed NO OUTLET. Park at the end of that spur, which is the trailhead for the Icehouse Canyon Trail, and don't forget to post a National Forest Adventure Pass on your car. This popular trailhead sometimes fills up by midmorning on busy weekends.

Description: Walk up the Icehouse Canyon Trail following the alder-shaded, boulder-filled streambed, which may be dry at its lowermost end. The first couple of miles along the canyon are a fitting introduction to a phase of Southern California scenery unfamiliar to many visitors and newcomers. Huge bigcone Douglas-fir, incense-cedar, and live oak trees cluster on the banks of the flowing stream, which dances over boulder and fallen log. Moisture-loving, flowering plants like columbine sway in the breeze. Some of the old cabins along the lower canyon survive, while others, destroyed by flood or fire, have left evidence of their existence in the form of foundations or rock walls.

Old newspaper reports suggest that an ice-packing operation existed in or near Icehouse Canyon during the late 1850s. The ice was packed down San Antonio Canyon on mules to a point accessible to wagons, whereupon it was carted, as quickly as possible, to Los Angeles for use in making ice cream and for chilling beverages. Whether ice was quarried in this canyon or in another, Icehouse Canyon's name is apt enough: cold-air drainage produces refrigerator-like temperatures on many a summer morning and deep-freeze temperatures in winter.

Chapman Trail (a longer, alternate route) intersects on the left (north) at 1.0 mile. At Columbine Spring (2.4 miles, the last water during the warmer months), the trail starts switchbacking up the north wall. After passing the upper intersection

of the Chapman Trail at 2.9 miles, you continue to pine-shaded Icehouse Saddle at 3.5 miles, where trails converge from many directions. The trail to Cucamonga's summit contours southeast, descends moderately, and climbs to a 7,654-foot saddle at 4.4 miles between Bighorn and Cucamonga Peaks. Thereafter, it switchbacks up a steep slope dotted with lodgepole pines and white firs.

At 5.8 miles, the trail crosses a shady draw 200 feet below and northwest of the Cucamonga Peak summit. An indistinct path goes straight up to the top, 6.0 miles from your starting point at the Icehouse Canyon trailhead. Return the same way, or take the alternate route, the Chapman Trail, if you'd like to explore a longer but scenic descent from Icehouse Saddle.

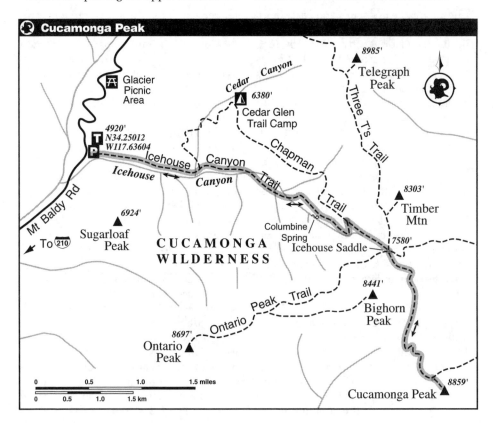

HIKE 34

The Three T's

Location	Eastern San Gabriel Mountains
Highlights	Great views and a ridgeline traverse
Distance	13 miles (one way with a short shuttle)
Total Elevation Gain/Loss	5,000'/4,000'
Hiking Time	8 hours
Optional Maps	Tom Harrison Maps Angeles High Country or USGS 7.5-minute *Mount Baldy*, *Cucamonga Peak*, and *Telegraph Peak*
Best Times	May–November
Agency	ANF/SGRD
Difficulty	Strenuous
Trail Use	Dogs allowed, suitable for backpacking
Permit	Cucamonga Wilderness permit required

Timber, Telegraph, and Thunder Mountains form the undulating northeast wall of San Antonio Canyon. This superb romp over the three T's begins up Icehouse Canyon and descends through the ski resort at Baldy Notch. For an easier hike that shaves off 3 miles and more than half the elevation gain, take the ski lift from the top of Mount Baldy Road up to the notch and do the trip in reverse.

To Reach the Trailhead: This trip requires a short car or bicycle shuttle. Exit I-210 at Mills Avenue in Claremont, and follow Mills north toward the mountains. After 1.8 miles Mills veers right and becomes Mount Baldy Road. An 8-mile climb up through San Antonio Canyon on Mount Baldy Road takes you to the small village of Mount Baldy, and a national-forest ranger station on the left where you can

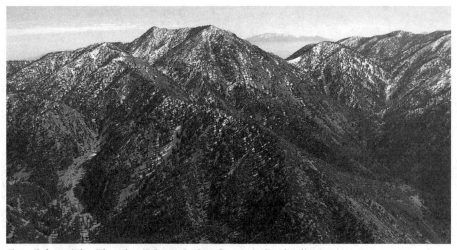

From left to right: Thunder, Telegraph, San Gorgonio (in the distance), Timber, and Icehouse Saddle

pick up the needed wilderness permit. Continue 4.2 miles up the road to Manker Flats, where you will leave one vehicle. Drive or pedal 2.7 miles down the hairpin turns, and turn left into Icehouse Canyon, where you park at the trailhead on the left.

Description: Follow the Icehouse Canyon Trail 3.5 miles to the signed five-way junction at Icehouse Saddle (see Hike 33). Turn left and climb north 0.7 mile toward Timber Mountain. The trail curves around the west side, so you will have to make a 0.2-mile detour to reach the true summit. Follow the trail 2.0 miles down to a saddle

and up to Telegraph Peak. Again, make a short detour on a use trail to the northeast to reach the summit, which is the highest point of the trip.

Return to the trail and drop steeply to a third saddle, and then climb back up to the final summit, reaching Thunder Mountain in 1.2 miles. From here, the Gold Ridge ski road leads 1.5 miles back down to Mount Baldy Notch.

From the notch, hike down the service road 3.2 miles to Manker Flats. Alternatively, the ski lift runs on weekends and is a tempting way to save your knees from wear and tear.

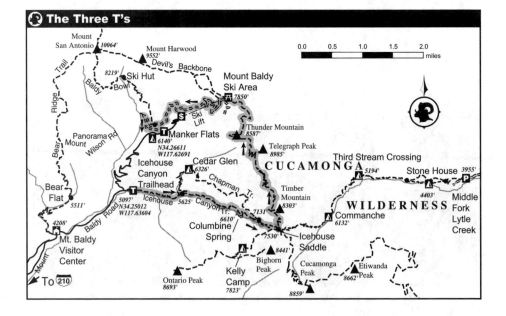

HIKE 35

Cougar Crest Trail

Location	Big Bear Lake, San Bernardino Mountains
Highlights	Pinyon-juniper forest and lake and mountain views
Distance	4.4 miles to PCT or 6.6 miles to Bertha Peak (out-and-back)
Total Elevation Gain/Loss	600'/600' or 1,450'/1,450'
Hiking Time	2½ hours or 3½ hours
Optional Map	USGS 7.5-minute *Fawnskin*
Best Times	April–November
Agency	SBNF/BBD
Difficulty	Moderate
Trail Use	Dogs allowed, good for kids (to Cougar Crest)

Big Bear Lake, with its popular resorts and ski areas, offers some fine hiking experiences for those willing to stretch their legs a bit. A number of old roads and trails lace the slopes south of Big Bear Lake (the mini-metropolis of that same name on the lake's south shore), but the sloping mountain rim that rises above the serene and mostly undeveloped north shore of the lake offers better hiking. Here, the Cougar Crest Trail ascends to a junction with the 2,600-mile-long Pacific Crest Trail—the world's longest maintained footpath.

To Reach the Trailhead: Arriving at Big Bear by way of Highways 330 and 18 from the city of San Bernardino (the most common approach), turn left on CA 38 as soon as you reach Big Bear Lake. Drive along the north shore for 5 miles to the large Cougar Crest trailhead on the left (north) side of the road near mile marker 038 SBD 53.50. Be sure to display your National Forest Adventure Pass in your car.

Description: From trailhead, head up the Cougar Crest Trail, formerly an obscure dirt road. Just up the trail, pass a spur on the right leading to the Big Bear Discovery Center. Traces of mining activity are evident as you climb upward along a

shallow draw filled with a delightful mix of outsized pinyon pines and junipers and occasional straight and tall Jeffrey pines. The sweet and pungent scents exuded by the wood and needles of these trees mingle intoxicatingly on a warm day.

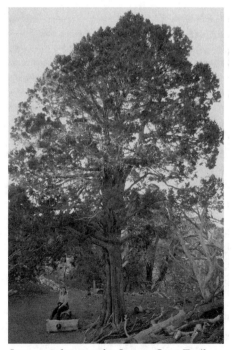

Incense cedar atop the Cougar Crest Trail

After a long mile, the old road becomes a narrow trail and begins to curl and switchback along higher and sunnier slopes. Big Bear Lake comes into view occasionally, its surface azure in the slanting illumination of a spring or summer morning or dotted with silvery pinpoints of light on a late fall day.

After about 2 miles, the trail reaches a divide, bends right, and for a short distance traverses a cool (or sometimes cold and icy), north-facing slope. At 2.2 miles

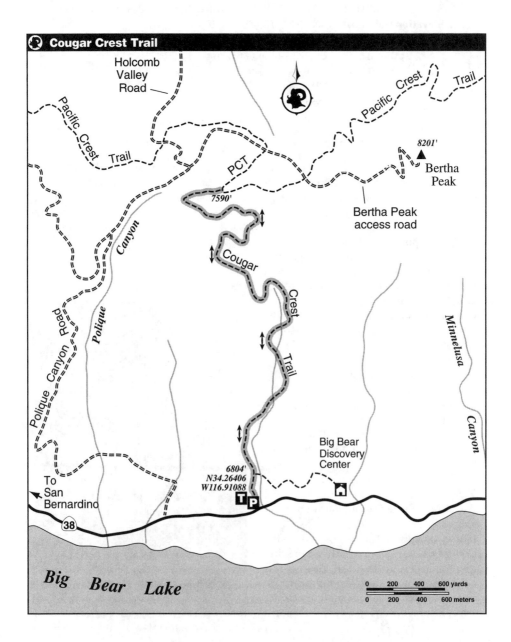

and 600 feet of climbing, the Cougar Crest Trail joins the Pacific Crest Trail, the latter reserved for hikers and horses (mountain bikes and other mechanical conveyances are prohibited on the entire PCT route between the Mexican and Canadian borders). Most hikers enjoy a snack by the pinyon pines and then turn around here.

If you wish to have a longer hike, bear right and start contouring east, high on the sunny, south-facing slope. Spread before you now is the lake (technically a shallow reservoir), which half-fills a 10-mile-long trough in the mountains, and various resort and residential communities spread along the shore and beyond. Behind the lake and about 12 miles distant, the rounded, often-snow-mantled ramparts of San Gorgonio Wilderness gleam.

The southern view does not significantly improve as you press on, though the high point ahead, Bertha Peak, will furnish a better view in other directions. When the PCT crosses a rock-strewn service road (2.6 miles from the start), leave the nicely graded trail and start climbing east on the road. A sweaty, 0.7-mile ascent takes you to a small microwave relay station atop Bertha Peak. Outside the relay station's perimeter fence you'll find a peak baggers' register, plus fine views over the treetops into Holcomb Valley and the Mojave Desert to the north.

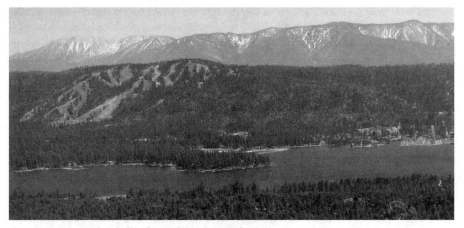

San Gorgonio on the skyline beyond Big Bear Lake

HIKE 36

Forsee Creek Trail

Location	San Gorgonio Wilderness, San Bernardino Mountains
Highlight	Peak bagging amid Southern California's highest mountains
Distance	13 miles (out-and-back) (to Trail Fork Camp)
Total Elevation Gain/Loss	3,700'/3,700'
Hiking Time	8 hours
Recommended Map	Tom Harrison Maps San Gorgonio Wilderness
Best Times	May–November
Agency	SBNF/SGD
Difficulty	Strenuous
Trail Use	Dogs allowed, suitable for backpacking
Permit	San Gorgonio Wilderness permit required

Tucked amid the tall, straight trunks of lodgepole pines at nearly 2 miles above sea level, the wind-sheltered and mostly bug-free Trail Fork Camp is a peak bagger's delight. Just above the trail camp lies the lightning-tortured roof of Southern California—San Bernardino Mountain—containing four named high points within reach of an easy, half-day stroll. Farther east lies the big daddy of Southern California summits—San Gorgonio Mountain—within reach of an all-day (16-mile round-trip) day hike involving only moderate elevation change.

The trek to Trail Fork Camp and the crest beyond is itself a challenging day hike. It's somewhat easier if you take one full day to hike in and a partial day to return. The high peaks of San Gorgonio Wilderness tend to create their own local storms in summertime, so be aware of thunderstorm forecasts before embarking on your journey. Raingear and a tent with a waterproof fly are musts during such conditions; better yet, consider canceling or postponing your trip if there is tropical moisture in the area.

A wilderness permit for day or overnight use is required for all but the very beginning of this trip. Permits are available on a first-come, first-served basis at the Mill Creek Ranger Station, at Mill Creek Road (CA 38) and Bryant Street, east of the town of Mentone. Some permits may be available by self-registration outside the door before the station opens.

To Reach the Trailhead: To reach the trailhead from I-10 at Redlands, take CA 38 east through Mentone (and past the Mill Creek Station), up onto the forested highlands of the San Bernardino Mountains. Just before mile marker 038 SBD 25.51, 18 miles beyond Mill Creek Station, turn right on Jenks Lake Road. After 0.3 mile turn right on a rough dirt road signed FORSEE CREEK TRAIL, and proceed cautiously another 0.6 mile to a large clearing used for parking.

Description: From the trailhead, make your way steadily uphill under shade-giving Jeffrey pines, incense-cedars, white firs, and black oaks, and a few sugar pines, quickly passing a side trail to Johns Meadow. Most summers, thin streams of water cascade down two or three gullies traversed by the first 2 miles of trail. After an hour or two of unrelenting labor, you leave the yellow-pine vegetation behind and enter a zone dominated by lodgepole pines. Much higher up, the lodgepole pines (with two needles per cluster) are joined by limber pines (with five needles per cluster and rubbery branch tips).

At 4.2 miles, Jackstraw Springs Trail Camp (which is prone to mosquitoes in the summer) lies down a side path to the right. At 6.2 miles, the trail bends sharply right and arrives at a junction. Just below, hidden in a clump of bushes, lies Trail Fork Springs—oftentimes the first trickle in the headwaters of Forsee Creek. Retrace your steps about 100 yards

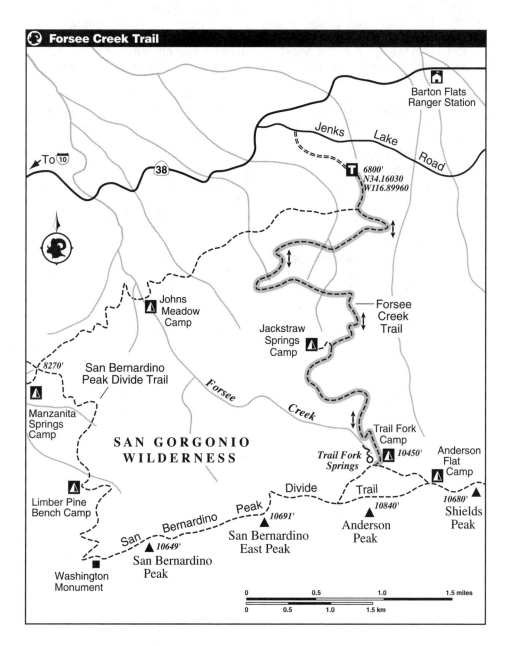

Forsee Creek Trail

Barton Flats
Ranger Station

Jenks Lake Road

To ⑩

38

6800'
N34.16030
W116.89960

Johns
Meadow
Camp

Forsee
Creek
Trail

Jackstraw
Springs
Camp

8270'

San Bernardino
Peak Divide Trail

Forsee

Creek

Manzanita
Springs
Camp

Trail Fork
Camp

SAN GORGONIO
WILDERNESS

Trail Fork
Springs

10450'

Anderson
Flat
Camp

Divide   Trail

10680'

Limber Pine
Bench Camp

San Bernardino Peak

10840'

Shields
Peak

10691'

Anderson
Peak

10649'

San Bernardino
East Peak

Washington
Monument

San Bernardino
Peak

| 0 | | 0.5 | | 1.0 | | 1.5 miles |
| 0 | 0.5 | | 1.0 | | 1.5 km | |

on the Forsee Creek Trail to find the steep, narrow side path leading east up to Trail Fork Camp. Several flat sites for camping can be found hereabouts amid the lodgepoles and weathered outcrops of banded metamorphic rock. A bald area on a flat ridge just northeast is the perfect spot to admire a view stretching north toward Big Bear Lake and to toast the last rays of the setting sun.

If time and energy permit, pay a visit to nearby Shields and Anderson Peaks, 0.7 mile and 0.4 mile away, respectively. On the crest between these peaks lie scraggly pines, many battered and stripped of their bark by lightning strikes. North of the crest, in protected pockets, uniformly spaced lodgepole pines grow tall and straight with dark "bathtub rings" around their waists indicating snow accumulations several feet deep.

An optional peak-bagging foray to the west might include both of the San Bernardino Peaks, plus the historic Colonel Henry Washington Monument, which commemorates the original San Bernardino baseline and meridian survey point, established in 1852. (The monument lies off-trail; you'll find it by walking 160 yards straight up the ridge from the southwesternmost switchback in the San Bernardino Peak Divide Trail.) For more than 150 years, all land surveys of Southern California have referred to Colonel Washington's initial baseline. Due west of the monument, starting from the foot of the mountain, today's Base Line Road stretches radially outward many miles across the flat, alluvial plain occupied by San Bernardino and several of its satellite cities. As viewed from the monument on clear days, Base Line Road seems to point toward a vanishing point in or beyond the San Gabriel Valley.

It is possible to return to the trailhead via a much longer (17.5 miles total) route that loops around via Johns Meadow. Descend the San Bernardino Peak Divide Trail north to an 8,270-foot trail junction near Manzanita Springs. Then head northeast on the often-steep, unmaintained, partially obscure trail toward Johns Meadow. East of Johns Meadow, the trail is maintained.

HIKE 37

Dollar Lake

Location	San Gorgonio Wilderness, San Bernardino Mountains
Highlight	Sparkling glacial tarn
Distance	13 miles (out-and-back)
Total Elevation Gain/Loss	2,700'/2,700'
Hiking Time	7 hours
Optional Map	Tom Harrison Maps San Gorgonio Wilderness
Best Times	May–November
Agency	SBNF/SGD
Difficulty	Strenuous
Trail Use	Dogs allowed, suitable for backpacking
Permit	San Gorgonio Wilderness permit required

Sparkling and silvery like a freshly minted silver dollar, Dollar Lake lies cupped amid a talus-frosted natural bowl, not far below the great divide of San Bernardino Mountain. Snow lingers late on the steep slopes overlooking the lake, sometimes into August. It's hard to believe that this splendid landscape, reminiscent of the High Sierra, exists here in Southern California, only 20 air miles from the suburban housing tracts of San Bernardino.

A day hike to Dollar Lake (via the South Fork Trail) in the San Gorgonio Wilderness is not only possible but rather straightforwardly easy for any well-conditioned Southern Californian willing to rise early and get to the trailhead by 8 or 9 a.m. A wilderness permit

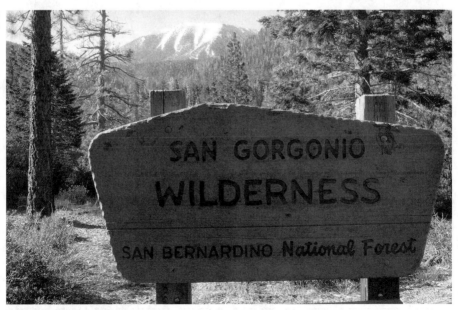

San Gorgonio Mountain

is required for day or overnight use of all but the lower part of the trail. A limited number of permits are available on a first-come, first-serve basis at the Mill Creek Ranger Station, at Mill Creek Road (CA 38) and Bryant Street, east of the town of Mentone.

To Reach the Trailhead: To reach the trailhead from I-10 at Redlands, take CA 38 east through Mentone (and past the Mill Creek Station), up onto the forested highlands of the San Bernardino Mountains. Just before mile marker 038 SBD 25.51, 18 miles beyond Mill Creek Station, turn right on Jenks Lake Road. Proceed 3 miles

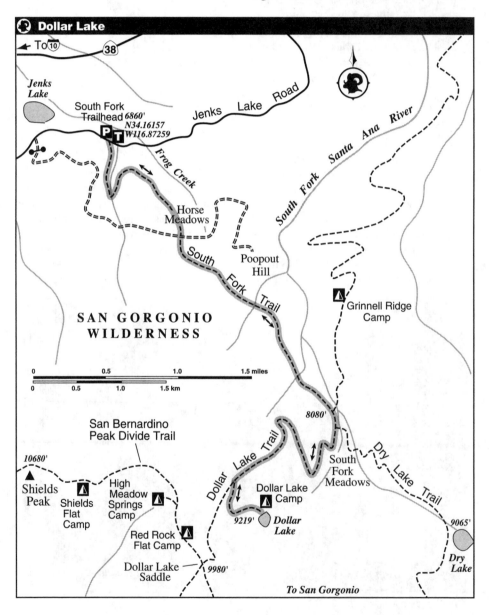

to the large South Fork Trailhead parking lot on the left. You'll need to display a National Forest Adventure Pass on your parked car.

Description: The South Fork Trail crosses Jenks Lake Road, heading south, and commences a moderate ascent up a shady canyon. Soon, the trail switches back, climbs out of the canyon, and climbs southeast toward a bracken-filled clearing—Horse Meadows. Near the meadow's upper edge, you cross a dirt road (1.5 miles). That road, now closed to traffic, leads to a spot known as Poopout Hill at the wilderness boundary. The short side trail to the left leads to a worthy viewpoint on the hill where San Gorgonio Mountain is framed between the trees.

Continue your ascent through the typical mid-elevation yellow-pine belt, consisting here of mostly of ponderosa pines and white firs. At around 4.0 miles, the trail draws close to the South Fork Santa Ana River. Remain on the right bank of the creek, staying right at the signed junction with the Dry Lake Trail. Off to the left is South Fork Meadows, where many small tributaries combine and funnel into the South Fork. Days or weeks later some of this water will travel down the wide Santa Ana River flood-control channel through Anaheim and Santa Ana. Much of the water seeps into gravelly or sandy soils downstream and recharges underground aquifers, that is, it never reaches the ocean. You stay to the right and do not cross the South Fork.

Your ascent continues on the crooked, mostly shaded Dollar Lake Trail. The yellow-pine belt fades while stout and straight lodgepole pines appear in greater numbers. At 5.9 miles, just past a large, manzanita-covered patch on the mountainside, you'll come to junction where a side trail starts slanting down toward Dollar Lake, a short half mile away. The San Bernardino Mountains are the only range of mountains in Southern California to show evidence of glaciation (prior to about 10,000 years ago), and the depression occupied by Dollar Lake is suggestive of this.

If your trip involves backpacking, the trail campground at Dollar Lake is a pleasant enough overnight stop. One mile above Dollar Lake (by trail) is Dollar Lake Saddle, and 4 miles southeast of that is the summit of San Gorgonio Mountain. Prior to the closing of the Poopout Hill trailhead in 1988, northern ascents of Gorgonio via either Dollar Lake or Dry Lake were the easiest, if not quite the shortest. Since then, the easiest and fastest way up the mountain has been by way of Vivian Creek (see Hike 38).

HIKE 38

San Gorgonio Mountain

Location	San Gorgonio Wilderness, San Bernardino Mountains
Highlight	Standing atop Southern California's highest spot
Distance	16 miles (out-and-back)
Total Elevation Gain/Loss	5,700'/5,700'
Hiking Time	10 hours
Optional Map	Tom Harrison Maps San Gorgonio Wilderness
Best Times	April–November
Agency	SBNF/SGD
Difficulty	Strenuous
Trail Use	Dogs allowed, suitable for backpacking
Permit	San Gorgonio Wilderness permit required

The barren, talus-strewn summit of San Gorgonio Mountain (or Greyback, after its steely gray appearance from the valleys below) receives dozens of hikers on most fine-weather weekends. No hiker, however, ever has an easy time of it. Either variation of the popular northern approach (via Dollar Lake or Dry Lake) requires more than 20 miles of round-trip hiking. On the southern approach by way of the Vivian Creek Trail, described here, you begin hiking at a point several hundred feet lower than the northern (South Fork) trailhead, but you save at least 5 miles of distance on the round-trip.

The Vivian Creek Trail, the original path to the top of San Gorgonio, was built around the turn of the 20th century. Today,

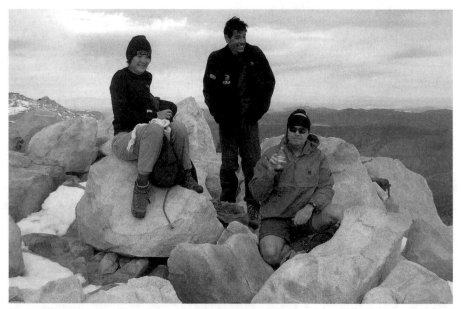

Happy hikers atop San Gorgonio

about eight distinct routes (or variations on routes) culminate at the summit. After 1988, when the north-side Poopout Hill trailhead closed, the Vivian Creek route once again become the fastest and easiest way up the mountain. The south-facing Vivian Creek route also has the advantage of a longer season; most snow on the upper parts of the trail is gone by May or June, a month or more before the northern routes are similarly clear.

Of those people who approach the summit by way of Vivian Creek, perhaps half do so over a two- or three-day period, hauling their overnight gear to camps such as Halfway or High Creeks and day hiking from there. Others, in excellent condition and traveling lightly, have taken as little as seven hours total, with a half hour spent at the top and some jogging on the way down. At a leisurely pace with plenty of breaks, a day-long summit hike could take a mind- and leg-numbing 14 hours. That approach is okay in June or July (assuming you start hiking at dawn), but you probably wouldn't want to try it during November, when daylight lasts 11 hours or less.

San Gorgonio Mountain lies within the heart of the San Gorgonio Wilderness. Whether day hiking or backpacking, you must secure a wilderness permit from the Mill Creek Ranger Station, at Mill Creek Road (CA 38) and Bryant Street, east of the town of Mentone. Apply up to 90 days in advance during the busy summer season when reservations for permits fill up quickly.

To Reach the Trailhead: To reach the trailhead from I-10 at Redlands, take CA 38 east through Mentone to Mill Creek Station, and up Mill Creek Canyon for another 6.2 miles beyond the station to a hairpin turn where you veer right onto Valley of the Falls Blvd. Proceed 4.5 miles through the cabin community of Forest Falls, all the way to the end of the road and a spacious trailhead parking lot. Be sure to display a National Forest Adventure Pass on your car.

Description: From the trailhead, walk east (uphill) past a vehicle gate and follow a dirt road 0.6 mile to its end. Go left across the wide, bouldery wash of Mill Creek, and find Vivian Creek Trail going sharply up the oak-clothed canyon wall on the far side. The next half mile is excruciatingly steep, and this pitch is worse on the return, when your weary quadriceps

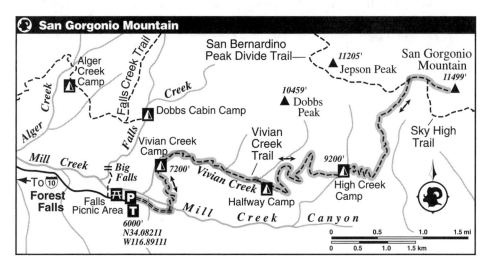

muscles must absorb the punishment of each lurching downhill step.

Mercifully, at the top of the steep section, the trail levels momentarily and then assumes a moderate grade up alongside Vivian Creek. A sylvan Shangri-La unfolds ahead. Pines, firs, and cedars reach for the sky. Bracken fern smothers the banks of the melodious creek, which dances over boulders and fallen trees. After the first October frost, the bracken turns a flaming yellow, made all the more vivid by warm sunlight pouring out of a fierce blue sky.

Near Halfway Camp at 2.5 miles, the trail begins climbing timber-dotted slopes covered intermittently by thickets of manzanita. Dobbs Peak, just below timberline, comes into view to the north, though the nearly treeless San Bernardino Mountain divide remains hidden. After several zigs and zags on north-facing slopes, you swing onto a brightly illuminated south-facing slope. Serrated Yucaipa Ridge looms to the south, rising sheer from the depths of Mill Creek Canyon. Soon thereafter, the sound of bubbling water heralds your arrival at High Creek at 4.8 miles and the trail camp of the same name. Be ready for a chilly night if you stay here; cold, nocturnal air often flows down along the bottom of this canyon from the 10,000-foot-plus peaks above.

Past High Creek Camp the trail ascends gently on several long switchback segments through lodgepole pines and, at length, attains a saddle on a rocky ridge. The pines thin out and appear more decrepit as you climb crookedly up along this ridge toward timberline. At 7.2 miles, the San Bernardino Peak Divide Trail intersects from the left. Stay right and keep climbing on a moderate grade across stony slopes dotted with cowering krummholz pines. Soon, nearly all vegetation disappears.

On the right you pass Sky High Trail, which bends around the mountain and descends toward Dry Lake and South Fork Meadows in the north. Keep straight and keep going. A final burst of effort puts you on a boulder pile marking the highest elevation in Southern California (7.8 miles from your starting point). From this vantage, even the soaring north face of Mount San Jacinto to the south appears diminished in stature.

Several campsites surrounded by enclosures of piled-up stones are scattered around the summit plateau. These comprise Summit Trail Camp, a fine place to stay overnight if the weather is calm and clear (most typically in September and October). At night, planets and stars gleam overhead, but they must compete for attention with the glow of millions of lights below.

HIKE 39

Aspen Grove

Location	San Bernardino Mountains
Highlight	Fall colors
Distance	1.8 miles (out-and-back)
Total Elevation Gain/Loss	350'/350'
Hiking Time	1 hour
Optional Maps	Tom Harrison Maps San Gorgonio Wilderness or USGS 7.5-minute *Moonridge*
Best Times	October
Agency	SBNF/SGD
Difficulty	Easy
Trail Use	Dogs allowed, good for kids

In October each year, the leaves of quaking aspens (*Populus tremuloides*) turn bright yellow for a few short weeks and then drop from the trees. Aspen Grove is one of only two places in California outside the Sierra Nevada where these splendid trees can still be seen. This hike follows Fish Creek through four groves of aspens. The willows in the creek also change color, adding to the festive fall display beneath the evergreen firs and pines. Call the Mill Creek Ranger Station for current foliage information. Neither of the recommended maps is perfectly accurate at portraying the maze of trails around Big Meadows, but the main trail form the Aspen Grove Trailhead is clearly marked.

To Reach the Trailhead: From Redlands drive east on CA 38 to the Heart Bar Campground turnoff just past mile marker 038 SBD 33.48. Turn right and follow Forest Road 1N02 for 1.3 miles. Then turn right onto 1N05, and proceed 1.6 miles to the signed Aspen Grove Trailhead. Low-clearance vehicles can normally make this trip unless the road has washed out.

Description: From the trailhead, walk south 0.3 mile down to Fish Creek. Cross

the creek and immediately reach a trail junction in a dense grove of aspen. It can be hard to get a perspective on the trees because you are right beneath them. Trails lead north and south from

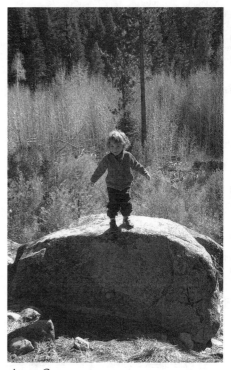

Aspen Grove

this junction along the west side of Fish Creek. Turn right (north) and follow the trail downstream. The forest is predominantly white fir, which is unusual in Southern California. In 0.25 mile, pass a second grove of aspens mixed with willows and cross back to the east side of the creek. In another 0.15 mile, look for a fine grove of aspens lined up on the far side of the creek.

In another 0.2 mile, cross Fish Creek three more times to reach the last grove of aspens. Although the trail continues, it is best to return the way you came.

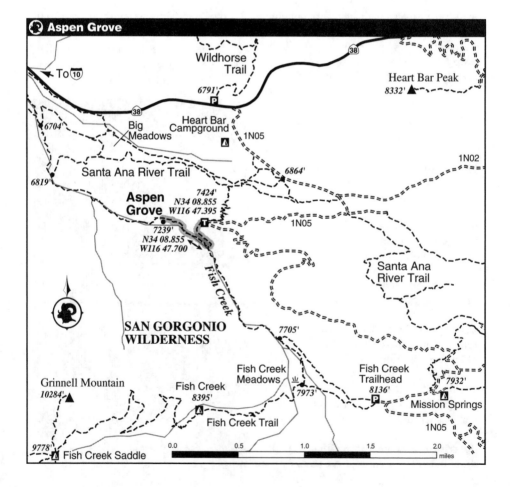

Aspen Grove

Wildhorse Trail

To 10

Heart Bar Peak
8332'

6791'

38

Heart Bar Campground
Big Meadows
1N05

6704'

1N02

Santa Ana River Trail

6819'

6864'

Aspen Grove
7424'
N34 08.855
W116 47.395

1N05

7239'
N34 08.855
W116 47.700

1N05

Santa Ana River Trail

Fish Creek

SAN GORGONIO WILDERNESS

7705'

Fish Creek Meadows
Fish Creek Trailhead
8136'

7932'

Grinnell Mountain
10284'

Fish Creek
8395'

7973'

Mission Springs

1N05

Fish Creek Trail

9778'
Fish Creek Saddle

0.0   0.5   1.0   1.5   2.0

miles

HIKE 40

Deep Creek

Location	Near Hesperia, the north slope of the San Bernardino Mountains
Highlights	Natural hot-spring pools alongside a mountain stream
Distance	3.8 miles (out-and-back)
Total Elevation Gain/Loss	950'/950'
Hiking Time	2½ hours
Optional Map	USGS 7.5-minute *Lake Arrowhead*
Best Times	March–November
Agency	SBNF/AD
Difficulty	Moderate
Trail Use	Dogs allowed

Deep Creek Hot Springs in the San Bernardino National Forest has been a minor magnet for hikers and nature lovers—eccentric and otherwise—for decades. Volunteers have spent years fashioning rock-bound basins that impound water ranging from about 96°F to about 102°F. Water flowing out of those basins quickly reaches chilly Deep Creek, which has carved a deep cleft in the north slope of the San Bernardino Mountains.

To Reach the Trailhead: To get to the most convenient portal for the hot springs hike, which lies outside the national forest boundary, go north on I-15 over Cajon Pass. Six miles north of the pass, exit east onto Main Street, and follow it 7.2 miles through Hesperia. Where Main Street curves south, veer left (east) onto Rock Springs Road. Cross the dry bed of the Mojave River, and follow the road

2.8 miles to a junction where its name changes to Roundup Way. Continue east for 4.4 miles, and then turn right (south) onto the good dirt Bowen Ranch Road.

Proceed 5.4 miles, passing various junctions, to a toll gate and 1920s-vintage cabin at the rustic, private Bowen Ranch. Pay the $4-per-person day-use fee at the gate, and be sure to pick up a copy of the hand-drawn "treasure" map that may help you navigate to the hot springs. Park your car at the ranch's overnight camping and parking area a short distance past the toll gate. Since the ranch lies outside the San Bernardino National Forest boundary, you do not need to display a National Forest Adventure Pass.

If you want to pitch a tent or stay in a vehicle overnight at Bowen Ranch, the charge is $5 per person. Note that US Forest Service regulations do not allow camping at the destination for this hike: Deep

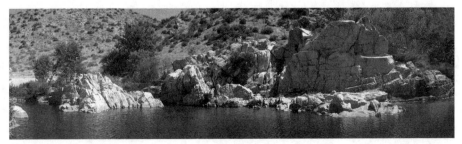

Deep Creek Hot Springs

Creek Hot Springs. For the purposes of planning your trip, note that Bowen Ranch does not have a phone, e-mail address, or website. Typically, the US Forest Service has no definitive information about either the Bowen Ranch or about stream or weather conditions at Deep Creek.

Description: Now you're ready to head out on foot toward the springs, almost 2 miles away and nearly 1,000 feet lower in elevation. After an initial 0.5 mile of downhill hiking, briefly jog left on a dirt road, then veer right on a signed trail entering San Bernardino National Forest land. You lose about 700 feet of elevation as you descend for another 1.3 miles into Deep Creek's canyon bottom.

About halfway down this stretch, where the trail splits, take the right fork to ensure an easier, more gradual descent.

Once you reach the canyon bottom you must decide how to cross the creek to reach the hot pools on the far side. In winter, the water is often swift and bone-chillingly cold. US Forest Service regulations allow nude bathing in the Deep Creek Hot Springs drainage area, and typically about half of the visitors do so. Camping, campfires, and glass containers are strictly prohibited.

Do realize that the uphill, post-soak hike back to the car can be enervating and possibly exhausting in the summer heat. Bring plenty of drinking water (not alcohol, which dehydrates the body) if the weather is warm! Inexperienced hikers have also gotten into deep trouble here when cold rain or snow is falling. The pools may be plenty warm, but inadequately equipped persons who can't get dry after a visit to the pools are at risk for hypothermia.

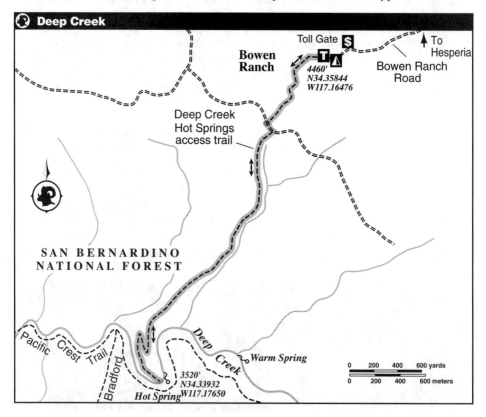

HIKE 41

Whitewater Canyon

Location	Whitewater Canyon Preserve, San Bernardino Mountains
Highlights	A desert river and possible bighorn sheep sightings
Distance	4.0 miles (out-and-back to Red Dome)
Total Elevation Gain/Loss	400'/400'
Hiking Time	2 hours
Optional Map	USGS 7.5-minute *Whitewater*
Best Times	8 a.m.–5 p.m., October–April
Agency	WCWP
Difficulty	Moderate
Trail Use	Dogs allowed, suitable for backpacking, good for kids
Permit	Notify a ranger before you leave a vehicle overnight

The Whitewater River is the largest waterway between the Mojave and Colorado Rivers. The Wildlands Conservancy has established an outstanding nature preserve in the river canyon at the site of the former Whitewater Trout Farm. This trip explores the desert and river along a short segment of the Pacific Crest Trail. The best time to visit is in the spring when wildflowers are in bloom and the river earns its name. Animals large and small visit the canyon for water and food; watch for prints and scat. Scan the cliffs above the preserve headquarters for bighorn sheep. This trip is a short out-and-back walk, but those desiring a longer trip can make many variations. If you're not staying overnight, be sure to be out by 5 p.m. when the gate closes.

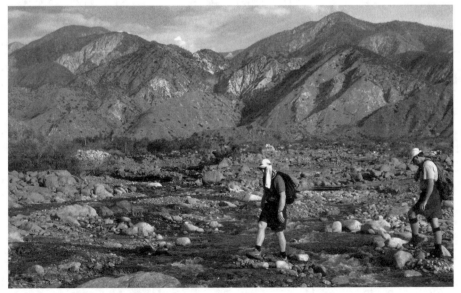

Crossing the Whitewater River

To Reach the Trailhead: From I-10 west of Palm Springs, exit north on Whitewater Canyon Road. Follow a frontage road that veers east and then immediately turns left into the canyon. Proceed 4.9 miles to the end of the road at the parking area for Whitewater Preserve.

Description: Sign in at the ranger station, then walk north along a rock-lined path from the trailhead kiosk. After passing a pair of palm trees, veer west and cross the Whitewater River wash. The trail varies from year to year as floodwaters reshape the canyon floor, but the path is usually marked. Even if it is hard to follow, watch for and eventually pick up the well-defined trail on the west side. Follow it through a grove of desert willows

to a junction with the Pacific Crest Trail at the mouth of a tributary canyon, 0.5 mile from the start.

Turn right and follow the PCT north. In 1.4 miles, reach a bend where the Whitewater River veers west. On the right side of the trail is a small volcanic lump called Red Dome. The PCT makes a poorly defined crossing of the wash here before heading over a ridge into the Mission Creek drainage. If you are out for a short hike, this is a good place to savor the river and then return the way you came.

If you arrange a ride or leave a bike at Mission Creek Preserve, 15 miles away via I-10 and CA 62, you can turn this trip into an enjoyable 8-mile one-way trip between the two Wildlands Conservancy preserves.

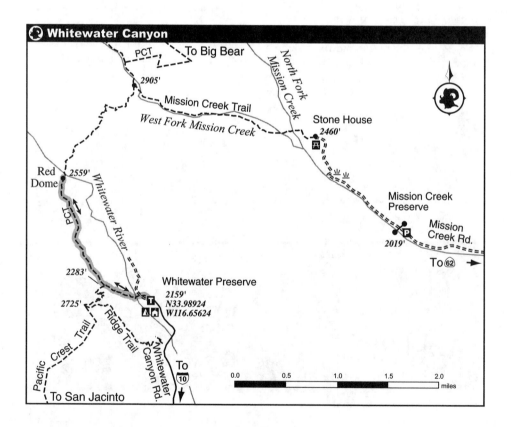

HIKE 42

Big Morongo Canyon

Location	Big Morongo Canyon Preserve, north of Palm Springs
Highlights	Riparian splendor amid the desert and excellent birding
Distance	1–3 miles (loop)
Total Elevation Gain/Loss	50'–300', depending on exact route
Hiking Time	½–2 hours
Optional Map	USGS 7.5-minute *Morongo Valley*
Best Times	October–May
Agency	BMCP
Difficulty	Easy
Trail Use	Good for kids

Nearly 300 species of birds have been spotted along a 6-mile stretch of Big Morongo Canyon, just outside the town of Morongo Valley. Wildlife frequenting the canyon includes bighorn sheep, bobcat, mountain lion, and mule deer. The 31,000-acre Big Morongo Canyon Preserve, administered by the federal Bureau of Land Management, encompasses the wettest parts of the canyon. The preserve sits astride a melding of coastal chaparral and desert habitats and is regarded as one of the most important wildlife oases in the California desert. The exotic freshwater marsh found here owes its existence to seepage of water up along a geologic fault associated with a great rift between tectonic plates—the San Andreas Fault Zone—not far to the south.

The uppermost (wet) part of Big Morongo Canyon Preserve lies about 2,000 feet above low-lying Palm Springs and the Coachella Valley, so the summer heat is intense but rarely intolerable here. Still, it's best to stick with the cooler months, or else confine your visit to early-morning or late-afternoon hours. The preserve is open daily from 7:30 a.m.–sunset.

To Reach the Trailhead: From I-10 near Palm Springs, drive 11.3 miles north on CA 62 to Morongo Valley. Just past the business district, turn right on East Drive, and look for the preserve entrance on the left.

Description: For a rewarding 1-mile stroll through contrasting habitats, walk past the visitor information display and pick up the Desert Willow Trail on your left. It guides you over a sun-blasted terrace dotted with prosaic-looking shrubs, such as honey mesquite, desert willow, and yerba santa. The latter exudes an unmistakable sweet-pungent odor. You dip to cross the Big Morongo Wash, and pass a spur trail, the Yucca Ridge Trail, 0.4 mile from the start.

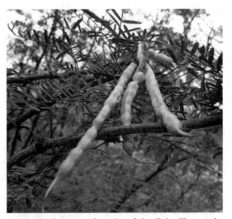

Mesquite beans, a favorite of the Cahuilla people

Continue on the Desert Willow Trail into the heart of Big Morongo's riparian oasis. You meander on boardwalks amid a junglelike assemblage of willows, cottonwoods, alders, and fan palms (the latter two apparently introduced, though they lie not far from the edge of their normal range). Watercress and water parsnip have overrun the surface of the shallow waters below your feet.

After 0.4 mile, you come to a T-intersection with the Marsh Trail. Off to the right a quarter mile is your parked car. To the left, you pass the Mesquite Trail before looping back to the trailhead.

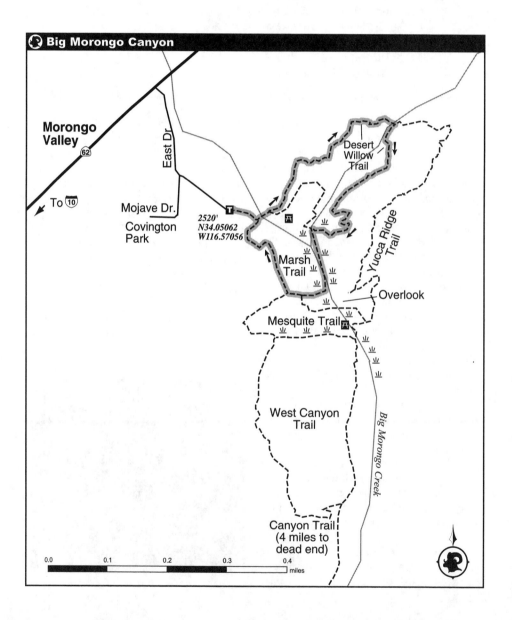

HIKE 43

Pushwalla Palms

Location	Coachella Valley Preserve
Highlights	Palm oases and a ridge walk
Distance	6.5 miles (loop)
Total Elevation Gain/Loss	1,000'/1,000'
Hiking Time	4 hours
Optional Map	Coachella Valley Preserve map
Best Times	October–March
Agency	CVP
Difficulty	Moderate

The 17,000-acre Coachella Valley Preserve, located on the San Andreas Fault between Palm Springs and Joshua Tree National Park, was established in 1986 to protect the sand dune habitat of the endangered Coachella Valley fringe-toed lizard. The crushed rock and clay in the fault zone is nearly impermeable to groundwater, forcing the water to the surface and creating a series of springs that support spectacular palm oases in the midst of the parched desert. This loop tour of the southeastern part of the preserve features three separate palm groves and expansive views from a narrow ridge.

To Reach the Trailhead: From I-10, exit on Ramon Road, and drive east (on the north side of the freeway) for 4.5 miles. Turn left on Thousand Palms Road, and proceed 2.1 miles to the visitor center parking area on the left. If you don't plan to stop at the visitor center for a map, you can save yourself a little walking by parking 0.3 mile back down Thousand Palms Canyon Road at a turnout on the east side.

Description: If you haven't already been to Coachella Valley Preserve, stop by the Palm House in the oasis next to the parking area. Docents can tell you about current conditions and wildlife. A sign on the south side of the visitor center

parking lot indicates the start of the trail to the Pushwalla, Horseshow, and Hidden Palm Oases. The trail leads across the desert and crosses Thousand Palms Road at the alternative parking turnout. At a signed junction just beyond, turn right and follow frequent signposts to steps

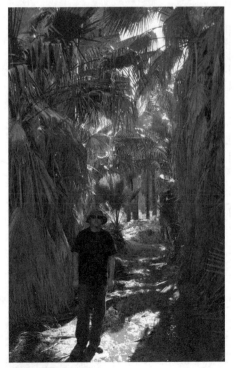

Pushwalla Palms

leading onto Bee Rock Mesa. At the crest of the ridge, a sign points east along the ridgetop toward Pushwalla Palms and south down to Hidden Palms. This trip heads to Pushwalla and will loop back to this point by way of Hidden Palms.

Follow the narrow and exposed ridge for a mile, enjoying the panoramic views. At a signed junction at the end of the ridge, stay right and follow the trail down off the ridge to another junction. Stay left for Pushwalla Palms; you will return to this junction later to take the other fork to Horseshoe and Hidden Palms. Descend a narrow gully and arrive at the oasis in Pushwalla Canyon. During the wet months, the canyon bottom will often have a trickle of water, though it is unsuitable for drinking. Turn left and explore up the canyon to find the two main palm groves.

Return through the narrow gully to the junction from which you just came and head west toward Horseshoe Palms, nestled at the foot of the ridge. The maze of trails through the valley can be confusing; follow the trail markers that eventually lead you onto an old jeep track down the middle of the valley. After passing Horseshoe Palms, come to a fork in the road at a hitching post. Take the trail on the right into Hidden Palms Oasis.

When the road ends, continue north on a trail that eventually rejoins jeep tracks. The maze of paths in this area can be confusing. At another fork beneath powerlines near the toe of the main ridge, veer right and return to the signed junction on Bee Rock Mesa. Descend the stairs and retrace your steps to your vehicle.

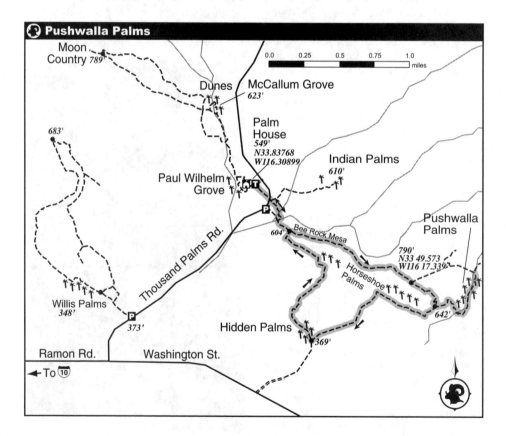

Pushwalla Palms

HIKE 44

Black Rock Panorama Loop

Location	Joshua Tree National Park
Highlights	Desert vegetation and views
Distance	6.5 miles (loop)
Total Elevation Gain/Loss	1,200'/1,200'
Hiking Time	4 hours
Recommended Map	Trails Illustrated Joshua Tree or USGS 7.5-minute *Yucca Valley South*
Best Times	October–April
Agency	JTNP
Difficulty	Moderate

Black Rock Canyon is near the western edge of Joshua Tree National Park and is connected to the main park by a long and strenuous footpath. While it lacks the outlandish rock formations characteristic of the main park, it does have an exceptionally lush and beautiful assortment of prickly desert vegetation. An extensive but poorly marked trail network fans out from the Black Rock Campground. The best moderate hike in this area, the Panorama Loop explores a series of washes, climbs up to a ridgeline with splendid views, and then returns via another wash system.

To Reach the Trailhead: From CA 62 in Yucca Valley, turn south on Joshua Lane at the sign for the Black Rock Campground (opposite CA 247, and 0.4 mile east of mile marker 062 SBD 12.00). Follow Joshua Lane as it curves east, then back south, and ends at a T-junction in 4.4 miles. Turn right, and then immediately turn left on Black Rock Canyon Road, which leads into the campground. Park by the Black Rock Backcountry Board on the east side of the road shortly past the entrance. The road is divided, and the trailhead is easy to miss.

Description: From the backcountry board, follow the trail east for 0.1 mile to a sandy wash. Follow the trail south in the wash, passing the California Riding and Hiking

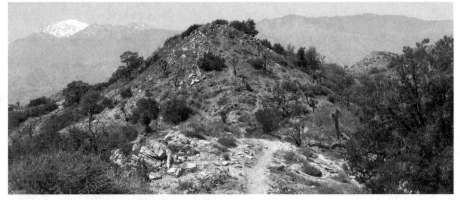

Ridgetop views of San Gorgonio Mountain

Trail, Short Loop Trail, Burnt Hill Trail, and West Side Loop. In 1.4 miles, the canyon narrows and you pass Black Rock Spring. Its tiny trickle is more of interest to desert animals and bees than to humans.

In another 0.2 mile, the loop splits at a signed junction. Navigation is easiest if you take the right fork and make a counterclockwise loop. In another 0.4 mile, pass a sign on the right pointing to

Warren Point. In 1.1 miles, reach a ridge. In another 0.3 mile, arrive at the highest point on the ridge, with excellent views of San Gorgonio and of the intricate canyons in the Little San Bernardino Mountains. The steep sandy trail veers left (north) down the ridge and then northwest down the canyon. In 1.2 miles arrive back at the split in the loop. Hike north down the wash back to the trailhead.

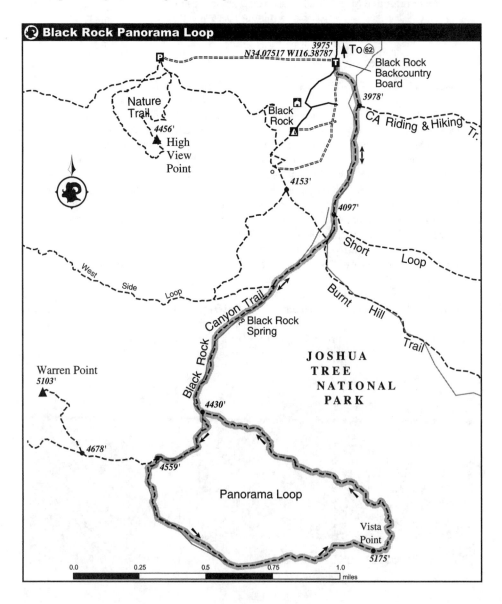

HIKE 45

Wonderland of Rocks Traverse

Location	Joshua Tree National Park
Highlight	Scrambling amid gigantic boulders
Distance	6 miles (one way)
Total Elevation Gain/Loss	200'/1,200'
Hiking Time	6 hours
Recommended Map	Trails Illustrated Joshua Tree or USGS 7.5-minute *Indian Cove*
Best Times	October–April
Agency	JTNP
Difficulty	Strenuous

More than a hundred million years ago, a molten mass of rock lay several miles underground, cooling and crystallizing by agonizingly slow degrees. As the mass solidified, it contracted slightly, and fractures developed within it. Over geologic time, this mass moved upward while older, overlying layers of rock were eroded away. As the younger rock neared the surface, groundwater seeping into the fractures chemically transformed some of the rock crystals into clay. Large, more-or-less rectangular blocks of rock with rounded corners became isolated from each other in a matrix of loose clay. Once exposed above the surface, the clay quickly washed away, leaving open crevices between the blocks. Various mechanical forces and chemical weathering further chipped away at the boulders and rounded them even more.

The products of all this uplift and shaping are the monzogranite boulders we see today spectacularly exhibited in the Wonderland of Rocks section of Joshua Tree National Park. Everywhere you look, your mind is dazzled by huge, pancake- or loaflike stacks of rocks (where horizontal fractures predominate), by rocks in columns or spires (where vertical fractures predominate), and by huge domes. Each unique structure has been fashioned by a particular set of events occurring over millions of years.

The one-way traverse across the Wonderland of Rocks described here is known by some as the Wonderland Connection. Make no mistake—this is no easy stroll. Its four-star rating is solely on account of the fiercely jumbled landscape you must cross during the latter part of the trip. You should be adept at both boulder-hopping and scrambling across tilted rock surfaces. Much of the travel involves meticulously lowering yourself downward over angular boulders—not recommended for the faint of heart. Camping is prohibited in the Wonderland area; you must plan your visit as a day trip.

To Reach the Upper Trailhead: From CA 62 in the community of Joshua Tree, take Park Boulevard into Joshua Tree National Park. Pay the national park fee (or show your annual pass) when you reach the entry station. Continue southeast another 6.2 miles to reach the Keys West backcountry board (kiosk) at a large parking area on the left (north) side of the road. This point is 0.7 mile east of Quail Springs Picnic Area and 2.3 miles northwest of Hidden Valley Campground.

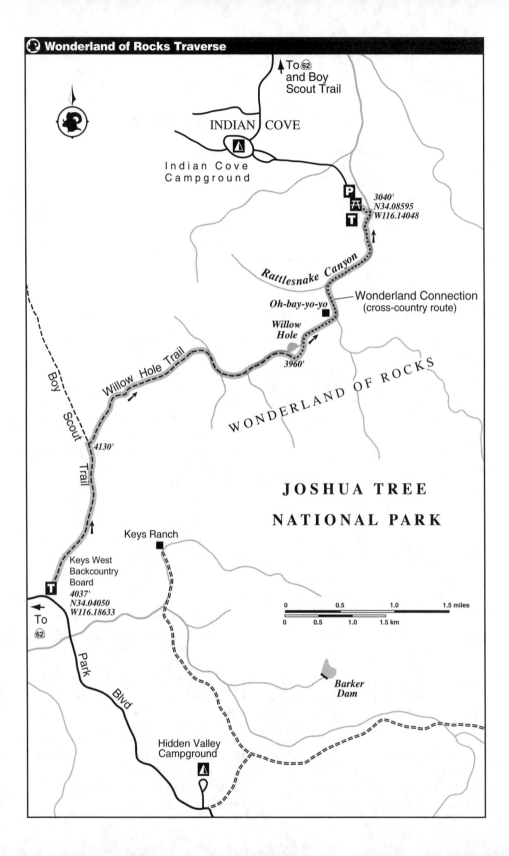

To 62
and Boy
Scout Trail

INDIAN COVE

Indian Cove
Campground

P
3040'
N34.08595
W116.14048
T

Rattlesnake Canyon

Wonderland Connection
(cross-country route)

Oh-bay-yo-yo

*Willow
Hole*

3960'

Willow Hole Trail

WONDERLAND OF ROCKS

Boy

Scout

4130'

Trail

JOSHUA TREE

NATIONAL PARK

Keys Ranch

Keys West
Backcountry
Board
4037'
N34.04050
W116.18633

T

To
62

Park

Blvd

*Barker
Dam*

Hidden Valley
Campground

0		0.5		1.0		1.5 miles
0	0.5		1.0	1.5 km		

To Reach the Lower Trailhead: The hike ends at the Indian Cove Campground and picnic area, just south of CA 62, 8 miles east of Joshua Tree and 5 miles west of Twentynine Palms. Drive all the way to the southeast end of the road to the picnic ground at the mouth of Rattlesnake Canyon, where the one-way hike ends.

Description: From the Keys West Backcountry Board, follow the Boy Scout Trail (a dirt road) 1.4 miles north across sandy flats dotted with Joshua trees to the Willow Hole Trail, intersecting it on the right. Follow the Willow Hole Trail northeast to where it enters a dry wash, and then continue downhill in the wash. The wash soon becomes a canyon bottom flanked by stacks of boulders. At 3.5 miles you arrive at Willow Hole—large pools flanked by a screen of willows.

Following a beaten-down path, you then work your way through the willows on the right, over a low ridge, and across a hard-to-identify gap between two rock piles. If you find yourself scrambling on difficult boulders, you've chosen the wrong path. Follow the narrow canyon bottom below, which carries water draining from the pools at Willow Hole during the wetter parts of the year. Your remaining route is entirely downhill, but negotiating a canyon section clogged with boulders impedes your progress.

At 0.7 mile beyond Willow Hole, a north-flowing tributary joins on the right. Look here for Oh-bay-yo-yo, a cavelike shelter beneath a huge boulder. Take care of this special spot and leave no trace.

Stay in the main canyon as it veers north and descends sharply for 0.3 mile to join Rattlesnake Canyon. Exercise care while descending this hazardous stretch. (It was here, during a prearranged rendezvous and car-key exchange between my party and a party traveling in the opposite direction, that one set of keys was dropped into the boulder maze and almost irretrievably lost. The lesson: Always have an extra key in a magnetic box on the car frame or hidden nearby.)

Once you reach Rattlesnake Canyon, only a bit more than a mile of hiking remains. The going is easy for a while as you follow the sandy wash downhill (northeast). Some cottonwood trees brighten the otherwise desolate scene of sand and soaring stone walls. As the canyon bends left for a final descent to the flats of Indian Cove below, you face more episodes of serious scrambling. Keeping to the left-side canyon wall, work your way around a slotlike canyon worn in the granitic rock. Down in the bottom of the slot are potholes worn by the abrasive action of flash flooding. A little more scrambling and a short walk down the canyon's sandy wash takes you to the end of the hike, the picnic area at Indian Cove.

If you can't arrange a vehicle shuttle, you can also return by way of the Boy Scout Trail that starts near the north end of Indian Cove. This option is 14 miles and takes about 10 hours of walking.

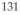

Boulder-choked ravine

HIKE 46

Ryan Mountain

Location	Joshua Tree National Park
Highlights	Panoramic mountain and desert views
Distance	2.8 miles (out-and-back)
Total Elevation Gain/Loss	1,000'/1,000'
Hiking Time	2 hours
Optional Maps	Trails Illustrated Joshua Tree or USGS 7.5-minute *Indian Cove* and *Key's View*
Best Times	September–May
Agency	JTNP
Difficulty	Moderate
Trail Use	Good for kids

Elongated Ryan Mountain rises above the boulder-studded plains of Lost Horse and Queen Valleys in Joshua Tree National Park. The view from the top is arguably the best in the national park, encompassing the blocky summits of San Jacinto and San Gorgonio, the intricately dissected Wonderland of Rocks, and a succession of shimmering basins and skeletal mountain ranges stretching east toward the Colorado River and south toward Baja California. The popular trail from the mountain's base to its top is well worn, yet steep and rocky enough to be a potential hazard for

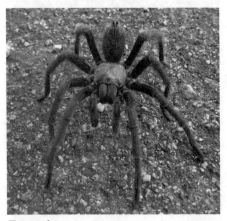

Tarantula

young children (and others) prone to tripping or stumbling.

To Reach the Trailhead: From the national park's headquarters and main visitor center on Highway 62 outside Twentynine Palms, drive 16 miles southwest on Utah Trail and Park Boulevard. Alternatively, starting from the town of Joshua Tree, drive 17 miles southeast on Park Boulevard. Your hike begins at the Ryan Mountain parking area, at mile marker 13 on Park Boulevard.

Description: From the parking area, head straightforwardly uphill along the north and west flanks of the mountain, amid scattered juniper and pinyon pine. Very soon, the geologic character of the rock underfoot changes. You cross the boundary between the White Tank monzogranite, the same rock you see exposed in boulder piles in the valleys below, and the Pinto gneiss, a much older rock into which the monzogranite rock was intruded (many miles underground) some 130 million years ago. The Pinto gneiss, which is foliated with layers of dark minerals, was metamorphosed (changed in form by intense heat and pressure) around 1.5 billion years ago, during an era when life on Earth consisted of nothing more than one-celled organisms.

If you can swing it, try a morning-twilight ascent of Ryan Mountain in the late fall or early winter. As the sun rises, look down and watch the interplay of light and shadow across the Joshua-tree dotted plains and on the monzogranite boulder piles, which rise like battlements out of the alluvium.

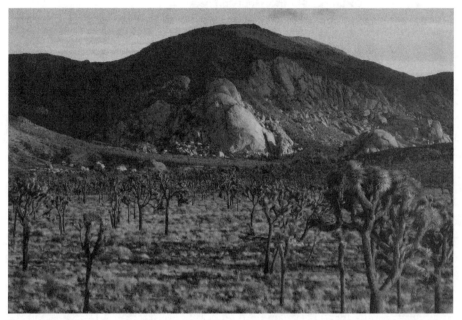

Ryan Mountain

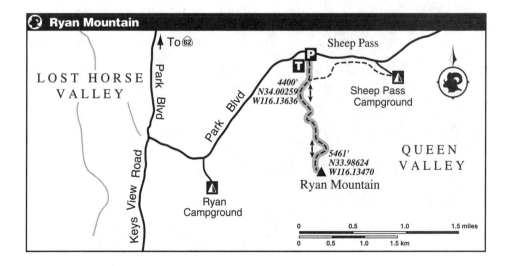

HIKE 47

Lost Horse Mine

Location	Joshua Tree National Park
Highlights	Mining history
Distance	4.2 miles (out-and-back)
Total Elevation Gain/Loss	500'/500'
Hiking Time	2 hours
Optional Maps	Trails Illustrated Joshua Tree or USGS 7.5-minute *Indian Cove* and *Key's View*
Best Times	October–April
Agency	JTNP
Difficulty	Moderate
Trail Use	Good for kids

The Lost Horse Mine, one of the few highly profitable gold mines in Southern California, yielded 10,000 ounces of gold between 1894 and 1931. The story of the mine was related by William Keys, a long-time resident of the area. Johnny Lang, a rancher, went looking for his horse that had vanished one night. He learned of the mine from a prospector and bought the rights to the mine for $1,000, naming it Lost Horse.

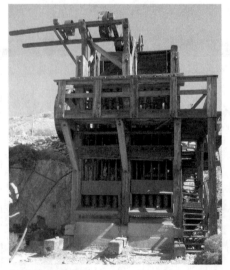

Lost Horse Mill

Five years later, J. D. Ryan joined the partnership and hauled in a massive steam-powered 10-stamp mill. The mill crushed the ore from the mine. The resulting powder was mixed with water to form a slurry, which was treated with mercury to separate the gold from the debris. The amalgam was then smelted to extract the gold, which was shipped in 200-pound bricks to Banning. To power the steam mill, Ryan ran a pipeline 3.5 miles from the well at his ranch to the mine. The hills around the mine are still sparsely vegetated because the junipers and yuccas were felled as fuel for the steam mill.

According to Keys, Ryan caught Lang stealing gold from the night shift and forced Lang to sell out. Lang later retrieved some of the bullion that he had secreted away near the mine, but he died of exposure along Keys View Road in the winter of 1925. Keys buried him near the Lost Horse Mine turnoff. As you hike this popular trail to the mine, imagine this Wild West drama unfolding, keep an eye out for hidden treasure, and take care that your hiking partner doesn't double-cross you.

To Reach the Trailhead: From the main Park Boulevard through Joshua Tree

National Park 0.8 mile east of mile marker 16, turn south on Keys View Road. In 2.5 miles, turn left at a good signed dirt road to Lost Horse Mine. The road, which is open for day use only, ends in 1 mile at a parking area with an outhouse.

Description: The wide trail, formerly a wagon road, begins at the east end of the parking area. It starts up the wash and then promptly veers left at a sign. This is a good place to learn to identify Mojave yucca (with hairlike threads on the edge of the blades) and nolinas (similar in stature, but with no hairs). In May 2009, the Lost Horse Fire burned this area. Started under suspicious circumstances, it incinerated much of the vegetation along the trail but thankfully did not damage the mine.

The trail gradually climbs to the southeast and crosses a low ridge in 1 mile. In another mile, reach a trail and old roadbed forking left toward the mine.

Lost Horse Mine is fenced off. The shaft formerly reached a depth of 500 feet, with lateral tunnels every 100 feet. As the wooden frame decayed and the tunnels began to collapse, a sinkhole started to form. The Park Service has plugged the shaft and shored up the mill, but stay clear of the fence for your safety. You can also explore the foundations of the old cabins and the cyanide-settling tanks.

Those looking for a longer hike can make this into a 6-mile loop. Continue southeast up the right fork of the main trail to a saddle in 0.2 mile, where you could make a short detour to the top of Lost Horse Mountain. Descend the steep and rugged remains of an old mining road into a beautiful system of ridges and gullies. Pass the remains of Lang Mine in 0.5 mile.

The trail climbs onto a ride, then it turns west along the south flank of Lost Horse Mountain. In another 0.5 mile, pass a chimney at Optimist Mine. The deep, unfenced mineshaft is above the tailing pile. In another 1.3 miles, the trail crosses and joins a dry wash leading through a secluded valley of Joshua trees. In 2.2 miles, reach a dirt road at an unmarked, easy to overlook junction. Turn right (east), and hike up the road 0.1 mile to the trailhead where you started.

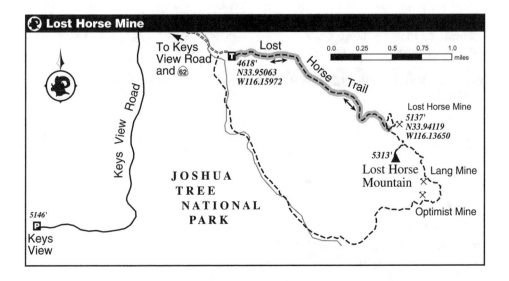

HIKE 48

Lost Palms Oasis

Location	Joshua Tree National Park
Highlights	A palm oasis and desert vegetation
Distance	7.5 miles (out-and-back)
Total Elevation Gain/Loss	700'/700'
Hiking Time	4 hours
Optional Maps	Trails Illustrated Joshua Tree or USGS 7.5-minute *Cottonwood Spring*
Best Times	October–March
Agency	JTNP
Difficulty	Moderately strenuous

Lost Palms Oasis showcases Joshua Tree National Park at its best. The trail leads you across cactus-clad hills before plunging into a deep canyon studded with the park's trademark quartz monzonite boulders that conceal the largest stand of California fan palms in the park. Lost Palms is in a day-use area; camping is prohibited.

To Reach the Trailhead: Drive east on I-10 for 32 miles past Indio, then exit north on Cottonwood Springs Rd. to Joshua Tree National Park. Proceed 7.2 miles to Cottonwood Visitor Center, where you pay your park admission fee. Turn right (east), and proceed 1.1 miles to the Cottonwood Spring Trailhead parking at the end of the road.

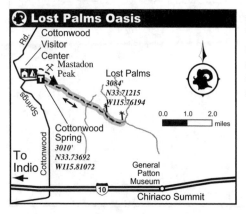

Description: A trail descends southeast from the trailhead into the small Cottonwood Spring Oasis, which was once home to Cahuilla Indians. The protein-rich bean pods from the thorny mesquite tree was one of their major food sources. Look for the deep mortars in the granite boulders where women ground the beans into flour.

Continue southeast to a signed junction at 0.6 mile. The left fork leads to Mastodon Peak, but this trail goes right. Walk across the flat desert past countless cholla cacti, yuccas, and ocotillos. Continue in and out of dry washes in the badlands before reaching another signed trail junction on the canyon rim, 3.5 miles from the start.

You may take a short detour to the right for an overlook of Lost Palms Oasis. The main trail to the left makes a steep and rocky descent into the oasis on the canyon floor. Your efforts are rewarded at the bottom of the canyon, when you can enjoy the splendid palm oasis.

HIKE 49

Ladder Canyon

Location	Mecca Hills, north of the Salton Sea
Highlights	Slot canyon and fault-churned landscape
Distance	4.3 miles (loop)
Total Elevation Gain/Loss	750'/750'
Hiking Time	3½ hours
Optional Maps	USGS 7.5-minute *Mecca, Mortmar,* and *Cottonwood Basin*
Best Times	October–April
Agency	BLM/PS
Difficulty	Moderately strenuous
Trail Use	Good for kids

Ladder Canyon is the informal name given to a slotlike ravine incised into the sedimentary strata of the Mecca Hills on the eastern fringe of the Coachella Valley. Several ladders at strategic spots within the canyon assist or make feasible passages over abrupt dry falls (drop-offs) along the bottom. On rare occasions—mostly during summer thundershowers—these drop-offs come briefly alive with cascading, muddy water.

Ladder Canyon is a tributary of the superbly scenic Painted Canyon, which worms it way into the Mecca Hills Wilderness, which is administered by the Bureau of Land Management. The famed San Andreas Fault Zone passes through here, giving you a glimpse of what hundreds of miles of horizontal displacement and tens of miles of stretching (over many millions of years) can do to a landscape consisting of little else but stark rock formations.

To Reach the Trailhead: The Mecca Hills lie about 120 miles east of Los Angeles. From I-10 east of Indio, turn south onto CA 86S. Drive 10 miles to 62nd Avenue near the town of Mecca. Drive east 2 miles to its end at Johnson Street, then turn right. Proceed another 2 miles, then turn left on 66th Avenue, which becomes Box

Canyon Road. Turn left onto Painted Canyon Road at a sign. This dirt road is usually passable by low-clearance cars unless it has washed out. Proceed 4.7 miles to the parking area in Painted Canyon.

Description: On foot, start hiking into the narrow canyon with sheer sandstone walls on the right (northeast), which is

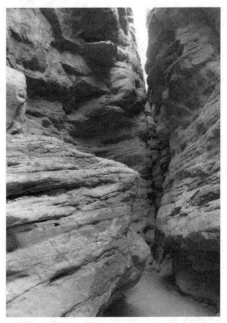

Ladder Canyon slot

upper Painted Canyon. All around you
are fantastic formations of sandstone and
shale (former sea bottom) that have been
tilted upward at steep angles due to tensional forces along the San Andreas Fault.
During the cooler part of the year, low-
angle sunlight partially illuminates the
canyon bottom, spotlighting scattered

smoke trees growing in the sandy wash,
making them appear like gray puffs of
smoke when seen from a distance.

At 0.4 mile, a slotlike ravine nearly
blocked by fallen sandstone boulders (and
possibly marked by a LADDER CANYON
sign) can be seen along the canyon wall
to the left. Some mild scrambling and

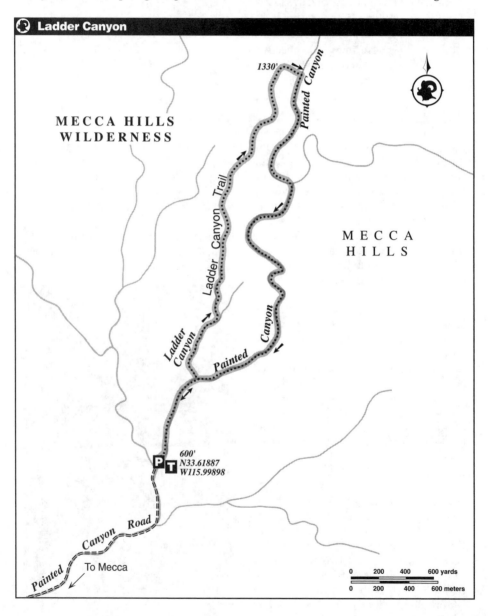

clambering up several near-vertical ladders allow you to gain elevation quickly. The original wooden ladders placed here are gradually being replaced by aluminum ones. Of course, the next major flood, probably years or decades away, will probably sweep all these ladders away.

At 0.8 mile from the start, there's a fork where the now-wider ravine divides into two nearly equal tributaries. Take the left fork for the easier route. (Using the right-fork tributary, you would quickly climb to the west rim of Painted Canyon and later rejoin the main route.) By 1.5 miles you reach the head of the left-fork ravine and find yourself just below and west of a rounded ridge (a large rock cairn lies on a knoll to the left). An informal trail swings up that ridge and follows its course steadily uphill in the direction of some radio towers about 2 miles north.

In the direction opposite the radio towers, a gorgeous view of the Coachella Valley and Salton Sea unfolds as you climb. The below-sea-level Salton Sea is the largest inland body of water in California—blue and inviting from a distance, but not especially picturesque or sweet-smelling up close. The sea has been the recipient of nearly a century's worth of irrigation runoff from the Coachella and Imperial Valleys (and more recently wastewater from the Mexicali region of northern Baja California), which has created a noxiously polluted body of water plagued by ever-increasing salinity levels. The vast, sunken landscape before you, flanked by mountains on both the east and west sides resulted from tensional forces that continue to pull apart the Pacific and North American tectonic plates in this part of California.

At 2.0 miles, in a saddle on the ridge, the trail turns abruptly right and darts down a rocky slope into the wide, sandy wash of upper Painted Canyon. Make a right and start to enjoy the entirely downhill remainder of the hike. Painted Canyon deepens as you descend, exposing a geological wonderland of primarily dark metamorphic rocks. At 2.7 miles, a deep tributary canyon comes in from the left—offering a good side trip of a half mile or more if you are curious and energetic. At 3.3 miles, a ladder facilitates easy passage over an otherwise frightening descent over a dry fall in the main canyon. The rest is easy going on a wide bed of coarse sand past the Ladder Canyon turnoff and back to your car.

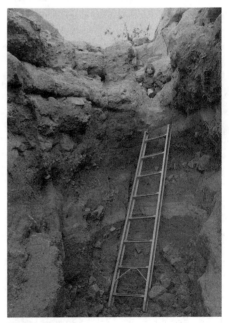

Ladder Canyon

HIKE 50

Murray Hill

Location	Santa Rosa Mountains
Highlights	Views, a peak, and some desert vegetation
Distance	7 miles (out-and-back)
Total Elevation Gain/Loss	1,700'/1,700'
Hiking Time	5 hours
Optional Map	Santa Rosa and San Jacinto Mountains National Monument
Best Times	October–March
Agency	SRSJMNM
Difficulty	Moderately strenuous

Prominent from many directions, pyramid-shaped Murray Hill offers panoramic views over the Palm Springs area and the Santa Rosa Mountains. It is best climbed on a clear cool day. Its diminutive name belies the fact that Murray Hill is a steep and strenuous hike that challenges and rewards the intrepid explorer. The summit is named for the Scottish rancher, Welwood Murray, who founded the Palm Springs Hotel in 1887 and drew attention to the area as a spa and resort. Murray Hill can be approached from the west, north, or south. This trip describes the western approach via the Garstin and Wild Horse Trails, but you can enjoy a longer loop or a one-way trip in combination with other trails. Many of the trails in this area were built by and named for members of the Desert Riders, an active equestrian group in the Coachella Valley.

To Reach the Trailhead: From I-10, take CA 111 south into Palm Springs. The road becomes North Palm Canyon Drive and then South Palm Canyon Drive. Most lanes turn left to become East Palm Canyon, but stay right (straight) and continue on South Palm Canyon Drive for 1.9 miles. Turn left onto East Bogart Trail, and follow it 0.9 mile over a bridge across Palm Canyon Wash. Then immediately turn left on Barona Road, and park at the end.

Description: The trail starts at an unlabeled post at the end of Barona Road and leads east. In 150 yards, it reaches a signed fork. The Henderson Trail veers left and heads northeast along the toe of the ridge, but turn right and follow Garstin Trail up steep switchbacks hewn from the hillside. Your efforts are rewarded by steadily widening views to the west.

Shortly before reaching the top of the hill, the trail forks. The right fork is recommended; it follows the ridgeline for 0.1 mile before rejoining its sister. Soon after, 1.2 miles from the start, come to a junction with Berns Trail on top of the ridge.

From here, Murray Hill stands prominently to the southeast. Your goal is to head there via the Wild Horse Trail without getting lost on the maze of poorly marked paths crisscrossing the mountains. Turn right and head toward Murray Hill. In 0.3 mile, stay right at a fork. Just beyond, at a four-way junction with the Thielman Trail, go straight onto the Wild Horse Trail. Continue 1.2 miles up the ridge to a junction. The right fork drops to Fern Canyon, but this trip stays left onto the Clara Burgess Trail, which climbs the fine ridgeline 0.8 mile to the summit of Murray Hill.

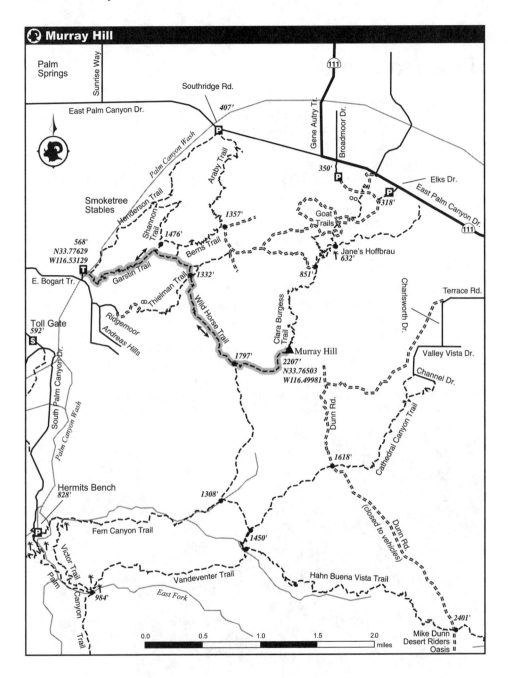

HIKE 51

Pines to Palms

Location	Santa Rosa Mountains
Highlights	Palm oasis and desert
Distance	15 miles (one way)
Total Elevation Gain/Loss	100'/3,500'
Hiking Time	7 hours
Recommended Map	Santa Rosa and San Jacinto Mountains National Monument
Best Times	October–March
Agency	ACBCI
Difficulty	Strenuous
Trail Use	Suitable for backpacking

Palm Canyon should be on every serious Southern California hiker's to-do list. The canyon separates the San Jacinto Mountains and Desert Divide on the west from the Santa Rosa Mountains on the east and offers magnificent scenery in all directions. As it descends from the pinyon pines of the mountains to the cacti of the desert, it takes you past most of the Seussian plant life of the Upper and Lower Sonoran zones. The enormous palm oasis at the north end (bottom) of the trail is a fitting conclusion to a long but rewarding day. Those looking for a more casual hike suitable for children will enjoy roaming the oasis from the trailhead at Hermits Bench.

This hike presents some logistical challenges. The northern trailhead at Hermits

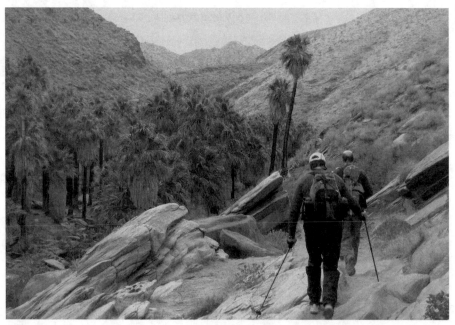

Palm Canyon

Bench is only open 8 a.m.–5 p.m. If you are not out before the gates close, the rangers will initiate a search. The drive between trailheads takes about 45 minutes, so if you leave a vehicle at Hermits Bench when it opens, drive to the upper trailhead, and begin walking at 9 a.m., you have at most 8 hours to complete the 15-mile trek. Some prefer to do the trip as an overnight backpack, with a trusty friend handling the drop-off and pick-up. Camping is prohibited on the reservation land comprising the northern half of the canyon (beginning about a mile north of Agua Bonita Spring).

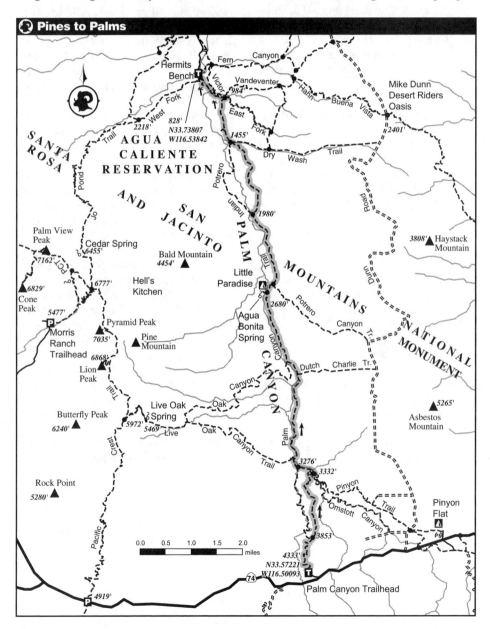

To Reach Hermits Bench (the Northern Trailhead): Position one car where the trip ends at Hermits Bench. From I-10, take CA 111 south into Palm Springs. The road becomes North Palm Canyon Drive and then South Palm Canyon Drive. Most lanes turn left to become East Palm Canyon, but stay right (straight) and continue on South Palm Canyon Drive for 2.8 miles to the tollgate at the entrance to Indian Canyons. Notify the ranger of your plans. Continue 2.5 miles to the trailhead parking at Hermits Bench.

To Reach Palm Canyon (the Southern Trailhead): Head back north and turn right onto East Palm Canyon Drive, which becomes CA 111. Go east and southeast 11 miles, then turn right on CA 74 and follow it 18 miles. Just past mile marker 074 RIV 77.85, turn right onto Pine View Drive, and proceed 0.2 mile to the end of the paved road.

Description: Walk north from the Palm Canyon Trailhead up a dirt road. In 0.1 mile, veer right at a blank steel trail marker. Hike north through ribbonwood and chaparral, enjoying the sweeping views of Palm Canyon's upper reaches. In 1.3 miles, come to a signed four-way junction and continue straight on jeep tracks leading north on the ridge. (The trail to the left also reaches Palm Canyon, but it may be overgrown and more difficult to follow.)

Your route hugs the rolling ridgeline and then switchbacks northeast down into Omstott Canyon. Turn left and follow the trail down the canyon. Go around a bend and meet the Palm Canyon Trail at a post, 2.5 miles from the fork.

The trail along upper Palm Canyon is narrow, lightly traveled, and faint in places. This land is used for cattle ranching, and several gates control the cattle; close them behind you. Stay on Palm Canyon Trail. Within 0.2 mile, pass a fork where the unmaintained Live Oak Canyon Trail leads west. Then pass Dutch Charlie Trail to the east and the faint Oak Canyon Trail veering southwest through the mesquite. (If you have time, you might try following it around a bend to Hidden Falls.)

The next section of trail is notable for its abundance of yuccas. In another 1.7 miles, reach a signed junction. Agua Bonita Spring is on the canyon bottom to the west, and water can be found here much of the year. Look for bedrock mortars where the Cahuilla once ground their food. In 0.3 mile, the Potrero Canyon Trail veers off to the right. Palm Canyon becomes deeper and more rugged. The rocky badlands to the west are called Hells Kitchen. In another 2 miles, reach a junction with the Indian Potrero Trail. Either fork is enjoyable, and they rejoin in 2 miles at a junction with the aptly named Dry Wash Trail.

Continue north for 1 mile to an enormous palm oasis at the junction with the Victor, Vandeventer, and East Fork Trails. Stay left on the Palm Canyon Trail for another mile, passing many more palms before climbing up to Hermits Bench.

HIKE 52

San Jacinto Peak: The Easy Way

Location	San Jacinto Mountains
Highlight	Broad view of Southern California from summit
Distance	11 miles (out-and-back)
Total Elevation Gain/Loss	2,600'/2,600'
Hiking Time	6 hours
Optional Map	Santa Rosa and San Jacinto Mountains National Monument or USGS 7.5-minute *San Jacinto Peak*
Best Times	May–November
Agency	MSJSW
Difficulty	Moderately strenuous
Trail Use	Suitable for backpacking
Permit	San Jacinto Wilderness permit required

San Jacinto Peak is a close second after San Gorgonio Mountain on the roster of Southern California high points, but its more sharply defined and imposing bulk makes it instantly identifiable from almost anywhere. Upon witnessing the sunrise from the summit one morning, the famed naturalist John Muir exclaimed, "The view from San Jacinto is the most sublime spectacle to be found anywhere on this earth!"

Despite his propensity for superlatives, Muir may have been right—we may never know. Since his visit more than a century ago, more than 20 million people have come to settle within a 150-mile radius around the mountain. Air pollution dims today's view, even on the clearest days. Still, hundred-mile visibility is not uncommon—out to the Channel Islands in the west, down to the northern Sierra of Baja California to the south, and east into Arizona. San Gorgonio and the San Bernardino Mountains rear up in the north, 15–20 miles away, blocking vistas of the Mojave Desert.

The north face of San Jacinto, which at one point soars 9,000 feet up in four horizontal miles, is one of the most imposing escarpments in the United States. Expert climbers have made the grueling ascent from the north in as little as 9 hours. Fortunately several easier, well-graded trails let you bag the summit from other directions with a lot less effort. Every summer, thousands of people take advantage of the easiest route of all, the 5.5-mile trail between the mountain station of the Palm Springs Aerial Tramway (8,516 feet) and the top of San Jacinto (10,804 feet). Well-conditioned hikers accustomed to high altitudes will find this a moderate trip. Others can still get plenty of pleasure out of shorter trips that don't stray very far from the mountain station. The slopes hereabouts feature some of the most inviting high-country forests and meadows south of the Sierra Nevada.

To prepare for your trip, call the Palm Springs Aerial Tramway, 760-325-1391, or visit pstramway.com, for information and operating hours. The tramway closes for a few days in August for maintenance; otherwise, it operates daily year-round.

To Reach the Trailhead: From eastbound I-10, take the Palm Springs exit (CA 111), and drive 8.5 miles to Tramway Road, on the right. Drive 4 miles up Tramway Road to where it ends in the parking lot for the lower terminus (Valley Station) of the Palm Springs Aerial Tramway. Purchase a round-trip ticket, and ride the tramway up to the Mountain Station, where you can find visitor amenities, such as a restaurant and gift shop.

Description: A paved pathway leads 0.2 mile down from the Mountain Station to the San Jacinto State Wilderness ranger hut in Long Valley, where you must obtain a wilderness permit for travel beyond Long Valley. From the ranger hut, follow the wide trail leading steadily uphill for 2 miles to Round Valley, mostly through a coniferous forest of Jeffrey pine, sugar pine, and white fir. Backpacking campsites are located in the Round Valley area and at Tamarack Valley, 0.5 mile north of Round Valley via a side trail. Continue your ascent, somewhat steeper now, through thinning lodgepole pines to a trail junction at Wellman Divide, 3.2 miles from the start. This is where you get your first impressive view—south over tree-covered summits, foothills, and distant desert and coastal valleys.

After an almost obligatory (common, anyway) water or snack break at Wellman Divide, continue your leisurely uphill grind toward San Jacinto Peak. You traverse north for more than a mile across a boulder-strewn slope covered by scattered lodgepole pines and a carpet of low-growing alpine shrubs. Abruptly, you change direction at a switchback corner, climb southwest for a while, and arrive (2 miles from Wellman Divide) on a saddle just south of the peak itself. Veer right, follow the path up along the right (east) side of the summit, pass a stone hut, and then scramble from boulder to boulder for a couple of minutes to reach the top.

Hopefully the weather will allow you to rest a spell in the warm sun, cupped amid the jumbo-sized rocks, and savor the lightheaded sensation of being on top of the world. Make sure that you leave the summit of San Jacinto Peak in time to catch the last downhill tram ride. The steep paved climb back to Mountain Station may feel like the hardest part of the entire hike.

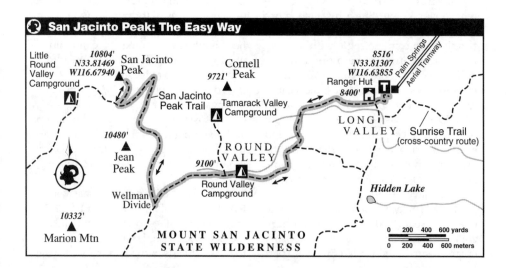

HIKE 53

San Jacinto Peak: The Hard Way

Location	San Jacinto Mountains
Highlights	Greatest elevation gain of any day hike in the Lower 48
Distance	20 miles (one way)
Total Elevation Gain/Loss	10,600'/2,600'
Hiking Time	13 hours or more
Recommended Maps	Santa Rosa and San Jacinto Mountains National Monument
Best Times	May–early June; October–early November
Agency	SRSJMNM
Difficulty	Very strenuous
Trail Use	Suitable for backpacking

This hike, known as the Cactus-to-Clouds Hike by Palm Springs hiking enthusiasts, is an absolute hoot—if you survive. For three decades now, ever-increasing numbers of adventurers have set foot in Palm Springs on a former American Indian trail hacked into the east slope of Mount San Jacinto. For some, the goal has been San Jacinto Peak, 14 trail-miles away and 10,400 feet higher. Other hikers have settled for Long Valley, where the Mountain Station of the Palm Springs Aerial Tramway sits—a "mere" 9 miles and 8,000 feet higher.

You must prepare for this hike with plenty of vigorous physical conditioning. Fortunately the San Jacinto and the nearby San Bernardino and San Gabriel Mountains have many great routes for you to train. Conditioning hikes should include 5,000 feet or more of elevation gain, plus exposure to elevations of 9,000 feet or more.

Because the climate encountered on the full climb ranges from a low-desert type to an arctic-alpine type, you should try this hike only during the most moderate seasons—either late spring or early fall. If you go too early in the spring season, you might encounter treacherous patches of icy snow below Long Valley. In fall, you must wait until typical morning temperatures on the lower trail sink to less than lethally

hot levels. The first snows usually arrive in November or December. For stable weather, it's hard to beat late October.

On a cool day during these moderate-season periods, you'll probably consume the better part of a gallon of water before your first dependable fill-up at Long Valley. In warm weather, you'll surely need a gallon or more. If you go all the way to San Jacinto Peak, remember that you must return to Long Valley and the tram station for a ride back down the mountain. The statistics quoted above in the capsulized summary include the round-trip from Long Valley to the peak and back. When you arrive at Mountain Station, you may need to purchase a one-way ticket for the tram ride down. Once you arrive at the bottom of the tram, you can call a taxi to get back to the starting point. Call the Palm Springs Aerial Tramway, 760-325-1391, or visit pstramway.com, for information about the tramway and its operating schedule.

A predawn start on the trail is mandatory, preferably two hours before sunrise, to beat the worst of the heat and ensure you have enough daylight on your return trip.

To Reach the Trailhead: Ramon Road, a major east-west thoroughfare through the south side of Palm Springs, intersects that city's main north-south drag, Palm

Canyon Drive, just south of the main business district. From that intersection, go 0.4 mile west on Ramon Road to where it dead-ends at the foot of Mount San Jacinto. Parking space can be found on the nearby residential streets, but carefully note any signs regulating curbside parking.

Description: Follow a dirt road north from the end of Ramon Road, and almost immediately you'll see the Carl Lykken Trail on the left. Pick up a self-issued permit for the Skyline Trail at the trailhead. Climb about 1 mile and 1,000 feet up this maintained riding and hiking trail to reach a rocky saddle. A rougher trail, originating at the Palm Springs Desert Museum, comes up from the east and joins the saddle as well. Another trail, also rough, takes off up the ridge to the west, past inscriptions that warn of the arduous ascent ahead.

That ridge-running trail is variously known as the Skyline Trail, Chino Canyon Trail, and Outlaw Trail. Other than some improvements made by a labor gang in 1933, and light-duty maintenance by contemporary users, the trail remains sketchy in places, especially near the top. The name Outlaw Trail refers to some rangers' quasi-disapproval of its use. Rescue attempts have been mounted in response to hikers getting into serious trouble, especially those attempting to hike the trail in the downhill direction. Do not hike the trail downhill from the top. You could lose your way and wander down the wrong ridge, and besides, a downhill ascent during the daytime means a temperature increase of as much as 60°F. Also, because the trail is so steep, the trail is at least as punishing on leg muscles in the downhill direction as it is in the uphill direction.

Vistas of Coachella Valley and the vast sweep of the Colorado Desert expand as you trudge uphill, step after step, curling up along one side of the sinuous ridge, then along the other. In a matter of a few hours, you will ascend through low-desert, high desert, and chaparral plant associations into a boreal zone of pines and firs.

At about 5 miles (from Ramon Road), the trail might be more difficult to follow amid the manzanita chaparral. If you lose the trail, back up immediately and try to find it. You must stay on the route in order to negotiate the steep, rocky, brushy terrain ahead. At about 6.5 miles (at 5,800 feet), the trail crosses a shallow ravine, veers left, traverses through some oaks just above the creek, crosses the ravine again, and then climbs out of the ravine toward a ridge. It wanders up this ridge, sparsely dotted with timber, to about 7,600

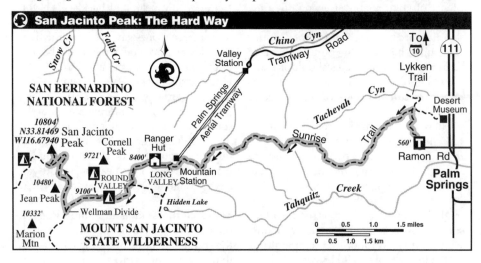

feet, where it veers right (northwest) and traverses several steep gullies on a deeply shaded (in the fall, at least) northeast-facing slope. The section ahead is very dangerous if it is covered by hard-packed snow or ice and you don't have an ice ax and crampons. As you near a sheer rock outcropping, the trail abruptly bends left (southwest) and climbs almost straight up a steep slope to the lip of terracelike Long Valley, at an elevation of 8,400 feet.

You've come 9 miles from Ramon Road and gained 8,000 feet. If you choose to bail out at this point, simply head north through Long Valley a few hundred yards to the tramway station. Otherwise, pick up a wilderness permit at the Long Valley ranger hut below the tramway station.

From the ranger hut, follow the wide trail leading steadily uphill for 2 miles to Round Valley, mostly through a coniferous forest of Jeffrey pine, sugar pine, and white fir. Continue the somewhat steeper ascent beyond Round Valley through thinning lodgepole pines to a trail junction at Wellman Divide, 3.2 miles from the ranger station.

Beyond Wellman Divide, a more leisurely uphill grind takes you inexorably upward toward San Jacinto Peak. You traverse north for more than a mile across a boulder-strewn slope covered by scattered lodgepole pines and a carpet of low-growing alpine shrubs. Abruptly, you change direction at a switchback corner, climb southwest for a while, and arrive (2 miles from Wellman Divide) on a saddle just south of the peak itself. Veer right, follow the path up along the right (east) side of the summit, pass a stone hut, then scramble from boulder to boulder for a couple of minutes to reach the top. The view is dizzying, not only because of the sheer height, but also because you have ascended into thin air to a level where about one-third of Earth's atmosphere lies below you.

Your journey is not over yet! Make sure that you leave the summit of San Jacinto Peak in time to catch the last downhill tram ride.

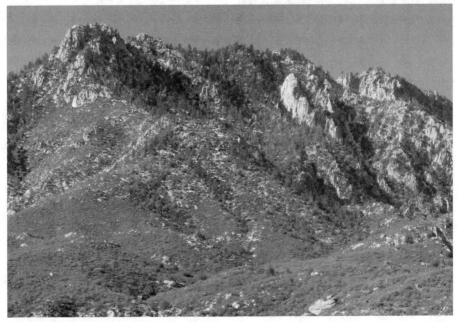

Upper reaches of the Sunrise Trail

HIKE 54

San Jacinto Peak: The Middle Way

Location	San Jacinto Mountains
Highlights	Broad vistas and an atmosphere reminiscent of the Sierra Nevada
Distance	15 miles (out-and-back)
Total Elevation Gain/Loss	4,400'/4,400'
Hiking Time	9 hours
Optional Maps	Santa Rosa and San Jacinto Mountains National Monument or USGS 7.5-minute *Idyllwild* and *San Jacinto Peak*
Best Times	April–November
Agency	SBNF/SJD
Difficulty	Strenuous
Trail Use	Suitable for backpacking
Permit	San Jacinto Wilderness permit required

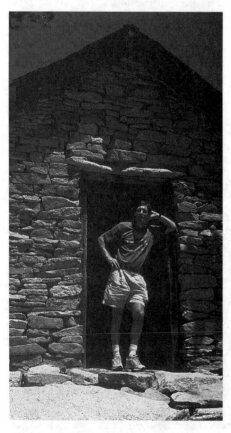

Stone hut below San Jacinto Peak

The San Jacinto Mountains, like many other units of the Peninsular Ranges (and much of the Sierra Nevada to the north) have gradually sloping west slopes and more steeply plunging east faces. Hike 53 tackled the desert-facing east slope of San Jacinto range. This route meanders in a far more leisurely fashion up the forested west slope of the San Jacinto Mountains. The comparison to the Sierra Nevada is an apt one: The climb from the yellow-pine botanical zone in Idyllwild toward the arctic-alpine zone atop San Jacinto Peak is similar to many trips in the western Sierra Nevada that take hikers up through various forest belts to timberline.

This hike (midway in difficulty compared to the previous two in this book) to San Jacinto Peak, follows the popular Devil's Slide Trail out of the resort community of Idyllwild. To control overuse, the US Forest Service has established quotas for this trail on summer weekends and holidays. Apply by mail; the quota fills up well in advance on popular weekends. Quotas or not, all hikers must obtain a wilderness permit (for either hiking or backpacking the route) at the US Forest Service ranger station in the center

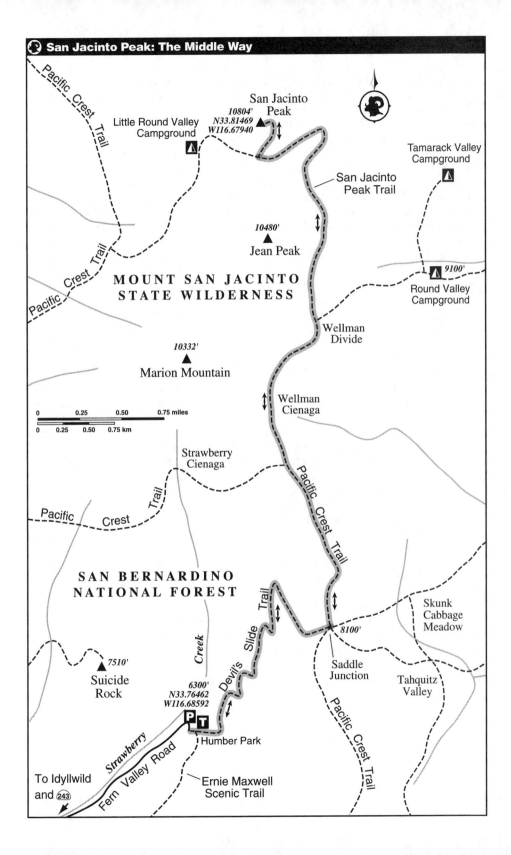

Pacific Crest Trail

San Jacinto Peak
10804'
N33.81469
W116.67940

Little Round Valley
Campground

Tamarack Valley
Campground

San Jacinto
Peak Trail

10480'
Jean Peak

Pacific Crest Trail

9100'
Round Valley
Campground

MOUNT SAN JACINTO
STATE WILDERNESS

Wellman
Divide

10332'
Marion Mountain

0   0.25   0.50   0.75 miles
0   0.25   0.50   0.75 km

Wellman
Cienaga

Strawberry
Cienaga

Pacific Crest Trail

Pacific   Crest   Trail

SAN BERNARDINO
NATIONAL FOREST

Skunk
Cabbage
Meadow

7510'
Suicide
Rock

8100'

Devil's Slide Trail

Creek

Saddle
Junction

Tahquitz
Valley

6300'
N33.76462
W116.68592

Pacific Crest Trail

Strawberry

P T
Humber Park

To Idyllwild
and (243)

Fern Valley Road

Ernie Maxwell
Scenic Trail

of Idyllwild. The station is located on the east side of CA 243, 1 block north of North Circle Drive. You will be driving past or very near this station on your way to the trailhead at Humber Park.

To Reach the Trailhead: Exit I-10 at Banning, and follow CA 243 south for 25 miles to reach Idyllwild's town center, and North Circle Drive on the left (east). Drive 0.75 mile northeast on North Circle Drive, veer right on South Circle Drive (crossing over Strawberry Creek), and take the first left, Fern Valley Road. Continue nearly 2 miles to the end of the road, where you will find parking space (perhaps not on weekends, unless it's early!) in the large lot at Humber Park. A National Forest Adventure Pass is required.

Description: Two trails diverge from the parking lot; the Ernie Maxwell Scenic Trail descends to the right (south), and the Devil's Slide Trail ascends to the left (east and north). You waste no time on that ascent as you switch back and forth along a zigzagging course, intermittently enjoying the shade cast by oak, pine, fir, and cedar foliage. Two rock-climbing destinations are in view as you climb: Suicide Rock generally on the left or west and the more imposing Lily Rock (or Tahquitz) on the right. During spring and early summer, rivulets of ice-cold water flow down several of the small ravines you cross on your way up.

At the top of the ridge, Saddle Junction (2.5 miles), you can take a breather on a nearby rock or fallen log. Five trails converge in this flat space. Opportunities for wilderness camping are east of here in the Skunk Cabbage Meadow and Tahquitz Valley areas. These wilderness camping sites could make a suitable base camp for a two- or three-day expedition to the peak and back.

For the next leg, follow the Pacific Crest Trail left (north) from Saddle Junction toward Wellman Divide. You ascend along a bouldered ridge, through statuesque Jeffrey pines and white firs, enjoying intermittent vistas east, south, and west. At a junction at 4.4 miles, the PCT swings left (west), contouring more or less across the south flank of Marion Mountain. Strawberry Cienaga, a permanently soggy area in the upper Strawberry Creek drainage and possible side trip, lies 1 mile down that trail. Our way, however, continues north through scattered lodgepole pines and white firs, past a boggy spot called Wellman Cienaga and reaches Wellman Divide at 5.4 miles.

At Wellman Divide, the trail to the right descends to Round Valley and Long Valley, while our way stays left (north), climbing moderately but inexorably toward San Jacinto Peak. You traverse north for more than a mile across a boulder-strewn slope covered by scattered lodgepole pines and a carpet of low-growing alpine shrubs. Abruptly, you change direction at a switchback corner, climb southwest for a while, and arrive (2 miles from Wellman Divide) in a saddle just south of the peak itself. Veer right, follow the path up along the right (east) side of the summit, pass a stone hut, then scramble from boulder to boulder for a couple of minutes to reach the top.

When it's time to go, retrace your route to the trailhead. Alternatively, you can loop around the west side of the mountain to make a terrific 20-mile tour of San Jacinto.

Tahquitz Peak

Location	San Jacinto Mountains
Highlight	Visiting a remote fire lookout with terrific views
Distance	7 miles (out-and-back)
Total Elevation Gain/Loss	2,000'/2,000'
Hiking Time	4 hours
Optional Maps	Santa Rosa and San Jacinto Mountains National Monument or USGS 7.5-minute *Idyllwild*
Best Times	April–November
Agency	SBNF/SJD
Difficulty	Moderately strenuous
Trail Use	Dogs allowed, suitable for backpacking
Permit	San Jacinto Wilderness permit required

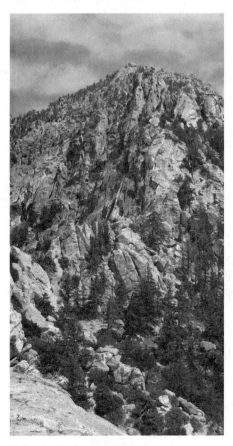

Tahquitz Peak

Tahquitz Peak (pronounced by those in the know as "talk wish") celebrates a legendary demon who, in the oral tradition of the Cahuilla Indians, used to dine on maidens and issue crackling bolts of lightning over the San Jacinto Mountains when displeased. At an elevation of 8,828 feet, the forest lookout tower perched atop the peak commands a view westward over haze and smog to the crests of the Santa Ana and San Gabriel Mountains. On rare days of crystalline visibility, you may glimpse the coastline at Santa Monica and Malibu, as well as the offshore islands of Santa Catalina and San Clemente.

You can directly approach Tahquitz Peak by way of the South Ridge Trail out of the mountain hamlet of Idyllwild. First, you'll have to obtain a wilderness permit from the US Forest Service station in Idyllwild's town center.

To Reach the Trailhead: Exit I-10 at Banning, and follow CA 243 south for 25 miles to reach Idyllwild's town center on the left, where you will find the US Forest Service station 1 block north of North Circle Drive. Continue south on CA 243 for 1 mile and turn left on Saunders Meadow Road. Continue to Pine Street, turn left (north), go 2 blocks, turn right (east) on Tahquitz View Drive, and go right on South Ridge Road, Forest Road 5S11. If your car is sturdy enough, drive up this potholed road for 1.5 miles to the South Ridge Trailhead.

Description: The no-nonsense South Ridge Trail ahead takes you steadily uphill along a viewful ridge, first through Jeffrey pine, live oak, and fir, then past thickets of low-growing chinquapin and stalwart lodgepole pines. Off to the left (north of the trail), you may see or hear some of the many rock climbers who gingerly make their way up the sheer face of Lily Rock (colloquially known as Tahquitz). Finally, after many switchbacks, you reach the fire lookout structure atop Tahquitz Peak, which may be staffed when you arrive. Visitors may or may not be invited to view the landscape

from the tower itself. The summit view encompasses the timbered slopes of the southern San Jacinto Mountains and innumerable valleys and ridges spilling west and south toward Southern California's coast.

After taking in the view, descend from the lookout the way you came. The following longer, looping return is perhaps a more suitable way to enjoy the mountain's charms on a two-day backpack: Head northeast, join the Pacific Crest Trail after 0.5 mile, and follow the PCT 1.3 miles north to Saddle Junction. (Nearby, to the east, are suitable wilderness campsites.) Descend Devil's Slide Trail 2.5 miles to Humber Park. There, you can arrange to be picked up. Or you can hoof it 2.6 miles down the gently descending Ernie Maxwell Scenic Trail to Tahquitz View Drive, not far away from the dirt road leading to your starting point.

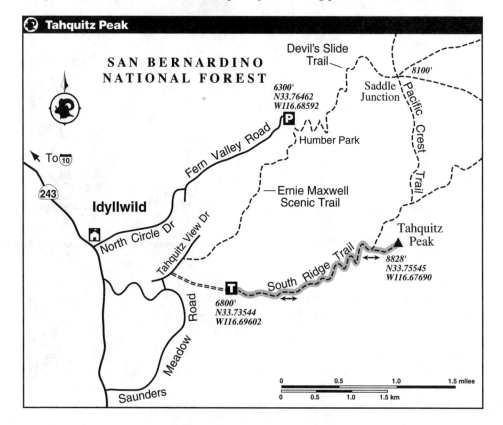

HIKE 56

Antsell Rock

Location	San Jacinto Mountains
Highlight	Rock scrambling up an impressive peak
Distance	4.2 miles (out-and-back)
Total Elevation Gain/Loss	2,300'/2,300'
Hiking Time	4 hours
Recommended Map	Santa Rosa and San Jacinto Mountains National Monument or USGS 7.5-minute *Idyllwild* and *Palm View Peak*
Best Times	April–June; October–November
Agency	SBNF/SJD
Difficulty	Strenuous
Permit	San Jacinto Wilderness permit required

The Desert Divide is a remote and lonely mountain backbone running south from San Jacinto and Tahquitz Peak to CA 74. Antsell Rock is the jewel of the Divide. Named by Edmund Perkins of the United States Geological Survey for an artist at Keen Camp Resort who was painting the peak, Antsell Rock stands high above the Divide, and its stony buttresses make an impressive sight from most directions. It is also one of the few mountaineers' peaks in Southern California that requires more than the usual plodding to reach the third-class summit. While this trip is short, it is certainly not easy.

Much of the divide is covered in dense chaparral. The legendary Sam Fink, a Santa Ana fire captain and Sierra Club leader, spent nearly a decade in the 1960s and 1970s chopping a route along the crest of the Divide. The Pacific Crest Trail now follows much of Fink's original route. Constructing the PCT required three years of drilling, blasting, and cutting, making it the most difficult stretch in Southern California to build.

This trip climbs from the Zen Mountain Center to the PCT, and then makes a rugged ascent up a gully to the summit rocks. The Zen Center graciously allows hikers to cross their property. Please help retain this privilege by being a courteous trail user. Avoid bringing large groups or large numbers of vehicles, and keep your voice down while crossing the center so as not to disturb meditators. Dogs are prohibited. The trail is not shown on topographic maps.

This trip is in the San Jacinto Wilderness, and you must obtain a free wilderness permit. Write to the Idyllwild Ranger Station to request one, or stop by on your way for a self-issued permit.

To Reach the Trailhead: From State Highway 74, 3.4 miles southeast of Mountain Center near mile marker 074 RIV 62.75, turn east onto Apple Canyon Road. Proceed 3.3 miles to its end at Pine Springs Ranch. Immediately before entering the ranch, veer right onto a good private dirt road leading to the Zen Mountain Center. In 1.1 miles, park in a small dirt lot on the left just before you enter the Zen Center.

Description: From the parking area, continue up the dirt road through the gate. Stay left at a fork by the office, then left again at a fork near the cabins. Continue up the dirt road toward the low point on the Desert Divide. In 0.3 mile, pass two water tanks. The unsigned trail begins here where the road switchbacks. It follows the spectacular canyon along a seasonal creek beneath enchanting incense-cedars and black oaks. In 0.1 mile, a spur on the right leads to the creek while the main trail begins to climb steeply to the left. Watch for Coulter pines with their enormous cones. The trail ascends the chaparral-clad slopes and reaches the crest in another 0.8 mile.

Turn left (west) and follow the PCT along the northeast side of Antsell Rock. In 0.5 mile, look for a gully marked with cairns in a grove of black oaks. A use trail up this gully leads to the summit of Antsell Rock. The jaunt is only 0.3 mile as the crow

flies, but it involves 800 feet of strenuous climbing. The steep and loose gully leads up to a prominent notch to the right of the rocky peak. The summit register can be found in this notch, so hikers uncomfortable with rock scrambling may stop here.

For one of the more delightful mountaineering experiences in Southern California, continue up to the true summit. Scramble up a weakness in the rock above the notch, and then go left around the corner to another tree-filled gully leading to the rocky summit ridge. Some third-class climbing (hands and feet) is required, but most parties would be comfortable without a rope.

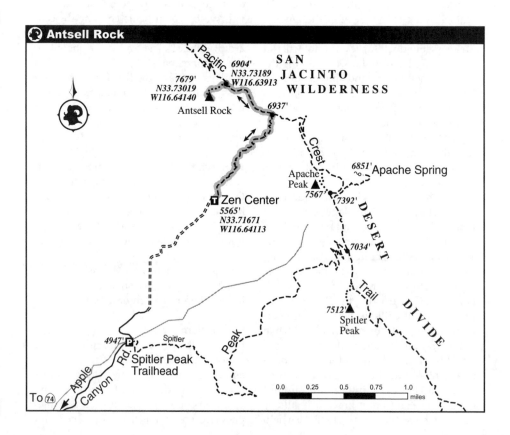

HIKE 57

Mount Rubidoux

Location	City of Riverside
Highlight	Views
Distance	3.3 miles (out-and-back)
Total Elevation Gain/Loss	450'/450'
Hiking Time	1½ hours
Optional Map	USGS 7.5-minute *Riverside West*
Best Times	All year, daylight hours, but hot in the summer
Agency	CRPR
Difficulty	Moderate
Trail Use	Dogs allowed, good for kids, suitable for biking

Mount Rubidoux is a prominent granite hill located west of downtown Riverside and south of the Santa Ana River. The mountain is named for Louis Rubidoux, who settled the area in the mid-1800s, but it was Frank Miller, one of Riverside's early promoters and the builder of the historic Mission Inn, who transformed Mount Rubidoux from an anonymous bump to a much-loved and inspirational park. Miller originally intended to develop the mountain for mansions, but his plan failed. Instead, Miller graded a road circling up the mountain that hikers, cyclists, joggers, and strollers enjoy today.

To Reach the Trailhead: Exit the 60 Freeway south on Rubidoux Boulevard. In 0.3 mile, turn left on Mission Boulevard. Follow it 1.5 miles across the Santa Ana River

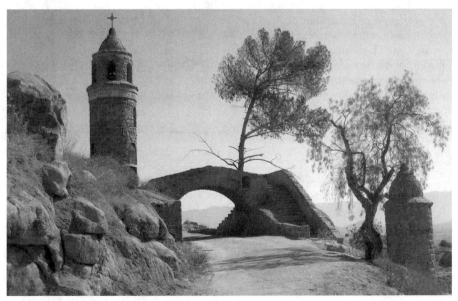

Peace Tower on Mount Rubidoux

to where it becomes Mission Inn Avenue, then turn right on Redwood Drive. Go 0.2 mile to Ninth Street, then turn right again and park along the street in 1 block near the corner of Mount Rubidoux Drive. The trailhead is located in a residential neighborhood with strict parking enforcement. Take care to observe the signed parking restrictions.

As this book was going to press, the July 2013 Mountain Fire was actively burning in this area. If you plan to visit soon after, call to confirm that the trail is open.

Description: There are two paved trails that wind up the mountain like intertwined corkscrews. The gentle route is 2 miles and loops the mountain twice, while the steeper route is 1 mile and loops the mountain only once. The two trails intersect twice.

This trip begins at the Mount Rubidoux Drive Trailhead and winds along the bottom of the mountain. Gnarly prickly pear cactus intermingles with coastal sage scrub and drifts downward into the backyard gardens of homes at the base of the mountain. Miller planted the yuccas, aloes, agave, and cacti that you see. In 0.5 mile, reach a signed four-way junction, and make a hairpin right turn to take the longer trail. As you climb, you will have views of downtown Riverside, Evergreen Memorial Cemetery, the Santa Ana River, and Flabob Airport, one of the older airports in America and a famous base for antique and home-built aircraft. Keep your eyes out for unusual planes on approach into the field.

Pass the short trail a second time as you cross under the Ben Lewis Bridge, then reach the Peace Tower, built by "friends of Frank Augustus Miller in recognition of his constant labor in the promotion of civic beauty, community righteousness, and world peace." Once you reach the top of the mountain, explore the amphitheater, the plaque honoring Father Junipero Serra, the flagpole, and the large cross. On a clear day you will have excellent views south over Riverside.

Return along the steeper trail, which leads west along the north side of the mountain and over the Ben Lewis Bridge. When you reach the signed junction on the south side, continue east along your original route back to the trailhead.

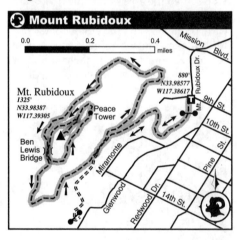

Lone Tree Point on Catalina

Location	Santa Catalina Island
Highlights	Island and sea vistas
Distance	6 miles (out-and-back)
Total Elevation Gain/Loss	1,800'/1,800'
Hiking Time	3 hours
Optional Maps	Catalina Island Conservancy Map or USGS 7.5-minute *Santa Catalina East*
Best Times	All year
Agency	CIC
Difficulty	Moderately strenuous
Trail Use	Good for kids

Santa Catalina Island, "26 miles across the sea" as the song goes, stretches 21 miles in length and up to 8 miles at its maximum width. The town of Avalon snuggles against a cove near the eastern end of the island, protected from prevailing winds that come out of the west and northwest. Avalon experiences the same almost-frost-free climate as the most even-tempered areas of the Southern California coastline, and it enjoys possibly the cleanest air of any spot near the Southern California coast. In the hills above Avalon you can find wild mountainsides smothered in Catalina's own unique assemblage of chaparral, spectacular ocean views, and some of the finest hiking in all of California.

Catalina was for most of this century owned by the Wrigley family (of chewing-gum and Chicago Cubs fame). In 1972 management of most of the island passed into the hands of the Catalina Island Conservancy, whose function is to preserve and protect the island's wild lands. Recreational use of the island, including camping, hiking, backpacking, and mountain biking (on select routes), is allowed on most of the island.

The languid pace of life on Catalina reflects its aloofness from the increasingly frantic business of living on the Southern California mainland. An overnight visit here is truly relaxing, whether you choose to lodge in Avalon or prefer to rough it at one of the several campgrounds spread around the island's coast and interior.

The hike described here, excellent during the spring wildflower season and on crisp fall or winter days, begins at Hermit Gulch Campground near Avalon and loops over the top of the hills overlooking Avalon and the ocean. (You'll need a

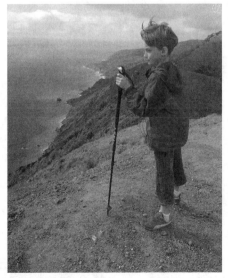

Lone Tree Point

free permit for this, available at the Catalina Conservancy office at 125 Claressa
Avenue in Avalon.) The highlight of the
hike is a side trip over to Lone Tree Point,
which commands an unparalleled view of
the clifflike Palisades falling sheer to the
ocean. You'll encounter a couple of very
steep grades on the fire road leading to
Lone Tree Point, so be sure to wear running shoes or boots with studs or lugs to
ensure that you have plenty of traction.
Small children will probably need some
assistance on that stretch.

You may see bison, boar, and deer—
all introduced to the island at one time or
another—on various parts of the island.
Recent efforts to remove many of these
nonindigenous and often destructive
animals have been quite successful. Spotting great herds of goats on the island is a
thing of the past.

To Reach the Trailhead: Ferries to Catalina depart terminals at San Pedro, Long
Beach, and Newport Beach. Air service is
also available from Long Beach. For more
information about camping, lodging, hiking, and biking on the island, as well as
transportation to the island, the following two phone numbers are most useful:
Catalina Island Conservancy, 310-510-
2595; and Santa Catalina Island Company,
310-510-2800. You may also visit Catalina
Island Conservancy's extensive website,
catalinaconservancy.org, for information
and links to other websites.

From the pier in Avalon, the Avalon
Canyon Nature Center and Hermit Gulch
Campground are 1.4 miles southwest up
Avalon Canyon. An inexpensive tram
makes the trip hourly from the end of
the pier, continuing to the canyon's end
at the botanical gardens. Alternatively,

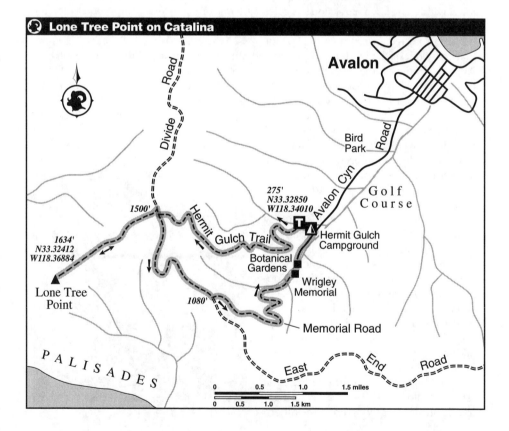

you can walk, bring, or rent bicycles, or take a taxi.

Description: From the top end of Hermit Gulch Campground, start your hike by following the well-built Hermit Gulch Trail up the ravine to the west. Before long, you leave the trickling stream in the canyon bottom and begin a twisting ascent up along a shaggy slope. During the springtime, red monkeyflower, shooting star, lupine, paintbrush, and other native wildflowers dot the trailside and adorn small clearings amid the tangles of chaparral. After 1.7 miles and an elevation gain of 1,200 feet, you meet Divide Road, the fire road along the eastern spine of the island.

Turn right, walk 0.1 mile, and then turn left onto a steep fire road signed LONE TREE TRAIL. Continue for 1.0 mile over several rounded barren hills, passing over the peaklet designated Lone Tree on most maps. That's where you'll find the best view of the ocean and shoreline. Sometimes you can gaze south over shore-hugging fog and spy the low dome of San Clemente Island, some 40 miles across the glistening Pacific. When visibility's best, you can trace the mainland coast as far south as San Diego, and also spy the long crest of the Peninsular Ranges, the chain of mountains running through Riverside and San Diego Counties into Baja California.

After taking in the visual feast, backtrack to Divide Road. From there you loop back to the starting point via a longer but more gradually descending route. Head south down Divide Road for 0.8 mile, then veer left on Memorial Road. Easy walking down this crooked dirt road takes you along a cool, north-facing slope covered by tall and luxuriant (by mainland standards) growths of scrub oak, manzanita, and toyon.

At the bottom of the hill you come upon Wrigley Memorial. Below that, you pass through the botanical gardens that Mrs. Ada Wrigley founded in the 1920s. Because of the virtually frost-free climate, an extensive array of California natives and exotics from distant corners of the world are able to thrive here. Once you are beyond the garden gates, it's but a couple hundred yards back to the campground.

HIKE 59

Hills for Everyone

Location	Chino Hills
Highlight	Woodsy canyon
Distance	4.5 miles (loop)
Total Elevation Gain/Loss	1,000'/1,000'
Hiking Time	2½ hours
Optional Map	Chino Hills State Park brochure or USGS 7.5-minute *Prado Dam*
Best Times	8 a.m.–sunset, November–May; closed several days after rains
Agency	CHSP
Difficulty	Moderate
Trail Use	Good for kids

Chino Hills State Park was established in 1984 on the hills dividing Orange County from San Bernardino County as a critical wildlife corridor between adjoining open spaces and as an escape for humans from the endless surrounding housing developments. Now comprising more than 14,000 acres of rolling hills, the park attracts an increasing number of hikers, mountain bikers, and equestrians.

In November 2008, more than 90% of the park burned in the Freeway Complex Fire, and the hike through Water Canyon recommended in earlier editions is no longer particularly attractive. Fortunately, much of the park has made a rapid recovery. This hiker-only trip makes a delightful loop through a woodsy canyon and a scenic ridge starting near the park headquarters. Winter

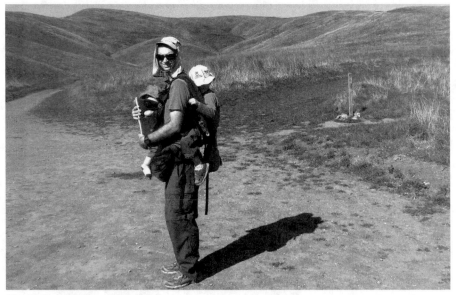

Tired hikers at Chino Hills

and spring are the most attractive times when the grass is green and the wildflowers emerge, but the park is enjoyable anytime that it is not too hot. Pick up a park map on your way in. The park is laced with dozens of miles of fine trails that will inevitably tempt you to return.

Note: **This trail was damaged in 2012 and is temporarily closed. Even more important, the park entrance may be temporarily closed for construction.** Check if it has reopened before you go, and be prepared for changes.

To Reach the Trailhead: Chino Hills State Park has a temporary north entrance that is as obscure as the park itself. From CA 71, 7 miles north of CA 91 and 5 miles south of CA 60, exit west on Soquel Canyon Parkway. In 1.0 mile, turn left on to Elinvar Drive, left again after 0.2 mile,

and then immediately right on the road signed CHINO HILLS STATE PARK.

In 0.7 mile, stop at the iron ranger to pay the day-use fee. The road eventually becomes paved and bends sharply right. In 3.0 miles from the park entrance, watch for the South Ridge and Telegraph Canyon Trailheads on the left, then in another 0.1 mile turn left into the parking and camping area. If you reach the historic Rolling M Ranch, you've gone 0.1 mile too far.

Description: From the day-use parking area, walk 250 feet back down to the main road. Turn right and walk another 250 feet, crossing the creek, to reach the gated dirt road signed TELEGRAPH CANYON TRAIL. Follow this path west for a mile. You may see evidence of the trees that burned in 2008. The grasslands, green

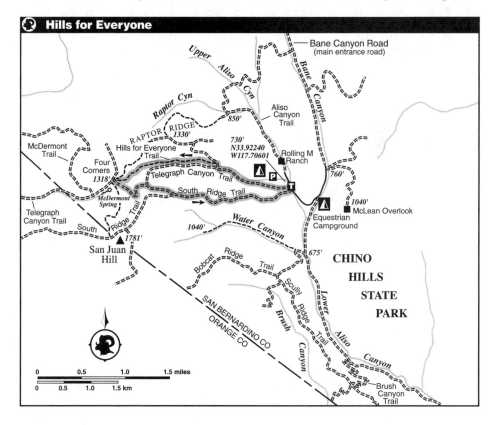

in the wet months and tawny the rest of the year, have rapidly recovered.

In 1.0 mile, take a dirt road on the right that crosses the creek on a bridge. Then make an immediate left onto a trail signed HILLS FOR EVERYONE. The trail, named after the volunteer group that helped establish the park, offers an intimate view of the canyon bottom. It is narrow and occasionally tilted or brushy, so it might not be a good choice for hikers with poor balance. Most of the oaks survived the inferno, making for an increasingly shady and beautiful walk as you continue upstream. Beware of poison oak that occasionally grows close to the trail, especially in the winter when it has lost its distinctive leaves. Watch for squirrels and raptors; if you are lucky, you might see deer, coyote, or other larger wildlife.

In 0.3 mile, the trail crosses a bridge to the south bank, where it takes an undulating course up the steep slope. Pass beneath a set of powerlines, then twice pass a second set zigzagging across the canyon. Cross the creek once more, and shortly afterward climb to the Four Corners Junction, 2.3 miles from the start.

Turn left onto the South Ridge Trail, another fire road that is popular with mountain bikers. Make a switchback to cross the canyon and climb to a low saddle, where you can enjoy a grand view over the Inland Empire to Southern California's tallest peaks, the Three Saints: San Jacinto, San Gorgonio, and San Antonio (also known as Old Baldy).

In 0.5 mile, pass a junction with the Telegraph Canyon Trail. Pass three more unmarked roads servicing the utility towers. After you crest another small hill, the campground and eastern part of the park come into view. In 1.8 miles, reach the paved park road. Turn left and make the short jaunt back to your vehicle.

HIKE 60

Santiago Oaks Regional Park

Location	City of Orange
Highlights	Oak woodland and a trickling stream
Distance	1–3 miles (many possible loops)
Total Elevation Gain/Loss	100'–400', depending on exact route
Hiking Time	½–1½ hours
Optional Maps	Santiago Oaks Regional Park brochure or USGS 7.5-minute *Orange*
Best Times	7 a.m.–sunset, all year; trails closed three days after rains
Agency	SORP
Difficulty	Easy
Trail Use	Good for kids, dogs allowed, suitable for mountain biking

What Santiago Oaks Regional Park lacks in sheer size its rare beauty more than adequately compensates for. The core of the park is made up of two former ranch properties acquired in the mid-1970s. A small Valencia orange grove and many acres of ornamental trees planted around 1960 on these properties complement the natural riparian and oak-woodland communities along Santiago Creek.

To Reach the Trailhead: From the 55 Freeway in the city of Orange, exit at Katella Avenue (Exit 15) and proceed east. Katella becomes Villa Park Road and again changes its name to Santiago Canyon Road on the eastern outskirts of Orange. Once you are 3.2 miles east of the freeway, turn left on Windes Drive, which leads into Santiago Oaks Regional Park.

As you approach the park entrance, subdivisions quickly fade from sight, and a lush strip of riparian vegetation (willows and sycamores) comes into view on the left. Pay your day-use fee at the entry station and request the park's excellent trail map. Park in the main lot and then stroll up past some oak-shaded picnic sites to the superb nature center, which is housed in a nicely refurbished 70-year-old ranch house.

Description: The best of this park's several miles of trails stay close to the wooded bottomlands of Santiago Creek. You might begin with the self-guiding

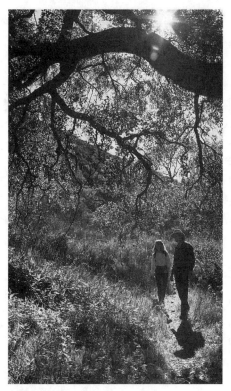

Oaks of Santiago Oaks

Windes Nature Trail and its extension, the Pacifica Loop, which starts alongside the nature center. Though only about 0.7 mile long, the trail is very steep in places, and it meanders up to the northern summit of Rattlesnake Ridge, an isolated, erosion-resistant block of mostly conglomerate rock. You can glimpse a slice of Pacific coastline from the high point of the trail, and a fenced lookout point nearby offers a view almost straight down on Santiago Creek and the rest of the park.

Back down by the nature center, you can walk upstream along the shaded creek bank to reach a small rock-and-cement dam dating from 1892. This dam replaced an earlier one, built in 1879, that was part of one of Orange County's first irrigation systems. Today, the surviving dam is a historical curiosity, dwarfed by

the large Villa Park flood-control dam a short distance upstream and Santiago Reservoir farther upstream.

North of the nature center, you can ford Santiago Creek and stroll along several paths amid the eucalyptus, pepper, and other exotic trees rooted to the gently sloping bench on the creek's far side. Its diverse habitats makes Santiago Oaks a delightful birding spot, with species ranging from the tree-dwelling western bluebird and acorn woodpecker to the water-loving great blue heron. On occasion, you may see vultures, ospreys, and some common hawks soaring overhead.

Longer-distance trails radiate outward from Santiago Oaks Regional Park toward Irvine Park to the southeast and up the slope east and northeast into Weir Canyon Park.

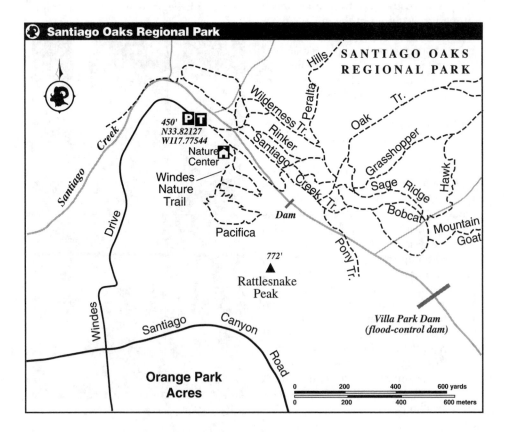

HIKE 61

El Moro Canyon

Location	Crystal Cove State Park
Highlights	Unspoiled coastal hills and canyon
Distance	6 miles (out-and-back)
Total Elevation Gain/Loss	900'/900'
Hiking Time	3½ hours
Optional Maps	Crystal Cove State Park brochure or USGS 7.5-minute *Laguna Beach*
Best Times	6 a.m.–sunset, all year
Agency	CCSP
Difficulty	Moderate
Trail Use	Suitable for mountain biking

Crystal Cove State Park preserves one of the last large, undisturbed parcels of open space along the Orange County coast, near Laguna Beach. Besides containing a 3-mile stretch of bluffs and oceanfront, the park reaches back into the San Joaquin Hills to encompass the entire watershed of El Moro Canyon—more than 4 square miles of natural ravines, ridges, and marine terrace formations. In the back-country (El Moro Canyon) section of the park alone, visitors can explore about 20 miles of dirt roads and paths open to hikers, equestrians, and mountain bicyclists.

Upper El Moro Canyon is far and away the most beautiful attraction in the park's backcountry. You stroll past thickets of willow, toyon, elderberry, and sycamore, all brightly illuminated by the sun; then you suddenly plunge into cool, dark, cathedral-like recesses overhung by the massive limbs of live oaks. In one such recess, several shallow caves, adorned with ferns at their entrances, pock a sandstone outcrop next to the road. Before the establishment of the California missions, American Indians gathered acorns, seeds, and wild berries in this canyon. These foods, coupled with the abundant marine life nearby, provided a balanced and healthy diet.

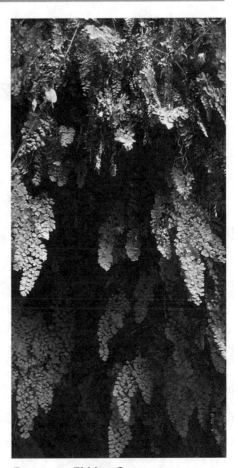

Fern grotto, El Moro Canyon

To Reach the Trailhead: From a point on Pacific Coast Highway (Highway 1) about 3 miles north of Laguna Beach and 4 miles south of Corona del Mar, turn east onto an access road. The road then veers right. Pay the hefty day-use fee (presently $15) at the entrance station, and request a copy of the excellent park map. Continue past the Moro Campground and down the hill, then turn left (east) and drive to the trailhead parking near a picnic area at the end of the road.

Description: From the east end of the parking lot, hike east across a bridge into shallow El Moro Canyon, where you join a wide trail that goes up the canyon. Other trails intersect left and right; you simply stay in the canyon bottom. At a point about 3 miles up the canyon, reach the head of the canyon, where the Elevator Trail starts climbing steeply to the ridge above. This is a good spot to turn around and head back the way you came, the easy way.

Should you wish to extend your hike, loop north and return to your starting point using any of several ridge-running trails. The densely packed mansions clinging to the ridge to the west give a hint of what this wilderness might have become if it were not set aside as open space.

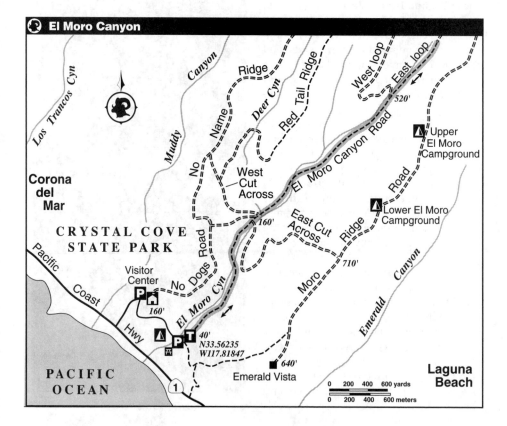

HIKE 62

Whiting Ranch

Location	Lake Forest and El Toro
Highlight	Red rock cliffs
Distance	4.4 miles (out-and-back)
Total Elevation Gain/Loss	500'/500'
Hiking Time	2 hours
Optional Map	USGS 7.5-minute *El Toro*
Best Times	7 a.m.–sunset, October–June
Agency	OCP
Difficulty	Moderate
Trail Use	Good for kids, suitable for mountain bikes

In 1991, Orange County opened its newest large open-space preserve, Whiting Ranch Wilderness Park. The park has grown to encompass some 4,300 acres along the rim of the communities of Lake Forest and El Toro. Ninety percent of it burned in the 2007 Santiago Fire, but this trip was scarcely touched.

Whiting Ranch's rounded hills look nondescript when viewed from the suburbs below, but they conceal some pleasant surprises, which you will discover by trekking out and back to Red Rock Canyon, the site of a spectacular erosional feature—sandstone cliffs banded with layers of ancient sand and mud. Late in the day, the sun's warm glow brings out a reddish tint in the rock.

To Reach the Trailhead: To reach the park's main entrance from I-5 in southern Orange County, take Lake Forest Drive east and north for 5 miles to Portola Parkway. Turn left, and follow Portola northwest for another half mile. Turn right at Market Place. The trailhead parking is on the left and a shopping center is on the right. The lot is open 7 a.m.–sunset. If you are using the Foothill Transportation Corridor (241) toll road, exit at either Lake Forest Drive or Alton Parkway.

Description: The trail starts at an interpretive kiosk near the outhouse. Take a trail map if you wish to explore the park beyond the route described here. Like most trails in the Whiting Ranch Wilderness Park, the wide dirt path ahead is open to mountain biking and horse riding, as well as hiking. You immediately plunge into a densely shaded ravine called Borrego Canyon through which

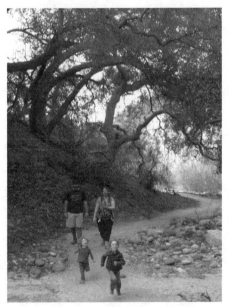

Boundless energy on the Borrego Trail

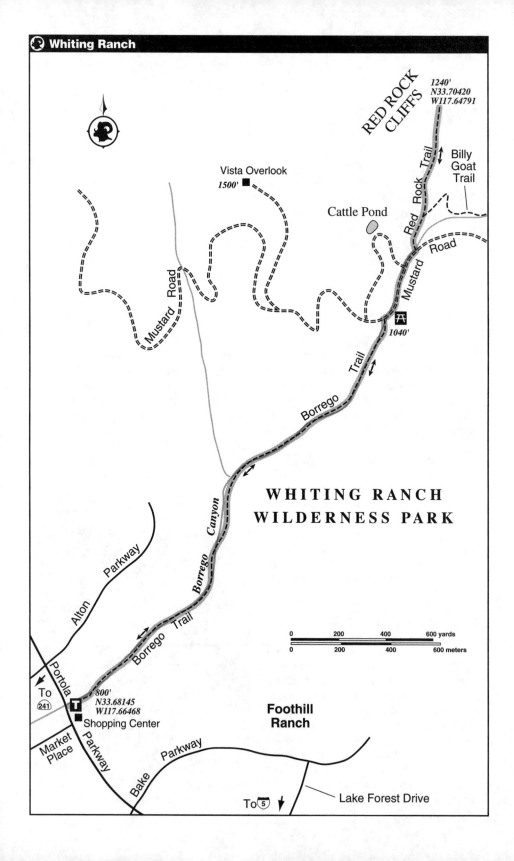

RED ROCK CLIFFS

1240'
N33.70420
W117.64791

Billy
Goat
Trail

Red Rock Trail

Vista Overlook
1500'

Cattle Pond

Mustard Road

Mustard Road

1040'

Borrego Trail

WHITING RANCH
WILDERNESS PARK

Borrego Canyon

Alton Parkway

Borrego Trail

| 0 | 200 | 400 | 600 yards |
| 0 | 200 | 400 | 600 meters |

Portola

To
241

800'
N33.68145
W117.66468

Foothill
Ranch

Shopping Center

Market Place

Bake Parkway

Parkway

To 5

Lake Forest Drive

flows a trickling stream. For a while, suburbia rims the canyon on both sides, but soon enough it disappears without a trace. The trek up the canyon feels Tolkienesque as you pass under a crooked-limb canopy of live oaks and sycamores and sniff the damp odor of the streamside willows. Often in the late fall and winter, frigid air sinks into these shady recesses overnight, and by early morning frost mantles everything below eye-level.

After 1.5 miles, you come to Mustard Road, a fire road that ascends both east and west to ridgetops offering long views of the ocean on clear days. Turn right on Mustard Road, and almost immediately come to a picnic site. Two trails fork to the left; the second, perhaps hard to see initially, leads into Red Rock Canyon.

Out in the sunshine now, you follow the Red Rock Trail (restricted to travelers on foot) up the bottom of a sunny canyon that narrows and steepens. The canyon burned in the Santiago Fire, but its vegetation is returning vigorously. In 0.7 mile, the trail ends at the base of the eroded sandstone cliffs, formed of sediment deposited on a shallow sea bottom about 20 million years ago. This type of rock, which contains the fossilized remains of shellfish and marine mammals, underlies much of Orange County. Rarely is it as well exposed as it is here.

After visiting Red Rock Canyon, you might decide to return via a more round-about and lengthy route. If a half-day's hike sounds about right, climb east on Mustard Road to the high point at Four Corners and then south on Whiting Road down to Serrano Canyon. At each of the numerous junctions, take the downhill fork. The woodsy descent through Serrano Canyon takes you back to Portola Parkway, and from there you follow the sidewalk a mile back to your starting point.

HIKE 63

Santiago Peak

Location	Santa Ana Mountains
Highlight	Best urban, mountain, and ocean views in Southern California
Distance	16 miles (out-and-back)
Total Elevation Gain/Loss	3,950'/3,950'
Hiking Time	8 hours
Optional Map	USGS 7.5-minute *Santiago Peak*
Best Times	October–May
Agency	CNF/TD
Difficulty	Strenuous
Trail Use	Dogs allowed

To the American Indians, it was Kalawpa ("a wooded place"), the lofty resting place of the deity Chiningchinish. Early settlers and surveyors named it variously Mount Downey, Trabuco Peak, Temescal Mountain, and Santiago Peak. Finally, mapmakers decided on the name that eventually stuck: Santiago. Today's bulldozer-scraped summit overrun with telecommunications antennae hardly pays sufficient homage to the peak's historic and scenic values. Witness, for example, this record of its first documented ascent in 1853, by a group of lawmen pursuing horse thieves up a canyon from the east:

> After an infinite amount of scrambling, danger, and hard labor, we stood on the very summit of the Temescal mountain, now by some called Santiago . . . where we beheld with pleasure a sublime view, more than worth the journey and ascent . . .

In 1861, while making a geologic survey of the Santa Anas, William Brewer and Josiah Whitney reached the same summit on their second try, using a northeast ridge. Their impressions echoed the sentiments of the earlier climbers: "The view more than repaid us for all we had endured."

The view that these early climbers described so enthusiastically remains spectacular—given, perhaps, a clearer-than-average winter day. In such conditions, you can trace the coastline from Point Loma to Point Dume, spot both Santa Catalina and San Clemente Islands, and scratch your head trying to identify the plethora of mountain ranges and lesser promontories filling the landscape inland.

Clockwise from northwest to southeast the major ranges on the horizon are the Santa Monica, San Gabriel, San Bernardino, Little San Bernardino, San Jacinto, Santa Rosa, Palomar, and Cuyamaca Mountains. To the south you might see several of the lower ranges along the Mexican border and perhaps glimpse the flat-topped summit of Table Mountain, a few miles inland from the Baja California coast. In the west and northwest, smog levels permitting, the flat urban tapestry spreads outward, spiked by the glass skyscrapers of downtown Los Angeles.

Don't underestimate the time required to bag Santiago Peak by way of today's most scenic approach, Holy Jim Trail. In winter, you'll need an early start to ensure that you return before sunset. And with summit temperatures roughly 20°F cooler than below, pack some extra clothing. Bring plenty of water too; Bear Spring, on the way to the summit, is *not* a potable water source.

To Reach the Trailhead: From the Foothill Transportation Corridor Toll Road (CA 241) in Rancho Santa Margarita, exit onto Santa Margarita Parkway. Drive 1.5 miles east, and turn left onto Plano Trabuco Road. Plano Trabuco Road becomes Trabuco Canyon Road 0.6 mile ahead at a sharp bend to the left. Curve downward into Trabuco Canyon for 0.8 mile, and at the bottom, turn right onto unpaved Trabuco Creek Road, which leads east toward Cleveland National Forest.

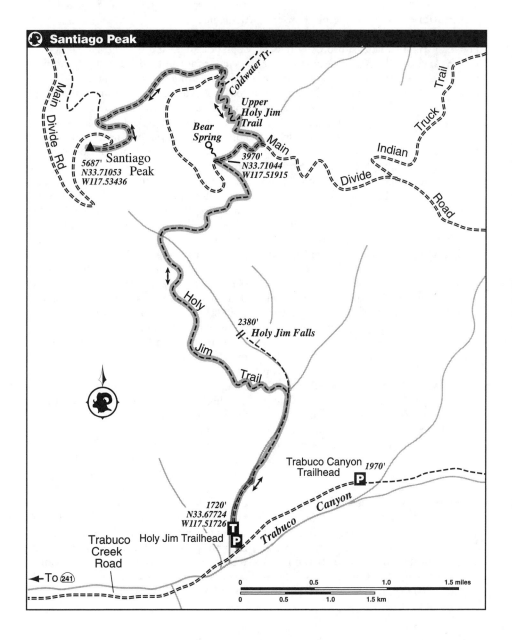

Driving this bumpy unpaved road may be an adventure itself, but the road is generally accessible to two-wheel-drive vehicles with moderate clearance. Proceed 4.7 miles east up the canyon to the Holy Jim Trailhead on the left. You must display a National Forest Adventure Pass on your car.

Description: The first segment of the trip follows a dirt road up and to the left above the trailhead kiosk. Proceed on foot (north) up along the east bank of Holy Jim Canyon's small stream, passing a number of cabins. More than a century ago this shady hollow was home to settlers who eked out a living by raising bees. Bee-keeper James T. Smith became so famous for his cursing habit that he was variously nicknamed "Cussin' Jim," "Lyin' Smith," "Greasy Jim," and "Salvation Smith." Dignified government cartographers invented a new name, "Holy Jim."

In 0.5 mile a gate marks the end of the dirt road and the beginning of the trail. Continue upstream another 0.8 mile, fording the stream seven times. Just past Picnic Rock, the trail crosses the stream at a signed junction. Our route switches back sharply to the left, while a lateral trail continues straight, going another 400 yards up along the stream to Holy Jim Falls. This little gem of a waterfall is worth the side trip if the stream is flowing decently. The Holy Jim Trail zigzags upward through dense chaparral on the west wall of Holy Jim Canyon. Well-traveled but minimally cleared of encroaching vegetation, the trail offers intimate glimpses of your immediate surroundings. You have a sense of motion and accomplishment as you ascend this trail.

Soon a few antenna structures atop Santiago Peak come into view, tantalizingly close, but about 3,000 feet higher. At 3.7 miles, the trail passes a small spring dug out of the hillside and then crosses the bed of Holy Jim Canyon at an elevation of 3,500 feet, far above the falls. You might be tempted at this point to short-cut to the summit by way of the scree-covered slopes; however, the loose rock and thickets of thorny ceanothus would surely cost you more time, effort, and grief than you ever imagined. (In April 2013, a pair of teenage hikers wandered off-trail, ran out of water, and called 911. An intense search took four days to locate the teens.)

So continue ahead on the trail, where soon you make a delicate traverse over a section prone to landslides. After another mile on sunny, south-facing slopes, you contour around a ridge and suddenly enter a dark and shady recess filled with oaks, sycamores, bigleaf maples, and big-cone Douglas-firs. By 5 miles, you come upon Main Divide Road, opposite Bear Spring (not potable).

From now on you simply turn left and follow the Main Divide Road (dirt road) uphill. Three more miles of steady climbing in sun and in shade bring you to Santiago's summit. Alternatively, from Bear Spring, you can turn right on Main Divide Road and go 0.4 mile to the obscure, unmarked Upper Holy Jim Trail that switchbacks vigorously up to rejoin the Main Divide Road at a hairpin turn halfway up the mountain.

You must walk around the antenna installation on the summit to take in the complete panorama. Modjeska Peak, 1 mile northwest and about 200 feet lower, isn't high enough to block the view of any far-horizon features. Collectively, Santiago and Modjeska Peaks form a familiar notchlike feature visible for miles around and known as Old Saddleback. The fine-grained rock of Old Saddleback is the prototype of the "Santiago Peak volcanics" exposed on many of the coastal mountain ranges extending south through San Diego County into Baja California. These metamorphosed volcanic-rock formations were originally part of a chain of volcanic islands that collided with our continent some 80 million years ago.

HIKE 64

Trabuco Canyon Loop

Location	Santa Ana Mountains
Highlights	Spring wildflowers, autumn color, and views
Distance	10 miles (loop)
Total Elevation Gain/Loss	2,700'/2,700'
Hiking Time	5½ hours
Optional Maps	USGS 7.5-minute *Santiago Peak* and *Alberhill*
Best Times	November–May
Agency	CNF/TD
Difficulty	Moderately strenuous
Trail Use	Dogs allowed

Wide-open views atop the Main Divide (Santa Ana Mountains) and passages through pockets of dense chaparral and timber make this one of the more varied and interesting hikes in this book. Depending on the level of maintenance the trails receive, passages may be overgrown by brush and poison oak. Wear long pants, or at least have them handy in your pack.

To Reach the Trailhead: From the Foothill Transportation Corridor Toll Road (CA 241) in Rancho Santa Margarita, exit onto Santa Margarita Parkway. Drive 1.5 miles east, and turn left onto Plano Trabuco Road. Plano Trabuco Road becomes Trabuco Canyon Road 0.6 mile ahead at a sharp bend to the left. Curve downward into Trabuco Canyon for 0.8 mile, and at the bottom, turn right onto unpaved Trabuco Creek Road, which leads east toward Cleveland National Forest. To reach the trailhead, continue 5.7 miles—all the way up this bumpy dirt road. The road is normally passable by two-wheel-drive vehicles with moderate clearance. A National Forest Adventure Pass is required to park at the road's end, which is where this hike begins.

Description: A trace of the now-retired road continues up-canyon—for hikers, equestrians, and skilled mountain bikers only. You travel past Orange County's biggest alder grove; fine specimens of live oak, bay laurel, and maple; a tiny community of madrone trees; and a wide variety of spectacular spring wildflowers. In late March and April, look for colorful displays of bush lupine, matilija poppy, paintbrush, wild sweet pea, red and sticky (yellow) monkeyflowers, prickly phlox, Mariposa lily, wild hyacinth, and penstemon along the sunnier spots traversed by the trail. Historically, Trabuco Canyon is significant for its mining activity and as the site of the killing of one of California's last wild grizzly bears in 1908.

After 1.0 mile the trail passes close to an old adit, one of several reminders of gold-and-silver-mining activity, which persisted until about 1925. Early miner Jake Yaeger built his cabin in the shade of a spreading maple down near the creek. You can see some scraggly bigcone Douglas-fir trees on a darkly vegetated slope to the south.

In 1.5 miles, pass an unmarked junction with a spur to the right that leads to a canyon overlook. In another 0.2 mile, reach a signed junction with the West

Horsethief Trail branching to the left; take it. Earlier, you may have spotted switchbacks carving up the treeless slope that now lies ahead. This improved section of the West Horsethief Trail replaces the original, straight-up-the-ridge route that American Indians used in prehistoric times and that horse thieves used in the Spanish days. After following a ravine bottom for a short while, the West Horsethief Trail begins to climb in earnest, zigzagging through dense chaparral. During the coolness of the morning, diligent effort will get you to the top of this tedious stretch fast enough; later in the day it could be a hot, energy-sapping climb.

After gaining 1,100 feet the trail straightens, begins to level out atop a ridge, and enters a vegetation zone dominated by manzanita and blue-flowering ceanothus. Cool mountain air washes over you, perhaps bearing the scent of the pines that lie ahead. Nearly coincident with the change of vegetation is a change in the rocks and soils underfoot. As you climb higher, light-colored granitic boulders and soil replace the dark-brown, crumbly metasedimentary rocks you saw earlier. Although the younger granitic rock doesn't crop out below, you may remember seeing granitic boulders down in the bed of Trabuco Canyon. These resistant blocks, originally weathered out of the granitic mass above, were swept down during flash floods.

At 3.3 miles into your trek, the West Horsethief Trail joins Main Divide Road (a truck trail) in a sparse grove of Coulter pines. Turn right and commence an easygoing passage along the "roofline" of Orange County. To the west lies Orange

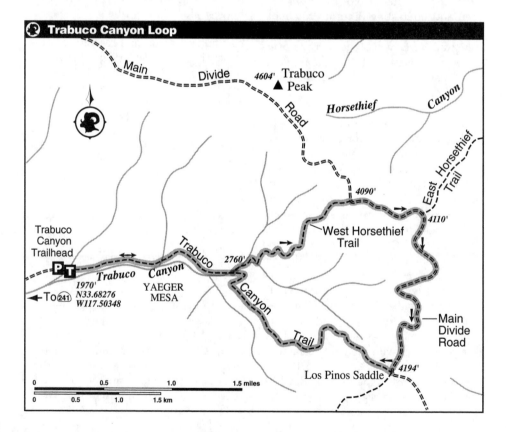

County's urban plain; to the east lies the more sparsely populated yet rapidly urbanizing Riverside County. The linear trough lying below you, north and east, was produced by movements along the Elsinore Fault.

The trail dips down and then climbs up again to reach Los Pinos Saddle amid a patch of Coulter pines and incense-cedars where the road swings hard left in 2.5 miles. At the northwest corner of a large, cleared area in the saddle itself, find and follow the Trabuco Canyon Trail. At the time of this writing, the trail sign is missing. Be careful not to take the Los Pinos Trail, which is just to the left. The Trabuco Canyon Trail angles downward along the uppermost reaches of the canyon's main fork. Thick stands of live oak and bigcone Douglas-fir keep the upper part of the trail dark and gloomy during the

fall and winter months and delightfully cool at other times. Flowering currant and ceanothus shrubs at the trailside brighten things up in the spring.

One mile below the saddle, the trail veers left, crosses a divide, and begins descending along a tributary of Trabuco Canyon. You may notice a spur trail on the right leading up a ridge to a hilltop vista. Walk by thickets of California bay (bay laurel), which exude an enigmatically pleasant and pungent scent. The trail then clings to a dry and sunny south-facing slope. Below, in an almost inaccessible section of the ravine, you may hear water trickling and tumbling over boulders half-hidden under tangles of underbrush and trees. Before long, you arrive back at the junction of West Horsethief Trail in shady Trabuco Canyon, and continue down to the trailhead.

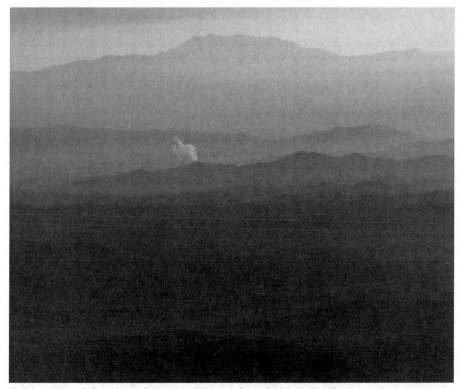

San Jacinto and the ridges of the Inland Empire from the Main Divide

HIKE 65

Bell Canyon Loop

Location	Caspers Wilderness Park, Santa Ana Mountains foothills
Highlights	Interesting geologic features and a wide variety of botanical features
Distance	3.3 miles (loop)
Total Elevation Gain/Loss	400'/400'
Hiking Time	1½ hours
Optional Maps	Caspers Wilderness Park brochure or USGS 7.5-minute *Canada Gobernadora*
Best Times	October–May
Agency	CWP
Difficulty	Moderate
Trail Use	Good for kids

The crown jewel of Orange County's regional park system, Caspers Wilderness Park is the county's largest park (8,000 acres), the least altered by human activities, and the most remote from population centers. ("Remote," of course, is a relative term in Orange County, more than two-thirds of which is urbanized). Beware of poison oak, which grows along this trail.

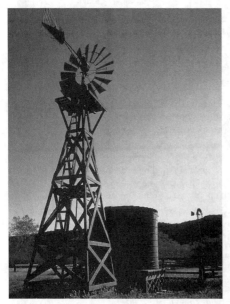

The windmill at Caspers Park

To Reach the Trailhead: From I-5 at San Juan Capistrano, drive east on Ortega Highway (CA 74) 7.6 miles to the park entrance station on the left. Pay the day-use (or camping) fee here, and drive past (or visit) the park's visitor center, which houses a small museum and an open-air loft with an expansive view of the Santa Ana Mountains. Continue 1 mile to the trailhead at the site of an old windmill, your starting point for this loop.

Description: The hike touches upon the best features of Caspers Wilderness Park, starting with a rather dizzying passage across the top of some curious white sandstone formations, rather like the breaks along the upper Missouri River or the barren cliffs of the South Dakota badlands. You'll loop up and over the main ridge that defines the west edge of the park, while enjoying views of much of Orange County's remaining rural and wild areas.

Start off on the path signed NATURE TRAIL. The trailhead is behind the equestrian parking area to the northwest and is difficult to see from the windmill. Follow the trail across the wide bed of Bell Canyon and into the dense oak woodland on the far side. After 0.3 mile, you'll spot a bench beneath a spreading oak tree. Just beyond, veer left on the Dick Loskorn Trail. This path meanders up a shallow draw and soon climbs to a sandstone ridgeline that at one point narrows to near-knife-edge width. At one point you step within a foot of a modest but unnerving abyss. The sandstone is part of a marine sedimentary formation called the Santiago Formation (roughly 45 million years old), which crops out along the coastal strip from here down to mid–San Diego County.

After climbing about 350 feet, you reach a dirt road, the West Ridge Trail. Turn right (north), skirting the fence of Rancho Mission Viejo, a landholding that encompasses much of southern Orange County. Before World War II, it included all of Camp Pendleton as well. To the left you look down on Cañada Gobernadora ("Canyon of the Governor's Wife,"

though a less literal meaning refers to the invasive chamise, or greasewood, that used to fill the canyon). Luxury housing is gradually overtaking the canyon's wide floor.

After 0.7 mile on the West Ridge Trail, turn right on the Star Rise trail to descend into Bell Canyon. Nearing the bottom, veer right on the Oak Trail. On this delightful trace of a trail you meander past California sycamores and ancient coast live oaks. In late autumn, you crunch through the crispy leaf litter and watch golden sunbeams dance amid the thousands of fluttering leaves overhead. In early spring, when these leaves are emerging, the sunlight filtering through them bathes the shadows in a jungle-green luminance.

The Oak Trail returns you to a T-junction with the Nature Trail, where you turn right to reach your starting point.

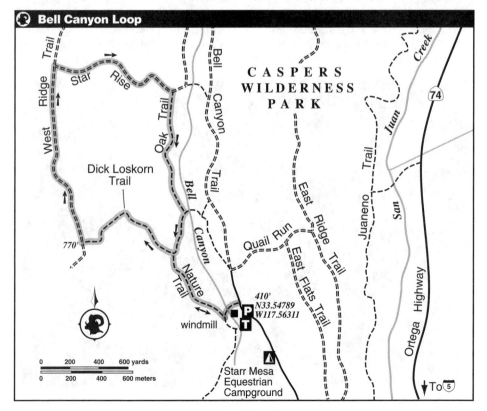

HIKE 66

San Juan Loop Trail

Location	Santa Ana Mountains
Highlights	Trickling stream and a small waterfall and pool
Distance	2.1 miles (loop)
Total Elevation Gain/Loss	350'/350'
Hiking Time	1 hour
Optional Map	USGS 7.5-minute *Sitton Peak*
Best Times	November–June
Agency	CNF/TD
Difficulty	Easy
Trail Use	Dogs allowed, suitable for mountain biking, good for kids

From San Juan Capistrano to Lake Elsinore, two-lane Ortega Highway stretches like a snake over the midriff of the Santa Ana Mountains, giving road warriors a taste of Orange County's wild, unfamiliar side. Even the most casual traveler can get to know the rugged and circumspect beauty of these corrugated mountains better by trying out the San Juan Loop Trail, right off the highway amid one of the most scenic spots in the range.

To Reach the Trailhead: From I-5 in San Juan Capistrano drive 19.5 miles east on Ortega Highway (CA 74) to reach the starting point, a well-marked trailhead parking lot on the left. (On the right is a humble but notable local landmark, the

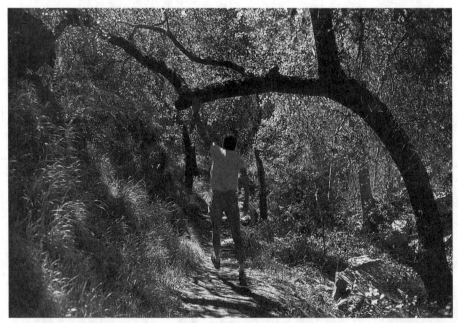

San Juan Loop Trail

Ortega Oaks Candy Store.) You'll need to post a National Forest Adventure Pass on your car.

Description: From the trailhead lot, a well-worn path takes off north along a slope overlooking the highway. Around a bend to the left, the trail starts threading the side of a narrow gorge that resounds (after the rainy season begins in fall or winter) with echoes of falling water. A spur path leads down toward the lip of the falls; from there you can boulder-hop over to the edge of a reflecting pool. A single gnarled juniper clings sentinel-like to a rock face overlooking this pool, very far from its normal, high-desert habitat 50 miles or farther north or east. If the mood strikes you, rest your bones amid the smooth contours of the water-polished granite, and settle in for a moment's quiet meditation.

Past the falls, you descend on ramp-like switchbacks through dense chaparral and presently reach the oak-dotted flood-plain of San Juan Creek. Stay left at a pair of unsigned junctions with Chiquito Trail; if you cross the creek, you're off-route. Ahead, you'll plunge into a veritable thicket of centuries-old coast live oak trees. Their overarching limbs mute the glare of the sun and sky. In the soft, filtered light, the ground glows with the seasonal greens, browns, and reds of ferns, poison oak, and wild grasses. Beware of several more unsigned use paths that branch off and rejoin the main trail.

Touching briefly upon the perimeter of Upper San Juan Campground, the trail veers sharply left to gain an open slope, again parallel to the highway. Continue for another 0.5 mile across this sun-struck slope, dotted with wildflowers in the spring, and arrive back at the trailhead.

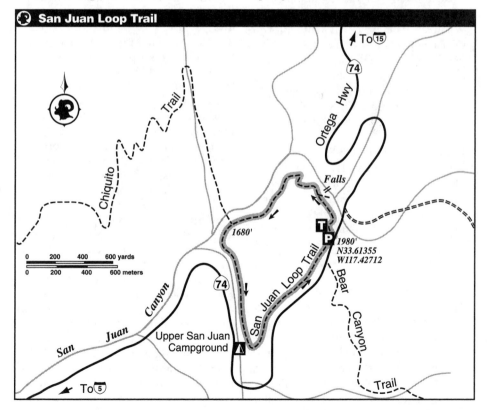

HIKE 67

Sitton Peak

Location	Santa Ana Mountains
Highlights	Coast and mountain views
Distance	9.5 miles (out-and-back)
Total Elevation Gain/Loss	2,150'/2,150'
Hiking Time	5½ hours
Optional Map	USGS 7.5-minute *Sitton Peak*
Best Times	October–May
Agency	CNF/TD
Difficulty	Moderately strenuous
Trail Use	Suitable for backpacking, dogs allowed
Permit	Day-use sign-in at trailhead; San Mateo Canyon Wilderness permit required to stay overnight

From below, Sitton Peak—a bump atop the rambling Santa Ana Mountains— looks imposing. On the summit, though, you feel decidedly on top of the world. When an east or north wind blows, cleansing the sky of water vapor and air pollution, 50-mile vistas in every direction are not uncommon. You must get a wilderness permit to camp overnight within the San Mateo Canyon Wilderness that encompasses most of this hike.

To Reach the Trailhead: From I-5 in San Juan Capistrano drive 19.5 miles east on Ortega Highway (CA 74) to reach the starting point, a well-marked trailhead parking lot on the left. On the right is a notable local landmark, the Ortega Oaks Candy Store. You'll need to post a National Forest Adventure Pass on your car.

Description: The signed Bear Canyon Trailhead is located on the south side of the highway just west of the candy store. Sign in at the day-use register a short distance up the trail. Hike through dense chaparral, including scrub oak, chamise, sugar bush, mountain mahogany, black sage, and buckwheat. Pass the San Mateo

Canyon Wilderness boundary 0.7 mile up the trail.

After 1.0 mile of moderate ascent, you come to an unsigned trail junction in a patch of oak woodland. Go right (the Morgan Trail forks left) and begin climbing more steeply along a chaparral-clothed slope. At 2.0 miles, you reach a four-way junction. The Bear Canyon Trail turns right and follows the bed of the old Verdugo Truck Trail. Note that the Bear Ridge Trail proceeds straight and rejoins the Bear Canyon Trail at Four Corners, offering an alternative return route. You soon pass (at 2.7 miles) oak-shaded Pigeon Spring, a seasonal trickle of water at the head of Bear Canyon. An old horse watering trough is here up a short spur to the left, with seeps nearby. Enjoy the shade—you won't find much more of it on the road ahead.

Continue south another half mile to reach a clearing misnamed Four Corners (at 3.2 miles), where four old roads and the newer Bear Ridge footpath join together. You can make an exposed camp here. Swing right on the road that climbs northwest, a disused section of the Sitton Peak Road. After a steady ascent of about 300 vertical feet, you reach a flat area (at 4.0 miles) just below a boulder-studded ridge (3,250 feet in elevation) to the north. Easily climbed, the ridge summit offers a view somewhat similar to the one from Sitton Peak. A few yards beyond, a spur leads south to a clearing by a lone oak where backpackers could camp.

Beyond the flat area the road descends another 0.5 mile to a saddle just below Sitton Peak. From this saddle, you leave the road and follow a steep climber's trail up through scattered manzanita and chamise on the east slope of the peak.

The view from the top is especially impressive to the west. Here the foothills and western canyons of the Santa Anas merge with the creeping suburbs of southern Orange County. Beyond lies the flat, blue ocean punctuated by the profile of Santa Catalina Island. Some 2,000 feet below, toylike cars on the highway make their way down the sinuous course of San Juan Canyon.

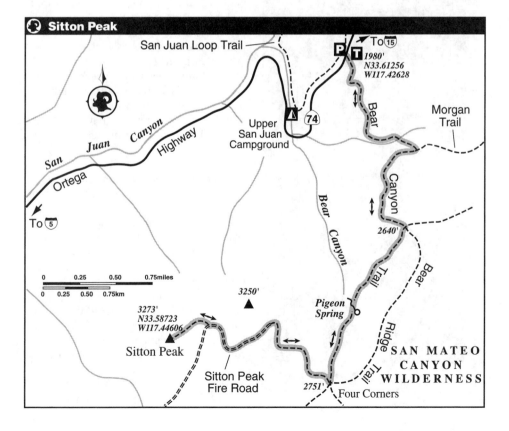

HIKE 68

Tenaja Falls

Location	San Mateo Canyon Wilderness
Highlight	Beautiful, multilevel waterfall
Distance	1.4 miles (out-and-back)
Total Elevation Gain/Loss	300'/300'
Hiking Time	1 hour
Optional Map	USGS 7.5-minute *Sitton Peak*
Best Times	December–June
Agency	CNF/TD
Difficulty	Easy
Trail Use	Good for kids, dogs allowed, suitable for backpacking

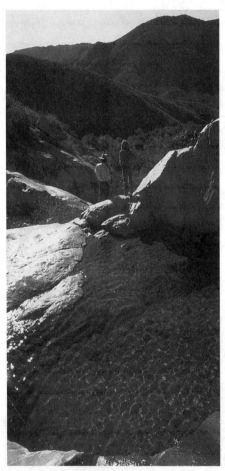

Upper pool, Tenaja Falls

With five tiers and a total drop of about 150 feet, Tenaja Falls is the most interesting natural feature in the San Mateo Canyon Wilderness section of Cleveland National Forest. In late winter and spring, water coursing down the polished rock produces a kind of soothing music not widely heard in this somewhat dry corner of the Santa Ana Mountains.

The only easy way to reach Tenaja Falls on foot is from the south, though the drive to that trailhead is rather lengthy by way of any approach. Beware of the plentiful poison oak growing alongside the trail.

To Reach the Trailhead *(from I-5)*: From I-5 in San Juan Capistrano drive 23 miles east on Ortega Highway (CA 74). Just past mile marker 74 RIV 6.50, turn right on South Main Divide Road. Proceed south to Wildomar Campground and off-road-vehicle (ORV) area. Beyond, new asphalt has transformed many miles of bone-shaking former truck trail into a decently paved narrow road. Continue a total of 16 miles (from Ortega Highway) to a large signed turnout on the right, overlooking the tree-covered bottom of San Mateo Canyon.

To Reach the Trailhead *(from I-15)*: Exit I-15 at Clinton Keith Road in Murrieta.

Proceed 6 miles south on Clinton Keith Road and 1.7 miles west on Tenaja Road to a marked intersection, where you must turn right to stay on Tenaja Road. Continue west on Tenaja Road for another 4.2 miles, then go right on the one-lane, paved Cleveland Forest Road. Proceed another mile, passing the Tenaja Trailhead, and continue 4.6 miles farther along the newly paved Old Tenaja Road to reach the Tenaja Falls Trailhead, a large turnout on the left, overlooking the tree-covered bottom of San Mateo Canyon.

Description: Don't forget to sign in at the self-registration box just down the trail, then head down to the canyon bottom, veer left a little, and cross the creek on remnants of an old concrete ford. Balance on rocks or wade through the water. Continue north on a steadily rising old roadbed

(now a wilderness trail), and you'll soon be treated to a fairly distant view of the falls. After 0.7 mile the road passes near the upper lip of the falls, where a few large oaks provide welcome shade.

Further exploration of the falls requires rock-climbing skills and extreme caution. The flow of water has worn the granitic rock almost glassy smooth. While scouting the middle tiers and pools, I found that slightly wet bare feet provided much more traction than the soles of my running shoes—don't be lured into dangerous situations though.

A somewhat safer way of approaching the lower falls is to scramble over the rough-textured rocks well away from the water. You might also backtrack down the road and then scramble down the slope into the brush-choked creekbed down near the base of the falls.

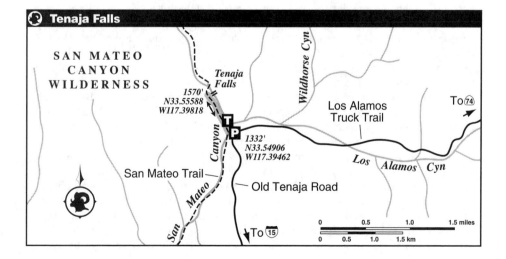

HIKE 69

Tenaja Canyon

Location	San Mateo Canyon Wilderness
Highlight	Riparian- and oak-woodland in a steep canyon
Distance	7 miles (out-and-back) (to Fishermans Camp)
Total Elevation Gain/Loss	1,100'/1,100'
Hiking Time	3½ hours
Optional Map	USGS 7.5-minute *Wildomar* and *Sitton Peak*
Best Times	November–May
Agency	CNF/TD
Difficulty	Moderately strenuous
Trail Use	Dogs allowed, suitable for backpacking
Permit	Day-use sign-in at trailhead; San Mateo Canyon Wilderness permit required to stay overnight

As the gloom of a late afternoon descended upon the deep-cut, linear furrow of Tenaja Canyon, dozens of orange-bellied newts waddled determinedly uphill and across the trail, oblivious to my footfalls. The cute faces and beady eyes of these little amphibians mirrored a mindless desire I cannot fathom: Sex in a bower of leaf litter and ferns? A bellyful of succulent tree-dwelling insects, ripe for the taking?

The Tenaja Trail rambles along a 10-mile stretch of the 62-square-mile San Mateo Canyon Wilderness, the largest parcel of designated wilderness near the Southern California coast. The wilderness consists mostly of steep, rough, and rocky chaparral country, softened by the strips of oak woodland and riparian vegetation that thrive along the larger canyon bottoms. This hike explores the south end of the Tenaja Trail, which follows Tenaja Canyon down to its confluence with San Mateo Canyon. The route takes you down and later all the way back up; if it's a warm day or you feel fatigued, you can always reverse your course at any time.

To Reach the Trailhead: To reach the Tenaja Trailhead, exit I-15 at Clinton Keith Road in the community of Murrieta.

Proceed 5.2 miles south on Clinton Keith Road to a sharp bend where the name changes to Tenaja Road. Continue 1.7 miles west to a marked intersection, where you must turn right to stay on Tenaja Road.

Go west on Tenaja Road for another 4.2 miles, then turn right onto the one-lane, paved Cleveland Forest Road. Proceed another mile to the trailhead parking area.

Description: Sign in at the self-registration box, and head downhill on the trail going west. A few minutes' descent takes you to the shady bowels of V-shaped Tenaja Canyon, where huge coast live oaks and pale-barked sycamores frame a limpid, rock-dimpled seasonal stream. Mostly the trail ahead meanders alongside the stream, but for the canyon's middle stretch, it carves its way across the chaparral-blanketed south wall, 200–400 feet above the canyon bottom.

After 3.7 miles of general descent, you reach Fishermans Camp, a former drive-in campground once accessible by many miles of bad road. Today the site, distinguished by its parklike setting amid a live-oak grove, serves as a fine wilderness campsite for an overnight backpack trip (for which you must get a wilderness permit). Its name hints at the fishing opportunities that nearby San Mateo Canyon Creek affords during and after the rainy season. A native species of steelhead trout was recently discovered in this drainage, surprising experts who thought that steelhead might be extinct south of Los Angeles County.

At Fishermans Camp, three other trails diverge. The San Mateo Trail, a narrow footpath, leads southwest downstream

many miles to the east boundary of Camp Pendleton. It also leads north upstream to meet Old Tenaja Road at the Tenaja Falls Trailhead. Just north of Tenaja Creek, the Fishermans Camp Trail (the old road) forks off the San Mateo Trail and climbs 1.6 miles directly up to Old Tenaja Road. If you positioned a vehicle at that trailhead, you can cut 2 miles and 500 feet of elevation gain off your trip by hiking out there. Otherwise, your quickest return route is back the way you came.

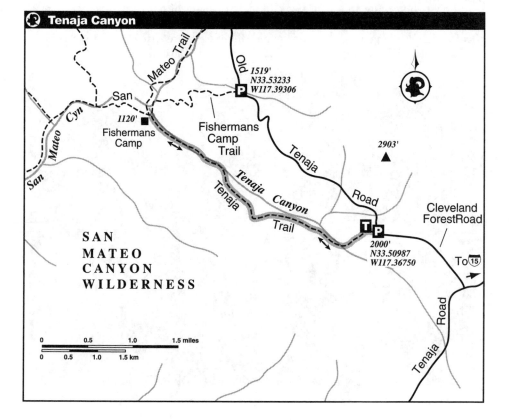

HIKE 70

Santa Rosa Plateau Ecological Reserve

Location	Near Temecula and Murrieta
Highlights	Green and golden hills, rare oaks, spring wildflowers, and vernal pools
Distance	6 miles (loop)
Total Elevation Gain/Loss	650'/650'
Hiking Time	3 hours
Optional Map	USGS 7.5-minute *Wildomar*
Best Times	November–June
Agency	SRPER
Difficulty	Moderate
Trail Use	Good for kids

A 200-mile-wide circle centered on the Santa Rosa Plateau Ecological Reserve in the southwest corner of Riverside County encompasses a megalopolis of some 20 million people. File this fact away in your mind, and then try to fathom its truth while walking amid the green and golden hills of this exquisitely beautiful reserve. Here is a classic California landscape of wind-rippled grasses, swaying poppies, statuesque oak trees, trickling streams, vernal pools, and a dazzling assortment of native plants (nearly 500 at last count) and animals. All who visit the reserve are struck by its timelessness and its insularity.

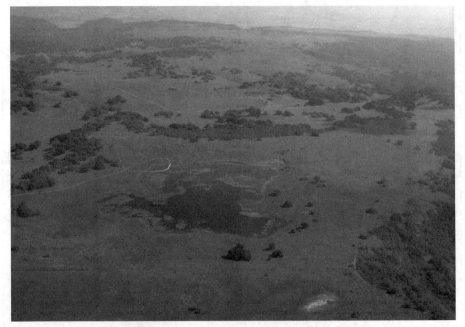

Aerial view of Santa Rosa Plateau

Starting with a nucleus of 3,100 acres, purchased by The Nature Conservancy in 1984, the reserve has expanded to enclose nearly 9,000 acres (about 14 square miles) today. The west half is laced with new hiking trails and well as old ranch roads, while much of the eastern part lies off-limits to all visitation due to its ecologically sensitive nature. The 6-mile loop described here visits the major accessible highlights of the reserve, which are most beautifully presented in the green months of March and April.

To Reach the Trailhead: The reserve can be reached in less than 90 minutes from either central Los Angeles or San Diego. Take I-15 to the Clinton Keith exit in Murrieta. Drive southwest on Clinton Keith Road, passing the reserve's visitor center (open weekends) at 5 miles. Keep going,

and note the sharp rightward bend at 5.2 miles where the road's name changes to Tenaja Road. At 0.7 mile past this sharp bend, park at the Hidden Valley Trailhead parking area (on either side of the road). There's a small day-use fee, payable here. Trails in the reserve are open sunrise–sunset.

Description: From the Hidden Valley Trailhead, head southeast on the Coyote Trail. After 0.5 mile, turn right on the Trans Preserve Trail. Follow it for 1.5 miles over rolling and sometimes wooded terrain, passing through part of the reserve's 3,000 acres of remnant native "bunchgrass prairie." Reserve managers have been implementing controlled burns to discourage the growth of non-native grasses and promote the recovery of native plants.

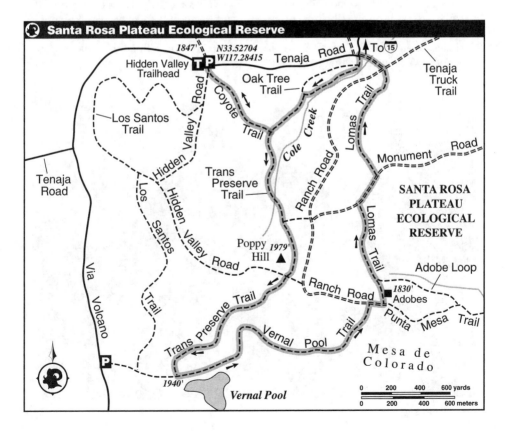

The last half mile of the Trans Preserve Trail rises to a plateau called Mesa de Colorado. At the top of the mesa, you turn left on the Vernal Pool Trail and soon visit one of the largest vernal pools in California (39 acres at maximum capacity). The hard-pan surface underneath vernal pools is quite impervious to water, so once winter storms fill them, the pools dry out mostly by evaporation. Unusual and sometimes unique species of flowering plants have evolved in and around this and other vernal pools throughout the state. When the watery perimeter of the pool contracts during the lengthening and warming days of spring, successive waves of annual wildflowers bloom along the drying margin. By July or August, all the water is gone, and only a desiccated depression remains.

Continue east on the Vernal Pool Trail, and descend from Mesa de Colorado to the two adobe buildings of the former Santa Rosa Ranch, 3.3 miles from the start. Constructed around 1845, these are Riverside County's oldest standing structures.

After a look at the adobes and a refreshing pause in the shade, make a beeline north on the Lomas Trail. Jog briefly right on Monument Road, then go left to stay on the Lomas Trail. At the junction with Tenaja Truck Trail ahead, go straight across toward the looping Oak Tree Trail. The left (streamside) branch is better— assuming that the creek is flowing. Both alternatives give you a close-up look at some of the finest Engelmann-oak woodland anywhere. The Engelmann oak tree, with its distinctive gray-green leaves, is endemic to a narrow strip of coastal foothills stretching from Southern California into northern Baja California. It's becoming one of the rarer of the state's oak species, primarily because its native range is squarely in the path of current and future suburban and rural development.

At the far end of the Oak Tree Trail loop, you come to the Trans Preserve Trail. Use it to reach the Coyote Trail, where a turn to the right and a retracing of earlier steps takes you a final half mile to your starting point.

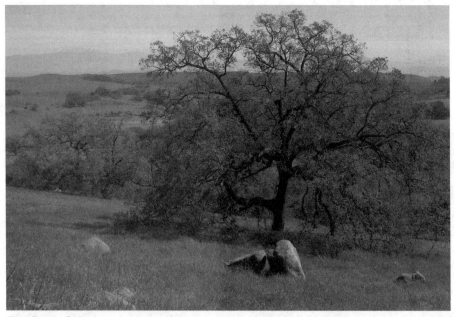

Engelmann Oak

HIKE 71

Dripping Springs Trail

Location	Agua Tibia Wilderness
Highlights	Spring wildflowers and valley and mountain views
Distance	14 miles (out-and-back to head of Castro Canyon)
Total Elevation Gain/Loss	2,900'/2,900'
Hiking Time	8 hours
Recommended Map	USGS 7.5-minute *Vail Lake*
Best Times	November–May
Agency	CNF/PD
Difficulty	Strenuous
Trail Use	Dogs allowed, suitable for backpacking
Permit	Sign-in at trailhead for day use; Agua Tibia Wilderness permit required to stay overnight

The 18,000-acre Agua Tibia Wilderness lies northwest of Palomar Mountain, straddling the San Diego and Riverside county line in Cleveland National Forest. Agua Tibia Mountain, one of the three distinct mountain blocks of the Palomar range, is the centerpiece of the wilderness that bears its name. Sparse groves of Coulter pine, bigcone Douglas-fir, incense-cedar, live oak, and black oak cover the highest elevations, while the lower slopes are scrub-covered and fluted by many steep canyons holding intermittent streams. The wilderness was named after one of these streams, Agua Tibia ("tepid water") Creek.

The Dripping Springs Trail, which is the primary route into the wilderness area, originates at Dripping Springs Campground. With only minimal interruptions, the trail ascends from the 1,620-foot elevation of the campground to a 4,400-foot crest near the high point of Agua Tibia Mountain, passing through belts of chamise chaparral, manzanita and ribbonwood chaparral, and finally oak and pine forest. In March or April of an average or better-than-average rain year, the blooming of annual wildflowers along the lower trail can be stupendous. The trail's upper part offers ever-widening, pseudoaerial views to the north, where the distant Transverse Ranges rise out of valley mists as if they were the rim of the world.

The Vail Fire of 1989 burned nearly all of the area traversed by the Dripping Springs Trail to a crisp. In 2000 the Pechanga Fire swept across the uppermost part of the trail, singeing many of the places the earlier fire had missed. After those fires, considerable efforts were devoted to clearing the Agua Tibia trails of new growth and fallen trees. The chaparral has fully recovered and only subtle signs of the devastating fires remain. The Dripping Springs Trail is regularly maintained

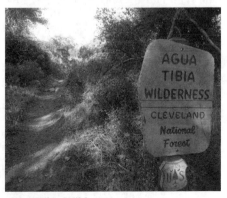

Agua Tibia Wilderness

and in reasonable condition, but the other trails in the wilderness can be brushy or blocked by fallen trees if a trail crew has not been through recently. Another thing to remember: Water tends to disappear quickly into the porous, decomposed granite soil, and flowing water tends to dry up quickly in the ravines. Bring all the drinking water you'll need.

To Reach the Trailhead: From I-15 in Temecula, drive 10 miles east on CA 79 to Dripping Springs Campground, on the right (south) side of the road (0.8 mile east of mile marker 79 RIV 10.0). The campground lies just behind the Dripping Springs Fire Station. If the campground is closed, you can park outside the gate and walk 0.4 mile past the campsites to reach the inner trailhead, where you sign in at a register before entering the national-forest wilderness area that lies just ahead. You'll need a National Forest Adventure Pass to park either inside or outside the campground.

Description: The trail mileages given below are keyed to the inner trailhead. From the campground, the Dripping Springs Trail immediately fords Arroyo Seco Creek and then begins a switch-backing ascent through sage scrub and chaparral vegetation, liberally sprinkled with annual wildflowers in early spring. After only 0.1 mile, there's a trail junction. The Wild Horse Trail, on the left, gains elevation relatively slowly, sticking to the slopes overlooking Agua Tibia Creek. Your way stays right, up the Dripping Springs route that is sure to give you a solid cardiovascular workout.

After a mile, the trail gains the top of a nearly flat ridge and then continues south toward a series of 10 ascending switchbacks that cross an old overgrown firebreak (stay on the zigzagging trail and don't take shortcuts). Vail Lake and Southern California's highest mountains—Old Baldy, San Gorgonio and San Jacinto—come into view. On a clear winter day, the snow-covered summits standing bold against the blue sky are a memorable sight.

At 3.5 miles (3,100 feet in elevation), the Dripping Springs Trail crosses the head of a small creek and continues upward amid new growths of manzanita and ribbonwood. At 4.5 miles, the trail descends a little and crosses an area of poor soil. A view opens up to the southeast and south. The white dome of the Hale Telescope at Palomar Observatory gleams on a ridge about 9 miles southeast. You can now see the pine- and oak-fringed summit ridge of Agua Tibia Mountain ahead.

Soon you follow sharp switchbacks again. The trail reaches a campsite nestled beneath the oaks and pines. The trail may become muddled here; look for ribbons marking the path. Just beyond, at 6.8 miles, a sign indicates the end of the Dripping Springs Trail and the start of the Palomar-Magee Trail, which turns right.

The Palomar-Magee Trail is an abandoned fire road along the Agua Tibia crest. The portion leading northwest from the junction has been completely obliterated, and the portion leading southeast is now a narrow footpath in a constant battle with encroaching chaparral.

If conditions permit, walk 0.2 mile south down the Palomar-Magee Trail to a point overlooking Castro Canyon. There, on most clear winter days, a clear panorama of north San Diego County, including conspicuous, undulating, linear I-15, spreads before you. On the far horizon to the west and south you can often see the Pacific Ocean and the mountains of Baja California.

If the trails have been recently maintained, it might be enjoyable to make a 20-mile loop by following the Palomar-Magee, Crosley, and Wild Horse Trails. Otherwise, return the way you came.

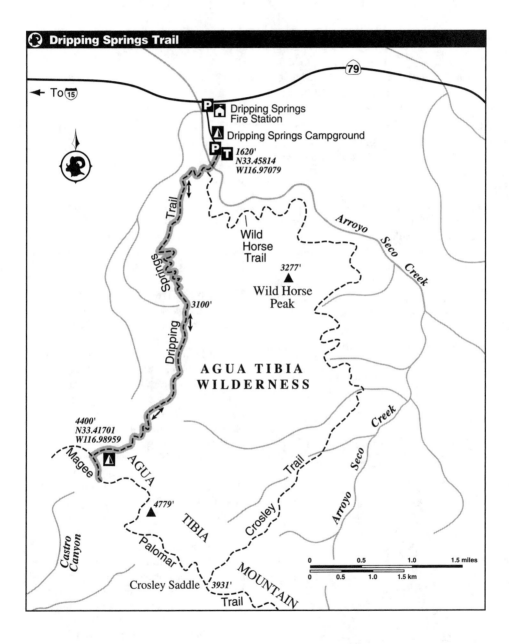

Dripping Springs Trail

79

← To 15

Dripping Springs Fire Station

Dripping Springs Campground

1620'
N33.45814
W116.97079

Trail

Wild Horse Trail

Springs

3277'
Wild Horse Peak

3100'

Dripping

AGUA TIBIA WILDERNESS

Arroyo Seco Creek

4400'
N33.41701
W116.98959

Magee

AGUA

Creek

Crosley Trail

Arroyo Seco

4779'

TIBIA

Castro Canyon

Palomar

Crosley Saddle   3931'

MOUNTAIN

Trail

| 0 | | 0.5 | | 1.0 | | 1.5 miles |
| 0 | 0.5 | | 1.0 | 1.5 km | | |

HIKE 72

La Jolla Shores to Torrey Pines Beach

Location	La Jolla
Highlights	Body surfing and remote beach backed by sheer cliffs
Distance	5.0 miles (one way)
Total Elevation Gain/Loss	Negligible (at sea level)
Hiking Time	2½ hours
Optional Maps	USGS 7.5-minute *La Jolla* and *Del Mar*
Best Times	All year
Agency	TPSR
Difficulty	Moderate

There are only a few places along the Southern California coastline where you can hike for miles and not see roads, railroad tracks, powerlines, or other signs of civilization. The Torrey Pines beaches are one such place. Here, for 3 or 4 miles, cliffs front the shoreline and cut off the sights and sounds of the world beyond.

Plan to do this beach walk at low tide. High tides, especially in winter, could force you to walk on cobbles at the base of the cliffs or oblige you to wade in the surf. At low tide, the Dike Rock tidepools are

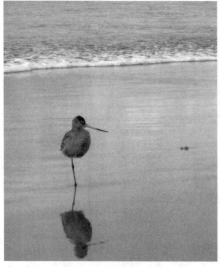

Sandpiper

accessible and the damp sand makes for easy walking. Beach sand is often carried away by the scouring action of the winter waves, but the currents usually replenish it as summer approaches.

To Reach the Trailhead: From I-5 north, take Exit 26A west on La Jolla Parkway (there is no exit from I-5 south, but you can also reach La Jolla from CA 52 west). The parkway eventually becomes Torrey Pines Road. In 2.0 miles, turn right (north) on La Jolla Shores Drive. In 0.5 mile, turn left on Calle Frescota and proceed 0.2 mile into the free parking area for La Jolla Shores Beach. The grassy park alongside is known as Kellogg Park.

If you're making this a one-way trip, leave a second car along North Torrey Pines Road (the Old Coast Highway 101), next to Torrey Pines State Beach, or in the adjacent pay lot at Torrey Pines State Reserve. This is a 7-mile car shuttle. It may be easiest to have someone drop you off at the start and pick you up later at the end. Another option is to use local buses to get from the finish back to the start: At Torrey Pines State Beach you can take the 101 bus south to La Jolla Shores Drive, from where a transfer to a Route 30 bus takes you to Calle Frescota near Kellogg Park. The buses do not make change, so bring dollar bills and quarters.

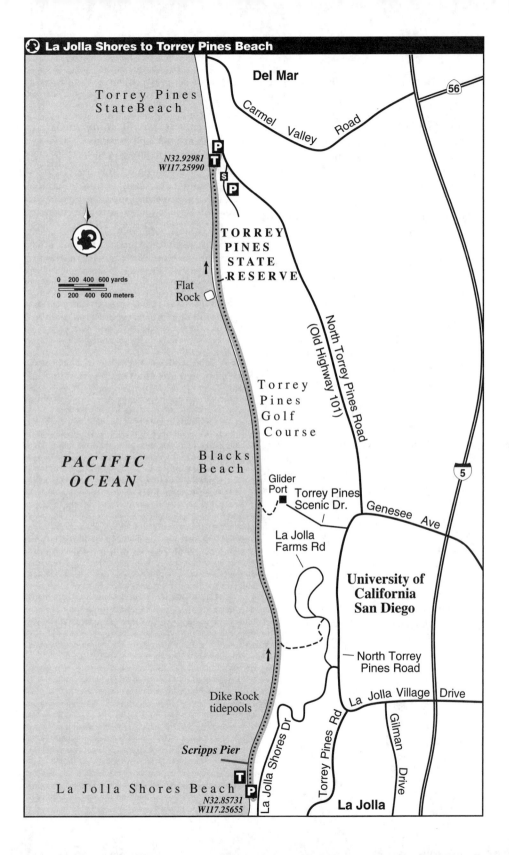

Description: Start your hike at La Jolla Shores Beach by walking north under Scripps Pier. At 1.0 mile, reach the Dike Rock tidepools. During low tide, you may discover sea stars, sea anemones, and hermit crabs in snail shells, as well as the ubiquitous mussels and limpets. This is part of the San Diego–La Jolla Underwater Park Ecological Preserve; enjoy the creatures and plant life, but do not disturb or collect anything. Once you are beyond the last of the cobbles and wave-rounded boulders, you can slip off your shoes and enjoy the feel of fine, clean sand underfoot.

You are now on Torrey Pines City Beach. A half mile past the tidepools, you'll see a paved road (closed to car traffic) going up through a small canyon. This is a safe way to reach (or exit) the beach. There's a limited amount of two-hour parking at the top along La Jolla Farms Road.

In another 0.7 mile, a precipitous trail ascends about 300 feet to the Torrey Pines Glider Port, where hang-gliders launch their craft. Look up to see antlike beachgoers lugging their gear up or down the zigzagging paths and hang-gliders soaring overhead. Nevertheless, the trail is signed DO NOT USE because of the unstable cliffs.

Beyond the glider-port trail, you may notice that some people have doffed more than just shoes. You're now on Torrey Pines State Beach, also known as Black's Beach, San Diego's unofficial nude-bathing spot. The city rescinded a clothing-optional policy for this beach in the late 1970s, but old traditions have never died.

Lifeguards patrol some areas of Black's Beach during busy periods, so you can feel fairly safe about jumping into the water, which may be warmer than 70°F in July through September. Shuffle your feet to alert stingrays of your presence. Elsewhere you swim at your own risk—watch out for rip currents focused by underwater Scripps Canyon, just offshore. This same canyon generates powerful surf that draws advanced surfers to the beach.

At 4.3 miles from Kellogg Park, you reach Flat Rock, where a protruding sandstone wall blocks easy passage. Follow the narrow path cut into the wall. If the tide is low, you can clamber onto Flat Rock and inspect an unusual tidepool on top of the rock. From a low shelf on the far side, the Beach Trail begins its ascent to Torrey Pines State Reserve's Visitor Center.

In the fifth and last mile, the narrow beach is squeezed between sculpted sedimentary cliffs on one side and crashing surf on the other. These are the tallest cliffs in western San Diego County. A close look at the faces reveals a slice of geologic history: the greenish siltstone on the bottom, called the Del Mar Formation, is older than the buff- or rust-colored Torrey Sandstone above it. Higher still is a thin cap of reddish sandstone, not easily seen from the beach—the Linda Vista Formation.

In the end, the beach widens, the cliffs fall back, and you arrive at Torrey Pines State Reserve's entrance along North Torrey Pines Road.

HIKE 73

Torrey Pines State Reserve

Location	Del Mar
Highlights	Rare vegetation, wildflowers, and ocean views
Distance	Up to 4 miles total (short loops)
Total Elevation Gain/Loss	Up to 600'
Hiking Time	Up to 2 hours
Optional Maps	Torrey Pines State Park brochure or USGS 7.5-minute *Del Mar*
Best Times	8 a.m.–sunset, all year
Agency	TPSR
Difficulty	Easy–moderate
Trail Use	Good for kids

The rare and beautiful Torrey pines atop the coastal bluffs south of Del Mar are as much a symbol of the Golden State as are the famed Monterey cypress trees native to central California's coast. Torrey pines grow naturally in only two places: in and around Torrey Pines State Reserve and on Santa Rosa Island, off Santa Barbara. Of the estimated 10,000 native Torrey pines now living, about one-third grow within

the reserve. A combination of drought and bark-beetle infestation killed about 15% of the reserve's Torrey pines during the late 1980s, but new seedlings planted in their place are thriving today.

Torrey Pines State Reserve would be botanically remarkable even without its pines. Three major plant communities can be found on the reserve's 1,750 acres: the sage-scrub, chaparral, and salt-marsh

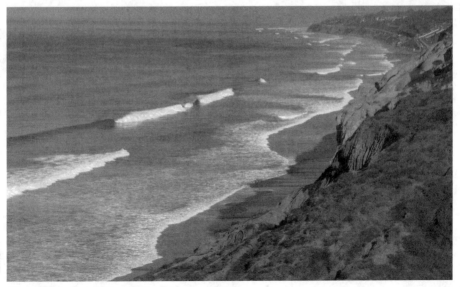

Ocean views from Torrey Pines Reserve

plant communities. More than 330 plant species have been identified within the reserve so far. That number is approximately 20% of all the known plants native to San Diego County. This is especially noteworthy because San Diego County is widely regarded as being the most geographically and botanically diverse county in the continental United States.

If you're interested in identifying plants and wildflowers typical of coastal and inland Southern California, come here in the spring. Excellent interpretive facilities at the reserve's museum make plant identification an easy task. Besides the exhibits, you can browse through several notebooks full of captioned photographs of common and rare plants within the reserve. You can also visit the native plant gardens surrounding the museum building.

A network of trails over the eroded bluffs will take you nearly everywhere in the reserve, except into most canyon bottoms. It's important that you stick to these trails and eschew shortcuts and cross-country travel. The thin soils are easily eroded without the protection of healthy vegetation. As you'll plainly see, there are already enough instances of erosion here, due to both natural and human causes.

To Reach the Trailhead: Exit I-5 at Carmel Valley Road (Exit 33), and drive west 1.5 miles to the Old Coast Highway 101 (which is named Camino del Mar to the north and North Torrey Pines Road to the south). Turn left, drive 1 mile to the Torrey Pines State Reserve entrance on the right, and pay the day-use fee for the reserve. Past the entrance a paved road goes up to a parking lot adjacent

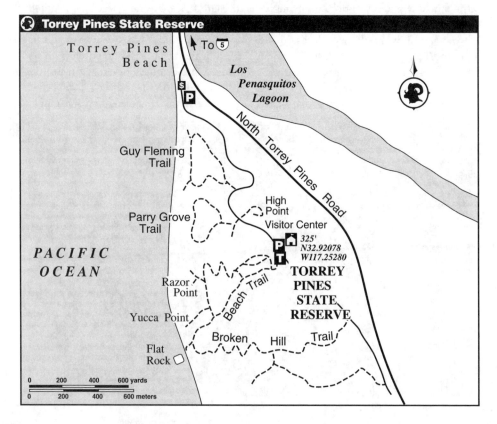

to the reserve office and museum. From there, you can walk to the beginning of any of the trails in 10 minutes or less. If that lot is full, you may be able to park in turnouts along the entrance road, in the beach parking lot at the reserve entrance, or along the shoulder of North Torrey Pines Road. The reserve has a finite carrying capacity. Access may be restricted on busy weekends, so get there early if you can.

Description: Pick up a handy trail map at the entrance station or the museum. After a stop at the museum for a bit of educational browsing, you might first explore nearby High Point, where your gaze encompasses a steep, off-limits section of the reserve known as East Grove. There, young Torrey pines are establishing a foothold on the bluffs and canyons in the aftermath of past wildfires.

Next, you might head south on the concrete roadbed of the "old" old coast highway (closed to car traffic) and pick up the Broken Hill Trail. The two east branches of this trail wind through thick chamise chaparral and connect with a spur trail leading to Broken Hill Overlook. You'll be able to step out (very carefully) onto a precipitous fin of sandstone and peer over to see what, except for a few Torrey pine trees here and there, looks like desert badlands. A third (west) branch of the Broken Hill Trail winds down a slope festooned with wildflowers and joins the Beach Trail at a point just above where the latter drops sharply to the beach.

The popular Beach Trail originates at the parking lot across the road from the museum. It forks repeatedly, passes a sandstone outcrop called Red Butte, and intersects with trails to Yucca Point and Razor Point. Fenced viewpoints along both of these trails offer views straight down to the sandy beach and surf.

The Parry Grove and Guy Fleming loop trails wind among Torrey pine groves hit hard by the late '80s drought. The Guy Fleming Trail is mostly flat, while the Parry Grove Trail starts with a steep descent on stairs. In spring, the sunny slopes along the Guy Fleming Trail come alive with phantasmagoric wildflower displays. Fluttering in the sea breeze, the flowers put on quite a show as several vivid shades of color dynamically intermix with the more muted tones of earth, sea, and sky.

Docent-led walks are featured on weekends. You can't picnic in the reserve, but after you hike, you can use the tables or the beach down near the entrance. Bring binoculars to watch the soaring ravens and red-tailed and sparrow hawks; you may sometimes even see hang-gliding humans.

HIKE 74

Los Penasquitos Canyon

Location	Northern San Diego
Highlights	An oak-shaded coastal canyon and a waterfall
Distance	6 miles (out-and-back or loop)
Total Elevation Gain/Loss	300'/300'
Hiking Time	3 hours
Optional Map	USGS 7.5-minute *Del Mar*
Best Times	All year
Agency	LPCP
Difficulty	Moderate
Trail Use	Good for kids, dogs allowed, suitable for mountain biking

Crickets sing, cicadas buzz, and bullfrogs groan. A sparrow hawk alights upon a sycamore limb, then launches with outstretched wings to catch a puff of sea breeze moving up the canyon. A cottontail rabbit bounds across the trail, and stops to take your measure with a sidelong stare. Los Penasquitos Creek slips silently through placid pools and darts noisily down multiple paths in the constriction known as the falls.

Despite the noose of suburban development tightening around it, Los Penasquitos Canyon Preserve still retains its gentle, unselfconscious beauty. The preserve's 4,000 acres of San Diego city- and county-owned open space stretch for almost 7 miles between I-5 and I-15,

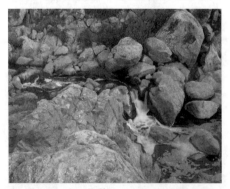

Los Penasquitos Falls

encompassing much of Los Penasquitos Creek and one of its tributaries, Lopez Canyon.

Visitor facilities at the preserve include parking and equestrian staging areas off Black Mountain Road on the east side and next to Sorrento Valley Boulevard on the west side. Near the east entry stands the Johnson-Taylor ranch house, now the preserve's headquarters, dating from 1862. In 1991, archaeologists announced that part of the ranch house is a surviving remnant of a house built in 1824 for Captain Francisco Maria Ruiz. Ruiz was commandant of the Presidio of San Diego and the recipient of the county's first Spanish land grant. The crumbling remnants of another adobe structure, also owned by Ruiz, stand under a protective roof at the west entrance to the preserve.

Farther afield, hikers, joggers, and equestrians have the run of the preserve. Take along a picnic lunch and a blanket. There are many fine places—sunny meadows, oak-shaded flats, and the sycamore-fringed streamside—to stop for an hour's relaxation. For starters, you can try the nearly level hike to the falls and back.

To Reach the Trailhead: Exit I-15 at Mercy Road/Scripps Poway Parkway (Exit 17), and go west on Mercy Road 1 mile to a traffic light at a T-intersection with Black Mountain Road. The main entrance to Los Penasquitos Canyon Preserve is straight across this intersection. Drive in, pay a small day-use fee, and park in the large parking lot. Alternatively, there is an entrance available at the west end of Canyonside Community Park; follow signs toward the ranch house and look for a gate on the left.

Description: On foot (or on wheels—the route sometimes swarms with mountain bikers), head west on a dirt road. In the first mile the road hugs Los Penasquitos Canyon's south wall, a steep, chaparral-covered hillside (penasquitos means "little cliffs"). Various paths fork off in both directions, but stay on the main dirt road.

As you pass near the Johnson-Taylor Ranch (screened from view by willows and dense vegetation along the creek), you'll notice several nonnative plants (eucalyptus, fan palms, feather-duster palms, and fennel, for example) introduced into this area over the past century. Efforts continue to remove these exotic species. Next, you enter a long and beautiful canopy of intertwined live oaks, accompanied by a lush understory of mostly poison oak.

Mileposts along the roadside help you gauge your progress. At mile 2 the trail winds out of the dense cover of oaks and continues through grassland dotted with a few small elderberry trees. Wildflowers such as wild radish, mustard, California poppies, bush mallow, blue-eyed grass, and violets put on quite a show here in March and April. Look, too, for the fuchsia-flowered gooseberry, quite unmistakable when in bloom.

At the 3-mile marker the road starts winding up onto a chaparral slope to detour around a narrow, rocky section of the canyon. At a signed junction for the waterfall viewpoint, make your way down to a narrow, rocky constriction along the canyon bottom. During winter and early spring, water in decent quantity tumbles through here. Polished rock 10 feet up on either side and deep, circular potholes testify to its sometimes violent flow. The outcrops of greenish-gray rock have been identified as Santiago Peak volcanics—the same hardened metavolcanic rock found farther north at Santiago Peak in the Santa Ana Mountains and farther south into Baja California.

You can make a loop by returning along a path on the north side of the canyon.

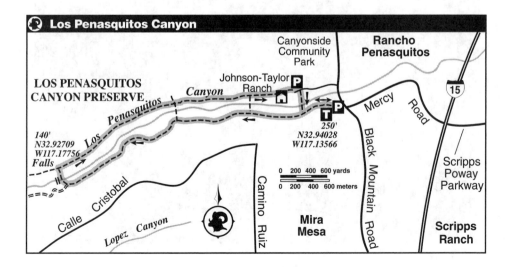

HIKE 75

Bernardo Mountain

Location	Escondido
Highlights	Wildflower-dotted hillsides, lake views, and bird-watching
Distance	7 miles (out-and-back)
Total Elevation Gain/Loss	1,000'/1,000'
Hiking Time	3½ hours
Optional Map	USGS 7.5-minute *Escondido*
Best Times	All year
Agency	SDRP
Difficulty	Moderately strenuous
Trail Use	Dogs allowed, suitable for mountain biking

Imagine a hiking, biking, and equestrian trail extending from the coast at Del Mar to the crest of the mountains in mid-San Diego County. Today, certain sections of this 55-mile-long route, known as the Coast to Crest Trail, are already open. These and other future sections of the trail will define the main axis of the San Dieguito River Park, now taking shape along the watersheds of the San Dieguito River and its main tributary, Santa Ysabel

Creek. Many pieces of the proposed park are in place today and open to the public, but fleshing out the entire 60,000 acres of parkland promises to involve much wrangling with landowners and long-term efforts by interested citizens and various local governments.

On this hike you'll travel one of the more accessible and scenic segments of the Coast to Crest Trail, overlooking scenic Lake Hodges, and you'll climb to the

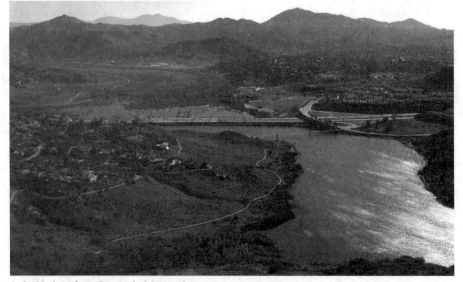

Lake Hodges from Bernardo Mountain

summit of Bernardo Mountain, which was purchased in 2002 for inclusion in San Dieguito River Park. Bird lovers will enjoy the diversity of birds that live on and near the lake.

To Reach the Trailhead: Exit I-15 at Via Rancho Parkway (Exit 27), and go east 0.2 mile to the first southbound street on the right, Sunset Drive. Drive to the end of Sunset Drive and park (free).

Description: From Sunset Drive, continue south on the Coast to Crest Trail, initially a concrete pathway parallel to the freeway. In 0.4 mile, the pathway turns sharply right and passes under the I-15 bridge that goes over the east arm of Lake Hodges. Depending on the amount of rainfall over the past year or two, the lake (a San Diego city reservoir) could be brimming with water at this spot or be completely dry, as it has been during recent droughts.

After swinging north on the far side (west side) of the freeway, the Coast to Crest Trail for a short time joins the crumbling pavement of the long-abandoned CA 395, the former inland highway running north from San Diego

into Riverside County and beyond. Soon, however, the pavement disappears, and you're on a dirt trail following the shoreline west. Pass the David Kreitzer Lake Hodges bridge, the world's longest stress-ribbon structure, completed in 2009. Take a short detour onto the bridge for fine views of the lake and mountain.

At 1.5 miles from the start, you cross Felicita Creek, a small perennial brook deeply shaded by oaks, sycamores, palms, and other water-loving vegetation. Rise out of the creek and ascend moderately, wrapping around the broad flank of Bernardo Mountain. The sunny slope on the right hosts an eye-popping assortment of wildflowers March through May. On the left, look for snowy egrets parasailing over the wind-rippled surface of the lake. Overhead, hawks and ravens can often be seen patrolling the afternoon skies, riding on thermals. Ospreys and golden eagles have been seen in this area as well—not to mention small and circumspect California gnatcatchers, which are classified as an endangered species.

At 1.7 miles, a few minutes past the creek crossing, make a very sharp right turn on the Bernardo Mountain Summit Trail heading north. You ascend slowly,

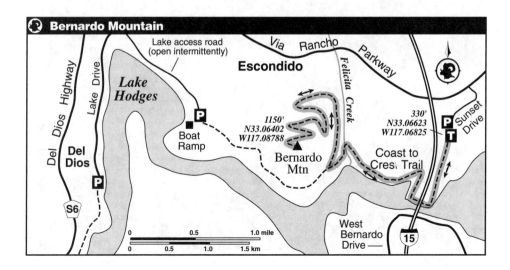

Bernardo Mountain

Lake access road (open intermittently)

Via Rancho Parkway

Escondido

Felicita Creek

Del Dios Highway

Lake Drive

Lake Hodges

Del Dios

Boat Ramp

1150'
N33.06402
W117.08788

330'
N33.06623
W117.06825

Bernardo Mtn

Coast to Crest Trail

Sunset Drive

S6

West Bernardo Drive

15

0   0.5   1.0 mile
0   0.5   1.0   1.5 km

with the oaks and sycamores of Felicita Creek just below you on the right and Bernardo Mountain rising on the left. By about 2.5 miles, you've swung around to the north side of the mountain. This area was burned bare by wildfire in October 2007, but the chaparral is rapidly regenerating as it has evolved to do. As the ascent quickens, stay left (uphill) at the next two trail intersections. Note the poorly marked junctions carefully so that you take the correct trail on your return.

You continue either rising or contouring in a zigzag pattern, passing a large water tank at 3.2 miles, and finally reaching the rocky summit at 3.6 miles. From this lofty vantage point you can clearly see the patchwork of urban, suburban, and wildland that inland north San Diego County has become. The white noise of traffic on I-15 wafts upward to you, but peering in certain other directions you see little apparent human impact on the landscape. Westward, down the valley below Lake Hodges, a slice of Pacific Ocean is visible on clear days.

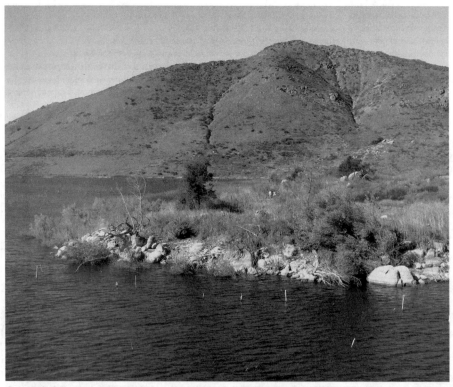

Bernardo Mountain

HIKE 76

Cowles Mountain

Location	Mission Trails Regional Park
Highlight	Best view of urban San Diego County
Distance	2.8 miles (out-and-back)
Total Elevation Gain/Loss	950'/950'
Hiking Time	2 hours
Optional Map	USGS 7.5-minute *La Mesa*
Best Times	All year
Agency	MTRP
Difficulty	Moderate
Trail Use	Good for kids, dogs allowed

Touted as one of the largest urban parks in the country, Mission Trails Regional Park, in San Diego's San Carlos district, preserves some of the last remaining open space close to the heart of this sprawling city. Cowles Mountain, centerpiece of the regional park, stands 1,591 feet above sea level and is recognized as the highest point within San Diego's city limits. Hundreds of people walk the main south trail to its summit daily. Since several newer trails have been laid out on the east and north slopes of the mountain in recent years, hikers can choose from among several summit routes. We describe the ever-popular south route, which consistently offers vistas stretching from the Pacific Ocean to Mexico.

To Reach the Trailhead: Exit I-8 at College Avenue (Exit 10), go north for 1.3 miles, and turn right (east) on Navajo Road. Continue 2 miles to the Cowles Mountain Trailhead (which has a parking lot and restrooms) on the northeast corner of Navajo Road and Golfcrest Drive. The lot is often full and additional parking is available along Golfcrest Drive.

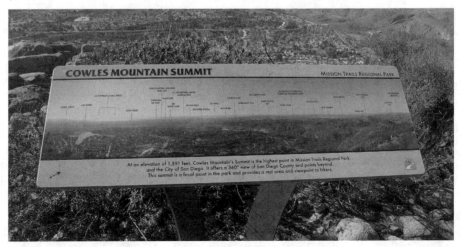

Cowles summit panorama

Description: From the trailhead you ascend steadily, zigzagging almost constantly up through low-growing chaparral punctuated by outcrops of granitic rock. Because the trail was cut into decomposed granite, it is quite susceptible to erosion. Don't shortcut the switchbacks, tempting as this may be, as this tramples plants and tends to destabilize the trail.

Nearly 1 mile up, a spur trail branches right toward a flat spot on the mountain's south shoulder. This site of ancient winter-solstice ceremonies by the ancestral Kumeyaay Indians has become a popular place to visit at dawn on or near the solstice (December 21). If you view it from the right spot, the sun's disk, just peeping over the mountains to the east, gets momentarily split into two brilliant points of light by a large outcrop atop a distant ridge.

Just beyond the spur trail, another trail branches right and eventually descends the east slope. Stay left and continue up the slope on the series of long switchback segments leading to the rocky summit of the mountain. A cluster of antennae somewhat obstructs the northward view, but otherwise the panorama is complete. With binoculars and the help of a large interpretive panel that identifies nearby and distant landmarks, you could spend a lot of time getting to know the region. In the rift between the mesas to the west, there's a good view of Mission Valley and the tangle of freeways that pass over and through it. Southwest, the towers of downtown San Diego stand against Point Loma, Coronado, and sparkling San Diego Bay. Lake Murray shimmers to the south. The chain of Santee Lakes contrasts darkly with pale hills to the north. In all directions you look out over the abodes of the nearly 5 million people now living in the combined metropolis of San Diego and Tijuana.

On the clearest days, the higher peaks of San Diego County stand in bold relief against the sky. Southward into Baja, you should spot the flat-topped Table Mountain behind Tijuana and the Coronado Islands offshore. Try looking for the dusky profiles of Santa Catalina and San Clemente Islands to the northwest and west, respectively.

Here's a suggestion for romantics and adventurers who don't mind descending the trail by flashlight: Catch the sunset from Cowles' summit when the moon is full. After the sun slides into the Pacific, turn around and enjoy the moonrise over the El Cajon valley!

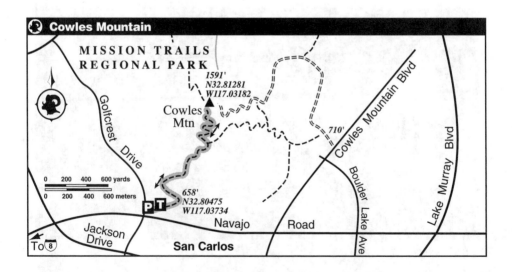

HIKE 77

Blue Sky Ecological Reserve

Location	Poway
Highlights	Riparian and oak woodland and spring wildflowers
Distance	5.0 miles (out-and-back)
Total Elevation Gain/Loss	800'/800'
Hiking Time	2½ hours
Optional Map	USGS 7.5-minute *Escondido*
Best Times	Daylight hours only, all year
Agency	BSER
Difficulty	Moderate
Trail Use	Good for kids, dogs allowed

The 700-acre Blue Sky Ecological Reserve near Poway protects one of the finer examples of riparian (streamside) vegetation in Southern California. As one of the most popular of the 119 California Department of Fish and Game wildlife reserves in the state, it focuses on both nature education and habitat preservation. Motorized vehicles and mountain bikes are banned—you'll be assured of peace and quiet and more frequent wildlife sightings as you stroll along.

To Reach the Trailhead: Exit I-15 at Rancho Bernardo Road (Exit 24), and drive east through Rancho Bernardo and Poway (where the road becomes Espola Road). In 3.1 miles, the road bends 90 degrees to the right. Just after that bend look for the Blue Sky reserve entrance and trailhead on the left. If you are coming from the south on Espola Road, the Blue Sky turnoff is 0.6 mile north of Lake Poway Road.

Description: The trail begins at the south end of the parking area. On foot, follow the unpaved Green Valley Truck Trail down and along the south bank of a creek. Traffic noise disappears, and frogs entertain you with their guttural serenades. Live oaks spread their limbs overhead, casting pools of shade, while

willows, sycamores, and lush thickets of poison oak cluster along the creek. On the left, about 0.25 mile out, a wide side trail diverges toward the creek. The canyon burned in the October 2007 Witch Fire, and many of the coast live oaks bear scorch marks. Stay on the trail as the vegetation regenerates. The creekside footpath rejoins the road in another 0.3 mile.

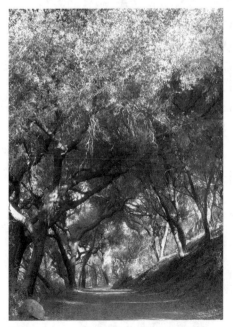

Live oaks over Green Valley Truck Trail

After a wet winter, usually by March, the canyon landscape turns an almost unbelievably bright shade of green. Mosses, ferns, annual grasses, and fresh new shrub growth coats everything, even the rocks. Wildflowers appear in great numbers by about April and start to fade by June, after the grasses have bleached to a straw-yellow color. More than 100 kinds of wildflowers have been identified here in a single year.

At 1.0 mile, a trail branching right (south) heads uphill to join the trail system of the Lake Poway Recreation Area. About 0.2 mile farther on the main road, pass an outdoor classroom with picnic tables and an outhouse. Just beyond, there's a major split. The right branch services a noisy pump station and is closed to the public. The left branch (Green Valley Truck Trail) fords the creek and starts climbing a dry south slope toward the Ramona Reservoir dam. In the next 1.3 miles of steady ascent, you gain about 700 feet of elevation and enjoy an ever-expanding view of Poway, Rancho Bernardo, and much of the rest of inland north San Diego County's rapidly urbanizing region.

Once you reach the dam you can turn around and return on the same route in much less time.

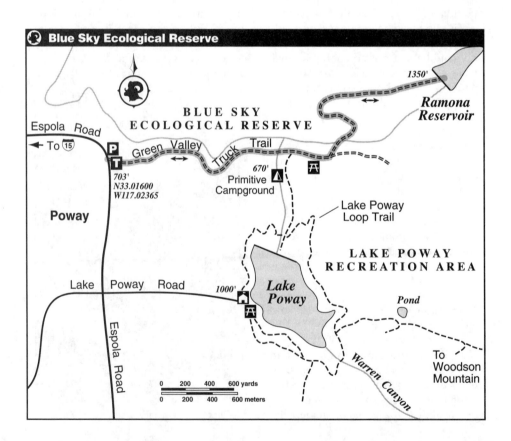

HIKE 78

Woodson Mountain

Location	Poway-Ramona
Highlights	Giant boulders and superb views
Distance	6 miles (loop)
Total Elevation Gain/Loss	1,500'/1,500'
Hiking Time	3 hours
Optional Map	USGS 7.5-minute *San Pasqual*
Best Times	October–June
Agency	LPRA
Difficulty	Moderate
Trail Use	Good for kids, dogs allowed

The native Kumeyaay people called it Mountain of Moonlit Rocks, an appropriate name for a landmark visible, even at night, over great distances. Early white settlers dubbed it Cobbleback Peak, a name utterly descriptive of its rugged, boulder-strewn slopes. For the past 100 years, however, it has appeared on maps simply as Woodson Mountain, in honor of a Dr. Woodson who homesteaded some property nearby well over a century ago.

The light-colored bedrock of Woodson Mountain and several of its neighboring peaks in the Poway/Ramona area is a type geologists call Woodson Mountain granodiorite. When exposed at the surface, it weathers into huge spherical or ellipsoidal boulders with smooth surfaces. The largest boulders have a tendency to cleave apart along remarkably flat planes, forming "chimneys" from several inches to several feet wide. Sometimes, one half of a split boulder will roll away, leaving a vertical and almost seamless face behind. It's no wonder that Woodson Mountain (or Mount Woodson, as it is popularly called) is regarded as one of the finest places to practice the craft of bouldering in Southern California.

This looping route up and over Woodson's summit takes advantage of the newer Fry-Koegel Trail along the mountain's bouldery north slope. Hikers have long had the opportunity of reaching the summit by either of two major routes, but there was never any easy way to avoid retracing steps.

To Reach the Trailhead: From I-15, take Poway Road 8.7 mile east to its end, then turn left and head north on Highway 67 for 3.0 miles to the California Division of Forestry Ramona Fire Station at mile marker 67 SD 18.00. Park on the often-crowded west shoulder of the road outside the fire station.

Description: The unsigned trail starts just south of the fire station entrance. It follows a well-beaten path south past the fire station to where it hooks up with a paved service road (closed to vehicular travel) curling up the mountain's east slope.

On most weekends, the sounds of nature along the road will be accompanied by the clink of aluminum hardware, plus the shouts of "On belay!" and other phrases in climbers' parlance. Even if you don't see climbers, chalk marks (from gymnast's chalk) on the larger boulders mark their favorite routes. Near the top of the mountain, the road passes narrowly between immense, egg-shaped boulders and split-boulder faces 20–30 feet high.

When you reach the top of the mountain, at 1.7 miles, you'll be amid a forest of radio antennae rising from the outsized boulders. Walk west past the last antenna to where the road turns into a dirt trail. Near here, look for the amazing cantilevered "potato-chip" flake of rock, the result of exfoliation and weathering, that has become a well-known attraction in recent years. From this vantage point overlooking Poway, north San Diego County's coastal region, and the great blue expanse of the Pacific Ocean, you can see Santa Catalina and San Clemente Islands on the clearest days. If you're weary, this is a good spot to turn back and return the way you came.

Otherwise, on ahead, you quickly pick up a rough trail that tilts downward, steeply at times, along Woodson's boulder-punctuated west ridge. Pass a junction with the old Fry-Koegel Trail and

then reach a four-way junction. It's worth the very short detour west up a rocky path to a viewpoint where you can enjoy a snack before continuing the descent.

Back at the four-way junction, turn northeast down the Fry-Koegel Trail through wildly tangled, mature chaparral, bound for the Mt. Woodson Estates subdivision at the north base of the mountain. Near the bottom, the trail meanders through spooky clusters of coast live oaks. Watch out for copious growths of poison oak through here.

Back in open air again, the trail detours around a block of new houses. Now fenced, it passes behind the Mt. Woodson Golf Club. Watch for a gap in the fence on the right where you can shortcut up to CA 67. If you miss it, you'll emerge on Archie Moore Road. In any event, a few minutes' walk along the highway shoulder takes you back to your car.

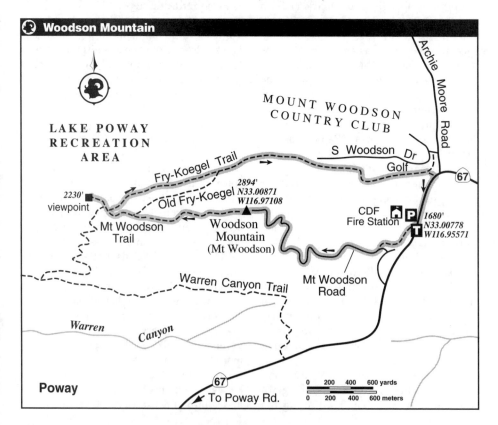

HIKE 79

Iron Mountain

Location	Near Poway
Highlights	Panoramic views
Distance	6 miles (out-and-back)
Total Elevation Gain/Loss	1,200'/1,200'
Hiking Time	3 hours
Optional Map	USGS 7.5-minute *San Vicente Reservoir*
Best Times	October–June
Agency	LPRA
Difficulty	Moderate
Trail Use	Good for kids, dogs allowed, suitable for mountain biking

North San Diego County's Iron Mountain thrusts its conical summit nearly 2,700 feet above sea level, frequently well above the low-lying coastal haze. On many a crystalline winter day, the summit offers a sweeping, 360-degree panorama from glistening ocean to blue mountains and back to the ocean again. Access to the summit—by foot, horse, or mountain bike—is now afforded by a key link in the City of Poway's ever-expanding multiuse trails system. Expect to have plenty of company on this extremely popular trail.

To Reach the Trailhead: The large and popular Iron Mountain Trailhead is located at the intersection of CA 67 and Poway Road at mile marker 67 SD 15.00, 8.7 miles east of I-15 by way of Poway Road or 15.0 miles north of I-8 by way of CA 67. There's a secondary trailhead on Ellie Lane, 0.7 mile north on CA 67 from the main trailhead, in case you want to try the extended route noted at the end of this description.

Description: From the main trailhead, the shortest way up the mountain (a little more than 3 miles one-way) takes you along signed pathways. Thick stands of chaparral stood along these trails until 1995, when a wildfire swept east from CA

67 and topped Iron Mountain's summit, burning everything in its path to a crisp. The mountain was swept by flames yet again in October 2003 by the 300,000-acre Cedar Fire, the largest blaze in contemporary California history. The chaparral, evolved to periodically burn and regenerate, has fully returned. Pass a four-way

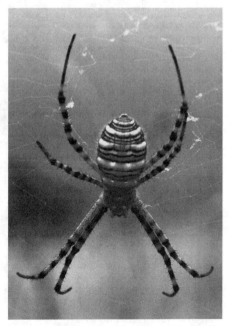

Early-morning spider, Iron Mountain Trail

junction with paths leading left to Ellie Lane and right to loop and rejoin the main Iron Mountain Trail. At 1.0 mile east of CA 67, just before the trail dips to cross a ravine, an obscure side trail goes north almost straight up a hill. If you care to make the short, strenuous side trip, you'll find a small pit where iron ore was once mined in small quantities. Dark, dense chunks of the ore lie strewn about—bring along a magnet to confirm their identity.

Once across the ravine, you commence a steeper ascent. At 1.4 miles you reach a trail junction in a saddle, where you turn right to head for Iron Mountain's summit, 1.5 meandering trail miles away. Numerous switchbacks on the trail's final half

mile take you back and forth across the ever-narrowing summit cone. On the summit you'll find a massive, pier-mounted free telescope thoughtfully provided for the purpose of scanning the near and far horizons.

Return the easy way by simply reversing your steps, or you can opt for a more challenging traverse over hill and dale to the north. The northern loop, which passes Table Rock and two old cattle ponds, adds 3 additional miles to the round-trip and involves several severe up and down pitches. You'll end up at the Ellie Lane Trailhead, 0.7 mile north of the main trailhead.

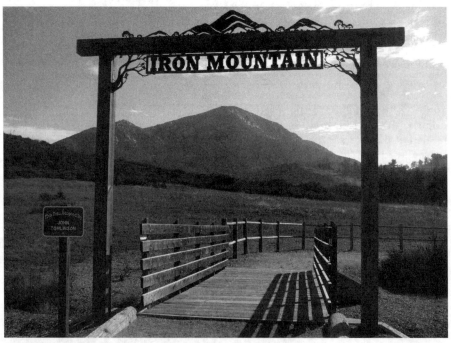

Iron Mountain Trailhead

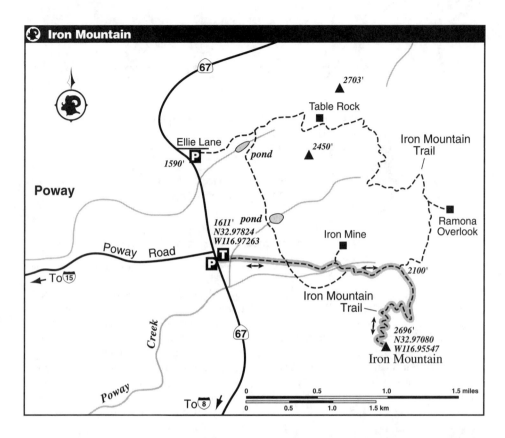

HIKE 80

El Capitan Open Space Preserve

Location	Near Lakeside
Highlights	Frequent vistas of coastal lowlands and ocean
Distance	12 miles (out-and-back)
Total Elevation Gain/Loss	4,000'/4,000'
Hiking Time	6 hours
Optional Maps	USGS 7.5-minute *San Vicente Reservoir* and *El Cajon Mtn.*
Best Times	7 a.m.–4:30 p.m., November–April
Agency	SDCP
Difficulty	Strenuous
Trail Use	Suitable for mountain biking, dogs allowed

As you walk along the granite-ribbed ridgeline, down the middle of the El Capitan Open Space Preserve, a binational panorama of ocean, islands, and innumerable mountain peaks lies in view. The broad San Diego River valley below curves beneath the sheer south face of El Cajon Mountain—the landmark informally known as El Capitan.

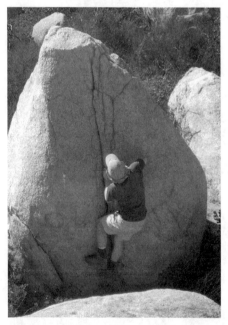

Working a boulder problem on El Cajon

This 2,800-acre preserve was pieced together out of former Bureau of Land Management (BLM) lands adjacent to the Cleveland National Forest. If you have the determination to tackle some really severe uphills and downhills, and get the benefit of a serious cardiovascular workout, try following the preserve's main route, an old, sometimes precariously steep road bulldozed by miners years ago. It twists and turns over a scrubby, boulder-punctuated landscape that in spring comes alive with a blue frosting of ceanothus (wild lilac) blossoms. Parts of this mining road are gradually being bypassed or improved and incorporated into the fledgling Trans-County Trail—a major multiuse pathway that will stretch east-west across San Diego County from Del Mar on the coast to Borrego Springs in the desert. Its ups and downs and lack of abundant shade make this hike surprisingly difficult. Many hikers underestimate the amount of drinking water they will need. Bring at least 3 quarts on a cool winter day and more when it's hot. The trails close at 4:30 p.m., necessitating a reasonably early start and a steady pace.

To Reach the Trailhead: From I-8, take CA 67 north for 5.8 miles, then turn east on Mapleview Street where the freeway portion of the highway ends. In 0.3 mile turn left (north) on Ashwood Street. Ashwood soon becomes Wildcat Canyon Road. Proceed north on it another 4.4 miles to a signed parking lot for the preserve on the right. (You can use the green mile markers by the roadside as your guide; slow down after mile marker 4.0.)

Description: From the lot, walk east 0.4 mile on the entry road to the private Blue Sky Ranch, past that ranch, to a trailhead with a large outhouse. The dirt road continues to the south, but it is more scenic to pick up the narrow trail, which starts a steep, zigzagging ascent up a cool, north-facing slope. You soon rejoin the old mining road, and the going gets easier for a while. (*Note:* These directions may change once a planned bypass trail is completed between the trailhead and the old mining road. You may observe a variety of side roads and trails, but stay on the main road all the way.)

As you reach a small summit (about 1.2 miles from the start) and start descending on the old mining road, the round top and sheer south brow of El Cajon Mountain (El Capitan) becomes visible in the middle distance. A very steep uphill pitch, commencing at about 3 miles, will surely reduce you to painfully slow uphill scrambling, if only for a few minutes. At a little less than 4 miles, you reach another significant summit. From this spot, a short side road leads north to some abandoned mines, shallow tunnels cut into a chalky hillside.

Similar to Sisyphus's struggle, your elevation gain is tragically interrupted just ahead. You sink 300 feet in less than a half mile on slippery, decomposing granite and then resume your uphill progress. At 4.7

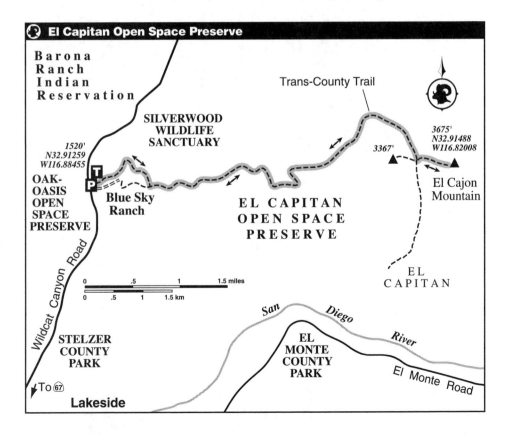

miles there's a rock-lined spring on the left, either brimming with iron-rich, nonpotable water or possibly dry. At 5.5 miles, the road arrives on a saddle between El Cajon Mountain's summit on the left (east) and a smaller 3367-foot peak on the right (west).

Turn left and follow a narrow path threading 0.5 mile through thick chaparral and around jumbo-sized granitic boulders to El Cajon Mountain's summit. (The route is slated to be improved and incorporated into the San Diego Sea to Sea Trail.) Although the summit is rounded and clogged with boulders, the view is panoramic in all directions. On a clear day as your gaze turns counterclockwise, you'll see San Jacinto, Palomar Mountain, Mount Baldy, Santiago Peak, Woodson Mountain, Iron Mountain, Black Mountain, Catalina and San Clemente Islands, Miramar Airfield, downtown San Diego and Point Loma, peaks of northern Baja, the El Capitan reservoir, and the Cuyamaca and Laguna Mountains.

Return to the saddle. Most hikers are satisfied at this point and return the way they came. If you are feeling energetic, however, you have two more options to explore. By turning right (west) and walking 0.2 mile, you reach a 3,367-foot summit, with evident remnants of a radio antenna installation. This rocky peaklet offers a nice panoramic view west and south.

The most difficult alternative is a 1.4-mile-long trek straight ahead (south) from the saddle, using a severely eroded and partially overgrown roadbed. This route takes you to the sheer brow of El Capitan. Walk out to the edge, beyond the end of the old roadbed, and descend over boulders 50 or 100 yards for a pseudo-aerial view of the San Diego River valley and El Capitan Reservoir, complete with toylike boats floating on its blue surface.

HIKE 81

Doane Valley

Location	Palomar Mountain State Park
Highlights	Verdant meadows and bubbling streams
Distance	3.0 miles (loop)
Total Elevation Gain/Loss	300'/300'
Hiking Time	1½ hours
Optional Maps	Palomar Mountain State Park brochure or USGS 7.5-minute *Boucher Hill*
Best Times	6 a.m.–sunset, all year
Agency	PSP
Difficulty	Moderate
Trail Use	Good for kids

This is a hike for inspiration. Here, at Palomar Mountain State Park, you'll find some of Southern California's finest montane scenery, complete with trickling streams, rolling meadows, and mixed forests of pine, cedar, and oak. The long, stomach-churning drive up the mountain's slopes is well worth the trouble once you get out of the car and start breathing in Palomar's sweet, tangy air.

Palomar Mountain is wonderful in every season. In summer, the mountain air and shady trails offer a respite from the heat of the valley. In fall, the black oaks turn brilliant gold before shedding their leaves. In the winter, a dusting of

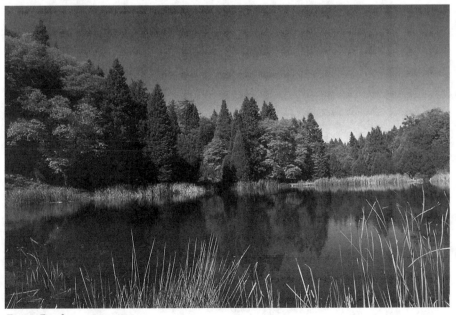

Doane Pond

snow can turn the mountain into a winter wonderland. And in spring, the creeks
run strong and the flowers and new buds
emerge. Palomar was slated to be closed
during California's 2012 budget woes, but
the state park thankfully remains open,
though woefully underfunded.

To Reach the Trailhead: Palomar Mountain State Park lies in far-north San Diego
County, about 20 miles east of I-15. From
most parts of San Diego County, it's fastest to use County Route S6 (Valley Center Road) to reach CA 76 near the foot of
Palomar Mountain. Continue east to mile
marker 76 SD 38.00, and turn left onto
County Route S6 again. Upon reaching
the crest in 6.9 miles, turn left and immediately left again onto County Route S7,
which becomes State Park Road. After
paying your day-use or camping fee at

the park entrance in 3.0 miles, continue
1.7 miles farther to the Doane Pond parking area at the end of the road, following
signs for School Camp and staying right
at all junctions. A restroom is available a
few yards down the Cedar Trail.

Description: You begin your hike by following the Doane Valley Nature Trail
across the road and downstream along
Doane Creek. Along the bank grow box-
elder trees, creek dogwood, wild strawberry, mountain currant, and Sierra
gooseberry. You pass a massive incense-
cedar tree towering more than 100 feet
high. If you weren't informed of its true
identity, you might think it was a giant
(sequoia) redwood.

After 0.3 mile, the nature trail curves
and climbs around a hill to connect with
Doane Valley Campground. At a trail

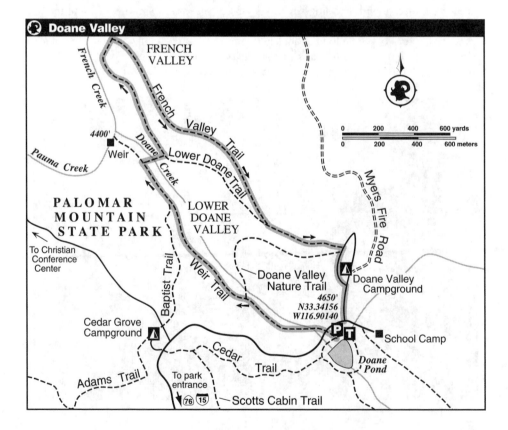

junction here, bear left on the Weir Trail, following Doane Creek through stately groves of white fir and incense-cedar. Walk all the way down to the weir at the end of the trail, and admire the stone-and-mortar structure above it. This small dam and gauging station were built in 1926 to test the stream's hydroelectric potential. The tests proved there was not enough flow to justify construction of a power plant. Today, the silted-in dam holds barely enough water to soak your feet in. Some years ago, park rangers were surprised to discover banana slugs (like those in California's central and northern coast ranges) in this drainage.

From the weir, backtrack 0.2 mile and take the Lower Doane Trail left across the valley to the French Valley Trail. Go left (north), passing into Lower French Valley. The setting is idyllic: rolling grasslands dotted with statuesque ponderosa pines, surrounded by hillsides clothed in oaks and tall conifers. The 2007 Poomacha Fire whipped across the park and cleared out the underbrush but left most of the mature trees intact. Land managers are coming to recognize that wildfire serves an essential natural role in the ecosystem and that decades of aggressive fire suppression have disrupted this role.

Several of the pine trees are riddled with holes, some of which are plugged with acorns. This is the handiwork of the acorn woodpecker, who uses the holes to store acorns filled with larvae. The birds retrieve these acorns and the grubs in leaner times. Listen for this woodpecker's repetitive, guttural call, and observe the distinctive red patch on its head and its white wing patch when it is in flight.

The trail abruptly turns sharp right and leads back above the meadow. Hike as far as the bank of French Creek, then head back toward your starting point along the upper part of the French Valley Trail. A shady glade beneath a grove of enormous live oaks invites you to rest your feet and contemplate the majestic trees. Beyond, you walk beneath the trunk of massive live oak. Until this tree toppled in 2009 at an age of about 1,000 years, it was the largest oak in San Diego County. Join Lower Doane Trail, pass a junction with the Nature Trail, arrive at Doane Valley Campground, and then turn right and walk through the campground to the parking lot where you began.

Doane Pond is located south of the parking area and is well worth the quarter-mile stroll. If you have more time to enjoy it, the park offers many more miles of scenic trails.

HIKE 82

Agua Caliente Creek

Location	Near Warner Springs
Highlights	Beautiful mountain stream
Distance	8 miles (out-and-back)
Total Elevation Gain/Loss	900'/900'
Hiking Time	4 hours
Optional Maps	Tom Harrison Maps San Diego Backcountry or USGS 7.5-minute *Warner Springs* and *Hot Springs Mtn.*
Best Times	November–May
Agency	CNF/PD
Difficulty	Moderately strenuous
Trail Use	Dogs allowed, suitable for backpacking

Until the early 1970s, the middle reaches of Agua Caliente Creek seldom saw the intrusion of humans. After the Pacific Crest Trail was routed through, it became a favorite resting spot for hikers heading north or south. This is one of only four places in San Diego County where the PCT dips to cross a fairly dependable stream, and it's the only place where the trail closely follows water for a fair distance. The stream—if not perennial—is at

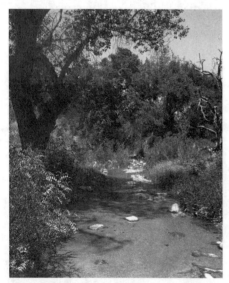

Agua Caliente Creek

least alive from the first rains of fall into early summer.

To Reach the Trailhead: From I-15 at Temecula, drive east on CA 79 for 37 miles to reach the resort community of Warner Springs. From the San Diego area, use CA 78 or CA 67 and 78 to reach Santa Ysabel, and then proceed north on CA 79 for 14 miles to Warner Springs. Just west of Warner Springs (toward Temecula), there's a turnout for parking at mile 36.7 on CA 79. Note the dirt road slanting over to where the PCT crosses under the highway.

Description: Join the PCT at the Agua Caliente Creek bridge at mile 36.6 on CA 79. Proceed upstream along the cottonwood-shaded creek, first on the left (north) bank and then on the right. In this first mile, the trail goes through Warner Ranch resort property on an easement. Near the Cleveland National Forest boundary, about 1 mile out, water flows or trickles from a canyon mouth (trail camping is allowed on the lands beyond this point if you get a permit). The trail detours this canyon by swinging to the east and climbing moderately onto gentle, ribbonwood-clothed slopes. After almost 2 miles of somewhat tedious twisting and turning in the chaparral, you join the creek again at the 3,200-foot contour. (Unofficial paths worn in by local equestrians intersecting the PCT may confuse navigation through here a bit.)

Gorgeous scenery begins when you reach the creek. In the next mile the trail (or at least remnants of the trail, since it washes out easily) crosses the stream several times and passes a number of appealing small campsites well up on the bank. Live oaks, sycamores, willows, and alders line the creek. The canyon walls soar several hundred feet on either side—clad in dense chaparral on the southeast side, dotted with sage and yucca on the northwest.

After a final crossing of the creek, the trail doubles back and begins a switchbacking (and not very scenic) ascent northwest toward Indian Flats Road. This is a good place to turn around and return the same way.

If you want to explore farther upstream along Agua Caliente Creek from where the trail ascends out of the canyon, you can either boulder-hop or wade. You'll face some serious scrambling around small waterfalls and personal battles with the ever-present alder branches ahead. Los Coyotes Indian Reservation property, which you must get permission to enter, lies about a mile ahead.

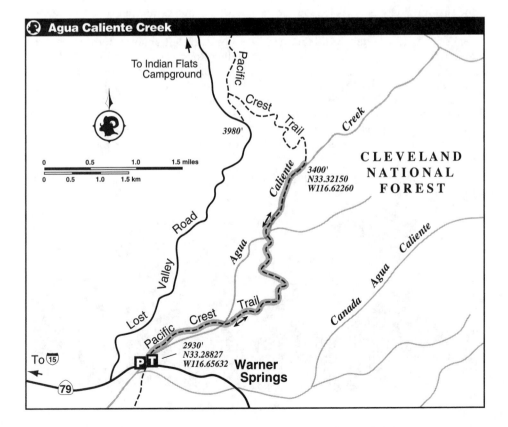

Agua Caliente Creek

To Indian Flats Campground

Pacific Crest Trail

3980'

Caliente Creek

Agua Caliente

Road

Valley

Lost

Pacific Crest Trail

CLEVELAND NATIONAL FOREST

3400'
N33.32150
W116.62260

Canada Agua Caliente

0   0.5   1.0   1.5 miles
0   0.5   1.0   1.5 km

2930'
N33.28827
W116.65632

P T

To 15

79

Warner Springs

HIKE 83

Eagle Rock

Location	Near Warner Springs
Highlight	Unusual rock formation
Distance	6 miles (out-and-back)
Total Elevation Gain/Loss	700'/700'
Hiking Time	3 hours
Optional Maps	Tom Harrison Maps San Diego Backcountry or USGS 7.5-minute *Warner Springs, Hot Springs Mtn.,* and *Ranchita*
Best Times	October–June
Agency	Vista Irrigation District (grants an easement but does not field questions from hikers)
Difficulty	Moderate
Trail Use	Good for kids, dogs allowed

Eagle Rock, perched on a hill overlooking Warner Springs Ranch, bears a stunning likeness to its namesake raptor. In April, the surrounding meadows explode with wildflowers. A walk along the oak-lined banks of Cañada Verde caps off this magnificent hike.

To Reach the Trailhead: Follow CA 79 to the south end of Warner Springs. Park in a turnout across from the California Department of Forestry fire station, 0.3 mile south of mile marker 79 SD 34.50.

If you wish to make a one-way trip with a shuttle, take a second vehicle to Barrel Spring by continuing south on CA 79. In 2.5 miles, turn left onto San Felipe Road (County Route S2). In 4.8 more miles, turn left again onto Montezuma Valley Road (County Route S22). In 1.0 mile, park at the Barrel Spring Trailhead in a large dirt lot on the right side near a PCT sign.

Description: Cross to the southeast side of the highway, and pass through a gate

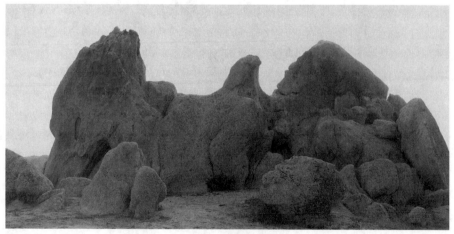

Eagle Rock

at a sign for the Pacific Crest Trail. Cross Cañada Verde ("green ravine") Creek, and pass through a second gate. The California Riding and Hiking Trail veers left toward Warner Springs, but your trip continues straight on the PCT.

In 0.1 mile, pass a third gate and hike up the oak-lined canyon. In 1.2 miles, the trail departs the canyon and veers south across rangeland. In another 1.8 miles,

reach a cluster of granite rocks. A signed trail curves around to the back side, where Eagle Rock is clearly recognizable.

If you set up a car or bicycle shuttle, you could continue on the PCT another 5 miles to its intersection with County Route S22 at Barrel Spring. In the springtime, San Ysidro Creek flows through a scenic canyon and delightful wildflowers carpet the meadows.

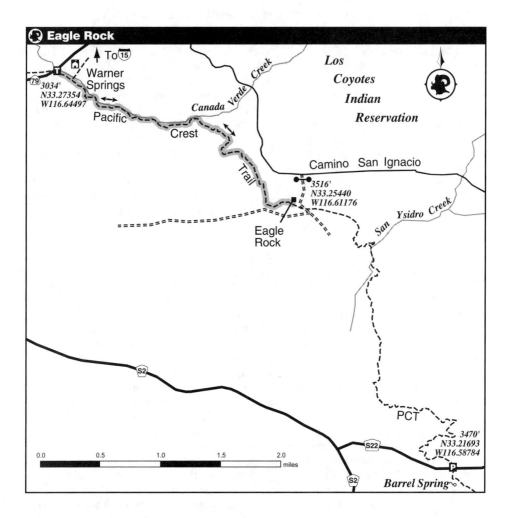

HIKE 84

Cedar Creek Falls

Location	West of Julian
Highlights	Beautiful cascade and punchbowl
Distance	5.5 miles (out-and-back)
Total Elevation Gain/Loss	1,000'/1,000'
Hiking Time	2½ hours
Optional Maps	USGS 7.5-minute *Santa Ysabel* and *Tule Springs*
Best Times	November–June
Agency	CNF/PD
Difficulty	Moderate
Trail Use	Good for kids
Permit	Day-use permit required from recreation.gov

The San Diego River and its upper tributaries drain the pastoral valleys and forested hillsides around Julian, and the rugged western slopes of the Cuyamaca Mountains. The water flows generally southwest through V-shaped canyons, and eventually reaches El Capitan Reservoir, not far from San Diego's eastern suburbs. Quite frequently the water encounters resistant layers in the underlying igneous and metamorphic rocks. In several places it tumbles over cataracts up to a hundred feet high. The grinding of stones trapped in pockets below these falls has created deep pools, or "punchbowls." Cedar Creek Falls, along with its punchbowl, is one of the more attractive and accessible of these wonders.

Before the construction of El Capitan Dam in the early 1930s, the falls were a popular destination for Sunday outings, and could be reached relatively easily on a road up the San Diego River Valley from Lakeside. Now, the drive to the Cedar Creek Falls trailhead, which takes San Diegans nearly as far as Julian, is far more circuitous—but scenic nonetheless.

This seemingly innocuous trail holds the dubious distinction of requiring more rescues and body removals than any other in San Diego County. It is dry

until Cedar Creek and can be extremely hot, resulting in regular incidents of heat stroke. Many dogs have died on the trail as well. Wear appropriate clothing, bring more water than you think you need, and, if it is hot, leave your pet behind. Several visitors have fallen to their death from the slippery cliffs above the falls, including a teenager in 2011. The falls also developed a reputation as a party spot, and thoughtless visitors trashed the canyon.

The trail was temporarily closed in 2011–12 because of all of these factors, but has reopened as of the time of this writing. The entire canyon above the falls is now closed; trespassing while it is closed is punishable by a hefty fine. Alcohol is prohibited, stay on the trail, and be sure to carry out your trash. In 2013, the forest instituted a day-use-permit system. Reserve your $6 permit through recreation .gov, or check with the Cleveland National Forest for current information.

A new trail making a western approach from Thornbush Road in Ramona may also be open by the time you read this; the quota will apply to that trail as well.

To Reach the Trailhead: From the town of Julian, on combined CA 78/79 drive west 1 mile. Near mile marker 78 SD 57.0, turn south on Pine Hills Road. After 1.5 miles, bear right on Eagle Peak Road. After 1.4 more miles, Eagle Peak Road veers right (Boulder Creek Road goes left).

Now you and your vehicle face 8.2 miles of mostly dirt road, parts of which become slippery and muddy in wet weather. However, if the road is in good condition, it is passable by ordinary low-clearance vehicles. In the end, you'll come to an intersection of gated roads (called Saddleback on detailed maps of the area) and a sign denoting the abandoned road ahead as the Cedar Creek Falls Hiking and Equestrian Trail. Park here so as not to block the intersection.

Description: Pass the gate and follow the abandoned roadbed leading west. As you head downhill on foot, look up the canyon in the north to see Mildred Falls,

arguably San Diego County's highest at more than 100 feet. Unfortunately, it's often little more than a dark stain on an orange-tinted cliff. When it is in flood, however, it is truly an awesome sight.

The old road winds farther west, offering a splendid view of the upper San Diego River canyon and then turns south for a long descent to the riverbed. At 1.6 miles, pass a spur on the left that used to reach the pool at the brink of the falls. This trail and the portion of Cedar Creek Canyon above the falls are now closed.

Instead, continue down another 0.7 mile to a junction on the floor of the San Diego River canyon by a shady grove of trees. Signs from the Helix Water District warn you not to trespass; instead turn left and follow the trail east into Cedar Creek Canyon. Cross the creek twice and reach the spectacular punchbowl in 0.5 mile.

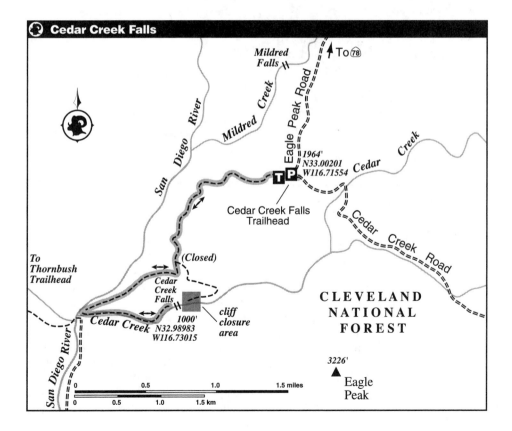

Volcan Mountain

Location	Near Julian
Highlights	Pastoral mountain landscapes
Distance	3.2 miles (to gate) or 5.0 miles (to summit)
Total Elevation Gain/Loss	900'/900' (to gate) or 1,300'/1,300' (to summit)
Hiking Time	2–2½ hours
Optional Map	USGS 7.5-minute *Julian*
Best Times	October–June
Agency	SDCP
Difficulty	Moderate
Trail Use	Good for kids, dogs allowed

Rising boldly above the apple orchards outside Julian, Volcan Mountain's oak- and pine-dotted slopes are swept by some of the freshest breezes found anywhere. Soughing through the trees like waves spending themselves against a sandy beach, these gusts bear the astringent dryness of the nearby desert, as well as the volatile scents of pine needles and sun-baked grass.

Named by early Spanish or Mexican travelers for its dubious resemblance to a volcano, Volcan Mountain (called the Volcan Mountains on topographic maps) is really a fault-block mountain, like many others in the Peninsular Ranges. The Elsinore and the Earthquake Valley Faults bracket the mountain on its southwest and northeast sides, respectively.

Off-limits to public use for the past century, Volcan Mountain is gradually falling into the public domain today. As funding becomes available, San Diego County and the San Dieguito River Park joint powers authority are purchasing privately owned land on the mountain. One such parcel, Volcan Mountain Wilderness Preserve—has already become an unsung crown jewel in the county parks system.

To Reach the Trailhead: From the center of Julian (on CA 78 and 79, 50 miles northeast of San Diego), drive 2.3 miles north on Farmer Road to Wynola Road. Jog right briefly, and then go left on the continuation of Farmer Road. Just ahead, on the right, a wooden sign announces the preserve. Park alongside Farmer Road.

Description: From your parked car, walk east on a dirt access road. After 0.2 mile, you come upon a carved entry structure and stonework designed by noted Julian artist James Hubbell. There's also a small, open-air kiva with a compass rose embedded in the floor, used during interpretive programs. The Elsinore Fault, a major splinter of the San Andreas, passes almost directly under this spot.

Just beyond this formal entrance, your wide path leads sharply up a hill overlooking an apple orchard. You soon swing sharply right and continue climbing in earnest along a rounded ridgeline leading toward the Volcan Mountain crest. Along the ridge, wind-rippled expanses of grassland alternate with dense copses of live oak and black oak. The rust-red bark of the many manzanita shrubs along the way perpetually peels, revealing a green undercoat. Look for the manzanitas ("little apples" in Spanish), the ripe, reddish brown berries that look and taste a bit like the apples hanging from the trees down in the valley below.

In 0.4 mile, a sign indicates the start of the Five Oaks Trail on the right. This delightful trail, named for the black, canyon, coast live, and scrub oaks and poison oak found in abundance along its course, is open only to hikers. It is slightly longer, but it offers better views and a more intimate experience and is the recommended route on the way up if you are on foot. It parallels the main path and rejoins it in 1.1 miles.

As you climb higher, the view expands to include parts of Julian, the dusky Cuyamaca Mountains to the south, and—on the clearest days—the blue arc of the Pacific Ocean in the west and southwest.

After 1.5 miles and 900 feet of climbing, reach the Midsummit Gate. The gate may be closed in the winter, making this your turnaround point.

If the gate is open, you can continue up the road. Shortly before reaching the ridgeline, pass through a splendid grove of incense-cedar and live oak. The path veers right upon reaching the ridge. Watch for a stone chimney on the right. This is the ruins of a cabin used from 1928–1932 by astronomers who were evaluating sites for the Hale Telescope, which was eventually constructed on Palomar Mountain instead.

The road makes a final climb to a loop on the summit of Volcan Mountain. Atop the mountain is the ruins of an airway light beacon built in 1928. Such beacons, spaced about 10 miles apart, were used to light the way for airmail pilots flying at night; they become obsolete with the development of radio navigation aids. On your descent, look for a white tower on a mountaintop to the north; this is the Very High Frequency Omnidirectional Radio (VOR) Beacon, which became the preferred means of navigation by the 1950s. The Global Positioning System (GPS) is gradually rendering VORs obsolete.

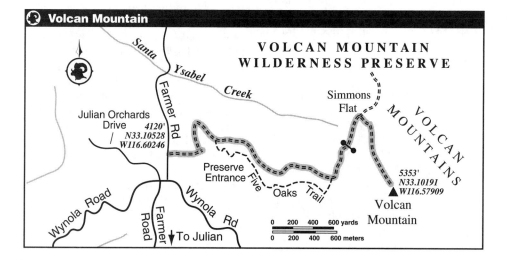

HIKE 86

Cuyamaca Peak

Location	Cuyamaca Rancho State Park
Highlights	Panoramic views and lessons in fire ecology
Distance	5.5 miles (out-and-back)
Total Elevation Gain/Loss	1,650'/1,650'
Hiking Time	3 hours
Optional Map	Cuyamaca Rancho State Park map, Tom Harrison Maps San Diego Backcountry, or USGS 7.5-minute *Cuyamaca Peak*
Best Times	All year
Agency	CRSP
Difficulty	Moderately strenuous
Trail Use	Dogs allowed, suitable for mountain biking

Cuyamaca Peak, San Diego County's second highest summit after Hot Spring Mountain, lies only a few miles from the county's geographical center. Its unique position and height make it the best land-based vantage point for studying the topography of the southernmost section of California. The 2003 Cedar Fire improved the view from the top by effectively removing most of the trees that used to block the panorama.

The one-lane, paved Lookout Road (Cuyamaca Peak Fire Road on some maps) is closed to public vehicles, but it provides a straightforward passage to the top of the peak for self-propelled travelers: hikers, runners, cyclists, and (rarely) cross-country skiers.

To Reach the Trailhead: You begin this hike at Paso Picacho Campground and Picnic Area on CA 79 0.2 mile north of mile marker 79 SD 9.00, about 12 miles north of I-8 near Descanso and about 11 miles south of Julian. Day-use parking is available here for a fee, next to the picnic sites. Walk through the campground to find the Lookout Road Trailhead near the southernmost campsites.

Description: Once you are walking on the Lookout Road, you will find the initial uphill grade to be only moderately steep. The dense pine, fir, cedar, and oak forest that grew on these Cuyamaca slopes before October 2003 was hard-hit by the fire.

After you cross the California Riding and Hiking Trail, which is called Fern Flat Fire Road to the south and Azalea Spring Fire Road to the north (1.2 miles), the paved road gets seriously steep and remains so for most of the remainder of the climb. The widening vista to the north and east includes Cuyamaca Reservoir and several desert mountain ranges. Notice how the aptly named Stonewall Peak to the east (just across CA 79) appears to shrink in stature as you continue your climb. In the final steep stretch, you climb past timber snags and suddenly arrive at the antennae-cluttered summit of the peak. A fire-lookout structure stood here until the late 1980s, when it was removed for lack of use.

During a Santa Ana condition in fall or winter and after major winter storms, Cuyamaca Peak becomes a grandstand seat for views stretching into at least five counties and one foreign state. To name some of the features visible within San Diego County: the Palomar Mountains (look for the tiny white speck, the Hale Telescope dome, on the summit ridge) northwest more than 30 miles away; Hot Springs Mountain, 26 miles almost due north over the summit of nearby Middle Peak; Granite Mountain, 11 miles to the northeast; the south end of the Santa Rosa Mountains, 40 miles northeast; and Whale Peak and the Vallecito Mountains, 18 miles east-northeast.

Close in, just 10 or so miles to the southeast, are the wooded Laguna Mountains. South and southwest along the international border are Tecate Peak and Otay Mountain, 25–30 miles away. The Pacific Ocean gleams in the west, with Point Loma, the Silver Strand, San Diego Bay, and Mission Bay visible at distances of about 35–40 miles. Along an arc from west to southwest, you'll spot coastal peaks like Black Mountain, Soledad Mountain, Fortuna Mountain, Cowles Mountain, Mount Helix, and San Miguel Mountain. Along a west-to-south arc, but closer in, you'll see El Cajon Mountain, Viejas Mountain, Lyons Peak, and Corte Madera Mountain.

To enhance your resting time on the peak, bring along a map of regional features and binoculars.

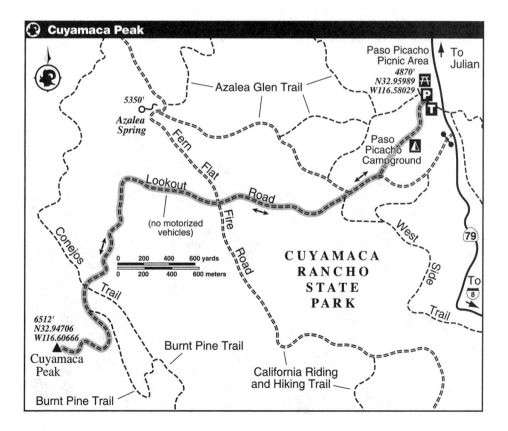

HIKE 87

Stonewall Peak

Location	Cuyamaca Rancho State Park
Highlights	Outstanding summit views
Distance	4.5 miles (out-and-back)
Total Elevation Gain/Loss	850'/850'
Hiking Time	2½ hours
Optional Map	Cuyamaca Rancho State Park map, Tom Harrison Maps San Diego Backcountry, or USGS 7.5-minute *Cuyamaca Peak*
Best Times	All year
Agency	CRSP
Difficulty	Moderate
Trail Use	Good for kids

Stonewall Peak's angular summit of white granitic rock is a conspicuous landmark throughout Cuyamaca Rancho State Park. Although Stonewall stands some 800 feet lower than nearby Cuyamaca Peak, its unique position and steep, south exposure provides a more inclusive view of the park area itself. The peak was named for the lucrative

Stonewall Jackson mine William Skidmore established on its northeast slope in 1870.

To Reach the Trailhead: You'll begin this hike at Paso Picacho Campground and Picnic Area on CA 79 0.2 mile north of mile marker 79 SD 9.00, about 12 miles north of I-8 near Descanso and about 11

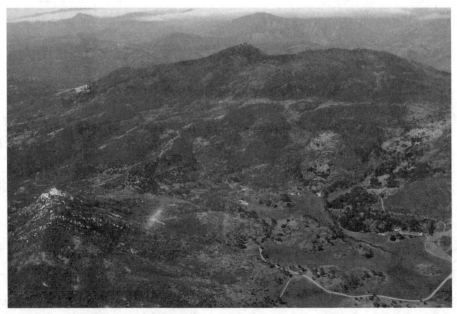

Aerial view of Cuyamaca and Stonewall

miles south of Julian. Day-use parking is available for a fee next to the picnic sites.

Description: Beginning across the highway from the entrance to Paso Picacho, the trail climbs steadily on a set of well-graded switchback segments up the west slope of Stonewall Peak. For many years to come, it will offer a fairly unobstructed view, since the majority of trees that grew here prior to the 2003 Cedar Fire did not survive.

About halfway up the trail, you can gaze down on Cuyamaca Reservoir to the north, its water level and extent varying according to the season and the year's precipitation. When it is full, water covers nearly 1,000 acres.

When you reach the top of the switchbacks, turn right and continue south toward the summit. Soon you arrive at the base of the granite cap that crowns the peak. The trail veers right onto that rock, and goes up some rough steps (with a guardrail) to the top. Small children may need assistance on this last airy segment.

The main Cuyamaca massif stands taller in the west, blocking views of the coastline, but the foreground panorama of the park's rolling topography is impressive enough. Patches of meadow along the streamcourses and the bald grassland areas below change color with the seasons: green in spring, yellow in summer, brown or gray in fall, and occasionally white with fallen snow in winter. The recovering forests below will probably appear different from year to year as they mature.

Swallows or swifts may buzz the Stonewall summit like miniature fighter jets, and larger birds, such as ravens, hawks, and even bald eagles, may cruise by. Eagles, along with egrets, herons, and ospreys, are sometimes attracted to the shoreline of nearby Cuyamaca Reservoir, especially in winter.

Descend 0.2 mile to the junction you passed on the way up. The way you came is the shortest way down. However, if you would like to make an enjoyable loop that is a mile longer, go straight on a trail that descends to the Los Caballos equestrian camp. Then turn left onto the California Riding and Hiking Trail and left again onto the Cold Stream Trail, which leads you back to the Stonewall Trailhead.

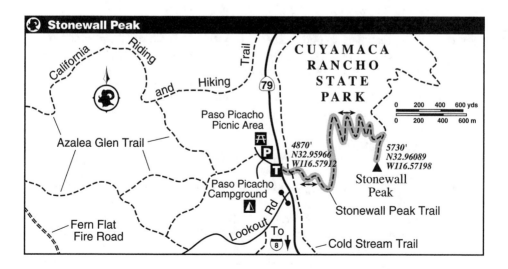

HIKE 88

Horsethief Canyon

Location	Pine Creek Wilderness
Highlights	Cascades and shallow pools
Distance	3.2 miles (out-and-back) (to Pine Valley Creek)
Total Elevation Gain/Loss	500'/500'
Hiking Time	2 hours
Optional Maps	Tom Harrison Maps San Diego Backcountry or USGS 7.5-minute *Barrett Lake* and *Viejas Mountain*
Best Times	November–June
Agency	CNF/DD
Difficulty	Moderate
Trail Use	Good for kids, dogs allowed, suitable for backpacking
Permit	Pine Creek Wilderness permit required to stay overnight

The croak of a raven cracks the stillness as we saunter down the green-fringed path. A groggy dragonfly flits through a beam of morning sunlight. Cool air, slinking down the night-chilled slopes, caresses our faces and sets aflutter the papery sycamore leaves overhead. Approaching the pools and cascades of Pine Valley Creek, we smell the moist exudations of mule-fat and willow trees. We cup the clear, cold water in our palms and dash it across our heads.

If you want this kind of escape from the city—and you want it relatively quickly—Pine Creek Wilderness, east of San Diego, is a great place to find it. The 13,000-acre wilderness, in the Cleveland National Forest, was created by an act of Congress in 1984 and now includes about 25 miles of hiking trails within its borders. Hiking in this wilderness does not require a permit, though you must obtain a permit to stay overnight. The quickest and most impressive route into it is by way of Horsethief Canyon.

Average or better winter rains followed by spring sunshine transform the place into a foothill garden, with water dancing down the larger ravines and careening off boulders in Pine Valley Creek, the large drainage bisecting the

wilderness. The tough chaparral vegetation coating the slopes gets to looking temporarily soft, the green of emerging annual grasses turns positively lurid, and the live oaks, sycamores, and cottonwoods send out new leaves and branches in a burst of growth.

Pine Creek Wilderness is only a dozen miles from the Mexican border. Migrants and smugglers sometimes pass through the area. The US Forest Service recommends hiking in a group and staying on designated trails.

To Reach the Trailhead: From I-8 at Alpine (Exit 30), follow Tavern Road 2.7 miles south, Japatul Road 7.3 miles east, and Lyons Valley Road 1.5 miles south to the trailhead. The large lot is adjacent to a sign for the Japatul Fire Station. From Jamul, in south San Diego County, drive east and north, using Skyline Truck Trail and Lyons Valley Road, to get to the same point.

Description: From the trailhead parking lot, hike east and then north along a gated dirt road for 0.25 mile. You then veer right down a ravine on the signed Espinosa Trail. After a fast 400-foot elevation loss over 0.5 mile, the path reaches an unsigned junction on the canyon bottom with a side trail leading north into the canyon. Turn right (east) to stay on the main path into the oak- and sycamore-lined Horsethief Canyon. True to its name, horse thieves stashed stolen horses in this corral-like cavern in the late 1800s in preparation for their passage across the international border.

The canyon bottom is dry most of the year. In July 2006, 16,000 acres in and around the Pine Creek Wilderness burned in the Horse Fire, which was started by an abandoned campfire. The chaparral has largely recovered, but charred limbs beneath the new growth offer a reminder of the conflagration. In 0.7 mile, pass an unsigned side trail on the right near Pine Valley Creek. Shortly thereafter, you arrive at the creek, which in winter and early spring brims with runoff from its headwaters in the Laguna Mountains.

Upstream from the pool, you can make your way alongside or over a jumble of car-size boulders and past several small cascades. Tangled willows and mule-fat (a willow look-alike) impede your progress.

Watch your step on slippery slabs of rock, and be aware of poison-oak thickets, possible rattlesnakes, and fast water if your visit comes immediately on the heels of a big storm. You can continue in this manner—straight up the canyon bottom—for 3 picturesque miles or more.

If you would rather make a loop hike, you can return to the junction you just passed and follow the unmarked trail south along Pine Valley Creek. This is not an official US Forest Service trail and is unmaintained, so be prepared to turn back if it has become overgrown. In 0.8 mile, after rounding the hill on the right, the trail starts to veer away from the creek. You may notice a lightly used track on the left returning toward the creek, but stay right and begin climbing the drainage on a long-abandoned roadbed. In 0.5 mile, cross the usually dry wash, then stay left at a junction with a faint now-closed trail. Upon reaching the ridgeline, the trail turns right and returns to the parking area. This variation is 4 miles for the complete loop.

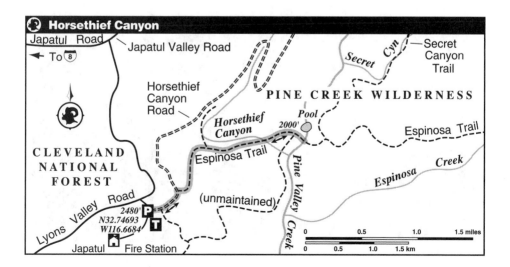

HIKE 89

Corte Madera Mountain

Location	South of Pine Valley
Highlights	Panoramic views
Distance	7 miles (out-and-back)
Total Elevation Gain/Loss	1,750'/1,750'
Hiking Time	4 hours
Optional Maps	USGS 7.5-minute *Morena Reservoir* and *Descanso*
Best Times	November–May
Agency	CNF/DD
Difficulty	Moderately strenuous
Trail Use	Suitable for backpacking, dogs allowed

On a clear day atop Corte Madera Mountain, you can see forever—or at least as far as Santa Catalina and San Clemente Islands to the west and the mile-high Sierra Juarez plateau in Baja California to the south. From many parts of San Diego, Corte Madera Mountain's sheer south face appears as an abrupt drop in the profile of the eastern horizon. On the summit, you stand near the edge of that 300-foot-high precipice.

You may see signs about seasonal closures to protect raptors nesting on the cliffs of Corte Madera. These closures impact rock climbers but do not presently affect visitors using this trail to the summit.

To Reach the Trailhead: To reach the hike's starting point, take I-8 to Exit 51/Buckman Springs Road, and go 3.5 miles south to Corral Canyon Road. Turn right (west), and go 4.8 miles on narrow pavement to a sharp hairpin turn. Unsigned, gated Kernan Road goes northwest from the hairpin. Park at a turnout just beyond Kernan.

Description: Begin at a trail marker to the left of the gate, and walk 0.5 mile uphill

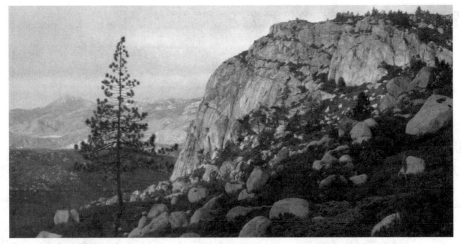

Corte Madera Mountain

on Kernan Road. Where the road bends right in a horseshoe curve, go left on the Espinosa Trail and continue northwest. The trail initially leads under coast live oaks along the creek and then climbs through scrub oak. In 1.0 mile, you top a saddle and intersect Los Pinos Road. Turn right and continue 0.3 mile to another saddle, a half mile southeast of boulder-studded, Coulter-pine-dotted Peak 4588. Decent camping can be found here. Leave the road, and find and follow a path that works its way up through manzanita and huge boulders past Peak 4588.

Continue following the path northwest, passing a clearing with fine views and more camping options. Climb over two more minor bumps. When the route occasionally becomes obscure, watch for cairns marking the trail. The view north includes a fabulous vista—available nowhere else on public land—of privately owned Corte Madera Valley. A beautiful lake and oak-studded meadows fill the valley. The name Corte Madera ("woodyard") apparently refers to the use of this area as a source of timber during the building of the San Diego area missions.

Finally veer southwest and climb to Corte Madera Mountain's summit, where you may find a cairn and summit register. From the southernmost point on the plateau you can peer over the abrupt face into the canyon drained by Espinosa Creek. To the southeast is Los Pinos Mountain, topped by a fire lookout, one of the few remaining in Southern California that is used on a regular basis.

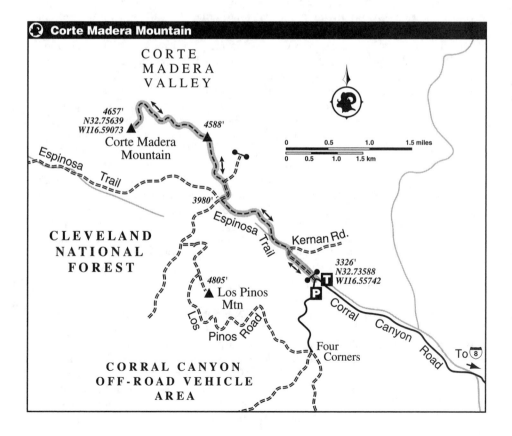

HIKE 90

Noble Canyon Trail

Location	Laguna Mountains
Highlights	Sparkling mountain stream and wildflowers
Distance	10 miles (one way)
Total Elevation Gain/Loss	750'/2,500'
Hiking Time	5 hours
Optional Maps	Laguna Mountain Recreation Area map, Tom Harrison Maps San Diego Backcountry, or USGS 7.5-minute *Monument Peak, Mount Laguna,* and *Descanso*
Best Times	October–June
Agency	CNF/DD
Difficulty	Moderately strenuous
Trail Use	Suitable for backpacking and mountain bikes, dogs allowed

The Noble Canyon National Recreation Trail is an extension and reworking of an older trail built across the Laguna Mountains in the 1930s by the Civilian Conservation Corps. Since its completion in 1982, it has become popular among hikers, equestrians, and especially mountain bikers. With transportation arrangements set up in advance, you can travel one-way along this trail in the relatively easy downhill direction.

The route is a good one for backpacking, with suitable campsites located at frequent intervals along the way, particularly on shady terraces midway through Noble Canyon. (Remember to establish your camp at least 100 feet from water). Water flows in the canyon bottom year-round, though it slows to a trickle before the first rains of autumn. Purification is necessary if you intend to rely on it for your drinking or cooking.

To Reach the Trailhead: To hike downhill, first stash a getaway vehicle at the lower Noble Canyon Trailhead at Pine Creek Road. From I-8, take Exit 45 for Pine Creek Road. Go north to a T-junction where you turn left on Old Highway 80. In 1.2 miles, turn hard right onto Pine Creek Road. Go 1.6 miles and turn right into the signed trailhead parking area. You must display a National Forest Adventure Pass to park here.

Now, drive up to the Penny Pines Trailhead in the Laguna Mountains. If windy, dirt Pine Creek Road gate is open (check with the Cleveland National Forest or drive up and look), you might be able to make this slow but scenic short-cut straight up the mountainside to the Penny Pines Trailhead. But the certain way is to return to Old Highway 80 and follow it 2.6 miles east to Sunrise Highway (County Route S1). Turn left and go 14 miles to the trailhead parking on the shoulder at mile marker 17.3. You must display an Adventure Pass in the vehicle you park here too.

Description: From the Penny Pines Trailhead, head west along the marked Noble Canyon Trail, along the southern border of the burn caused by the 2003 Cedar Fire. The catastrophic blaze was ignited by a lost hunter whose signal fire got out of control. Driven by fierce Santa Ana winds that were simultaneously fanning 14 other

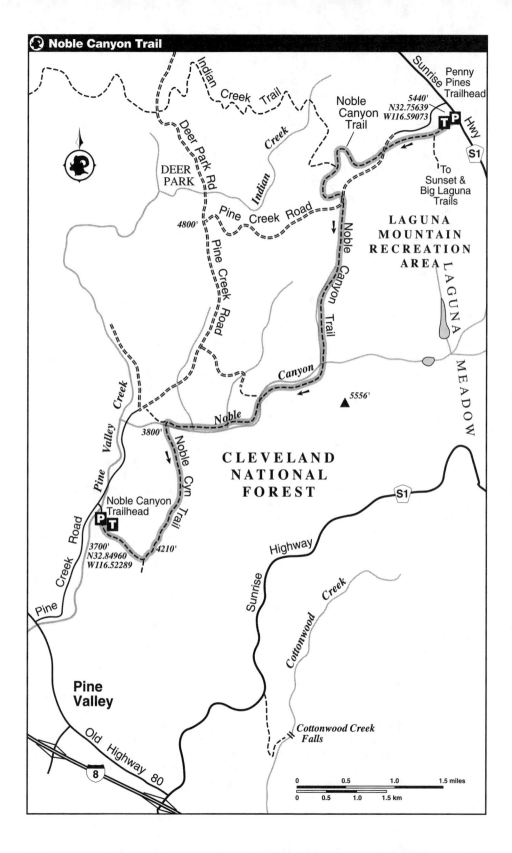

Indian Creek Trail

Deer Park Rd

Deer Creek

DEER PARK

Indian Creek

Pine Creek Road

4800'

Pine Creek Road

Sunrise Hwy

Penny Pines Trailhead

Noble Canyon Trail

5440'
N32.75639
W116.59073

T **P**

S1

To Sunset & Big Laguna Trails

LAGUNA MOUNTAIN RECREATION AREA

Noble Canyon Trail

Canyon

Noble

Canyon

3800'

Noble Cyn Trail

5556'

▲

LAGUNA MEADOW

S1

CLEVELAND NATIONAL FOREST

Noble Canyon Trailhead

P **T**

3700'
N32.84960
W116.52289

4210'

Pine Valley Creek

Pine Creek Road

Pine

Highway

Sunrise

Cottonwood Creek

Pine Valley

Cottonwood Creek Falls

Old Highway 80

8

0	0.5	1.0	1.5 miles
0	0.5	1.0	1.5 km

major wildfires in Southern California, the Cedar Fire grew to consume 280,278 acres, killing 15 people and destroying 2,232 homes. The Laguna Mountains were another of the casualties of the fire, and you can see some of the scars and recovery process along this leg of the hike.

Pass a spur on the left leading to Laguna Meadow. As you rise a bit along the north slope of a steep hill, your view to the north extends to the distant summits of San Jacinto Peak and San Gorgonio Mountain. You descend to cross dirt Pine Canyon Road three times in quick succession and then climb and circle around the chaparral-clad north end of a north-south-trending ridge. This seemingly out-of-the-way excursion avoids privately owned inholdings in the national forest, and it opens up interesting vistas to the north and west. Three varieties of blooming ceanothus brighten the view in springtime. At 2.2 miles, pass the Indian Creek Trail on the right, then cross to the south side of Pine Creek Road.

Next, you descend into the upper reaches of Noble Canyon, where you exit the Cedar Fire burned zone. After a wet season, the grassy hillsides show off springtime blooms of blue-purple beard tongue, scarlet bugler, woolly blue curls, yellow monkeyflower, Indian paintbrush, wallflower, white forget-me-not, wild hyacinth, yellow violet, phacelia, golden yarrow, checker, lupine, and blue flax.

The trail sidles up to the creek at about 3.0 miles and stays beside it for the next 4 miles. At 4.3 miles, past a canopy of live oaks, black oaks, and Jeffrey pines, the trail briefly braids, and you cross the creek and emerge into a steep, sunlit section of canyon. The trail cuts through chaparral on the east wall, while on the west wall only a few hardy, drought-tolerant plants cling to outcrops of schist rock.

Back in the shade of oaks again, you soon cross a major tributary creek from the east that drains the Laguna lakes and Laguna Meadow above. Pause for a

while in this shady glen, where the water flows over somber, grayish granitic rock and gathers in languid pools bedecked by sword and bracken fern. Look for nodding yellow Humboldt lilies in the late spring or early summer.

You continue through oak woodland and riparian vegetation for some distance downstream. Mixed in with the oaks, you'll discover some incense-cedar and California bay trees. The creek is screened by a typical growth of willows and sycamores. The understory vegetation includes dense thickets of poison oak, Indian-basket bush, wild rose, and wild strawberries.

If you look carefully, you may discover some mining debris, the remnants of a flume and the stones of a disassembled arrastra (a horse- or mule-drawn machine for crushing ore), dating from gold-mining activity in the late 1800s. Old cabin foundations are also in evidence.

Crossing to the west side of the creek at 5.7 miles, you break out of the trees and into an open area with sage scrub and chaparral vegetation. A fork on the right eventually leads to an old roadbed, but your trip turns left and continues downstream. The trail contours to a point about 100 feet above the creek and then maintains this course as it bends around several small tributaries, open to the midday sunshine nearly the whole way. Yucca, prickly-pear cactus, and even hedgehog cactus—normally a denizen of the desert—make appearances here. Keep an eye out for an old hillside adit in a while, but remember that abandoned mines are never safe to explore.

At 7.7 miles, the trail switches back, crosses the Noble Canyon Creek for the last time, and veers up a tributary canyon to the south. Cross a low saddle and veer right (west) at an unsigned junction in 1.7 miles. Cross the ridgeline and descend along a particularly rocky course (tough on mountain bikes, but not too bad for hikers) directly to the Noble Canyon Trailhead near Pine Creek Road.

HIKE 91

Garnet Peak

Location	Laguna Mountains
Highlights	Outstanding desert views
Distance	2.4 miles (out-and-back)
Total Elevation Gain/Loss	500'/500'
Hiking Time	1½ hours
Optional Maps	Laguna Mountain Recreation Area map, Tom Harrison Maps San Diego Backcountry, or USGS 7.5-minute *Monument Peak*
Best Times	All year
Agency	CNF/DD
Difficulty	Moderate
Trail Use	Good for kids, dogs allowed

Although Garnet Peak isn't the highest peaklet along the Laguna Mountain rim, its exposed position makes it a good place to view both the pine-clad Laguna plateau and the raw desert below. Especially rewarding is a predawn pilgrimage to observe the sunrise from its summit. Around the winter solstice, the sun's flattened disk peeps up over the desert wastes of northwestern Sonora, Mexico, some 150 miles away. On the clearest mornings at that time of year, you might witness the famed green flash, an event occasionally seen on the horizon at sunset on the coast, but seldom seen at sunrise anywhere.

To Reach the Trailhead: Just east of Pine Valley, exit I-8 at Sunrise Highway (County Route S1) and turn north. As you drive uphill, observe the green mile markers posted at half-mile intervals along the Sunrise Highway shoulder. They increase from approximately mile 13 at the I-8 and Sunrise Highway interchange. Find a place to park off the pavement of Sunrise Highway near mile 27.8, and find the

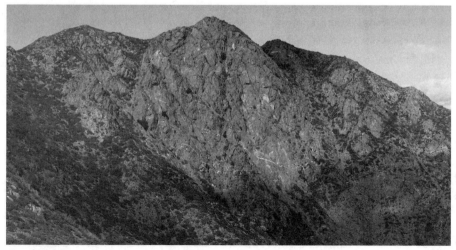

Garnet Peak

start of the Garnet Peak Trail on the right (east) side of the highway. Be sure to post a National Forest Adventure Pass on your parked car.

As this book was going to press, the July 2013 Chariot Fire burned through this area. If you plan to visit soon after, call to confirm that the trail is open.

Description: Follow the Garnet Peak Trail 0.5 mile north through burned timber to where it crosses the Pacific Crest Trail. The area you are traversing was where the eastward-moving Cedar Fire of 2003 met the edge of the burn area of 2002's Pines Fire and essentially died due to lack of fuel.

Continue north, away from the burned timber and onto a rocky path that slants up along the shoulder of the peak. Ceanothus, manzanita, and yucca have recovered vigorously, evolved to prosper in the never-ending cycle of fire and regeneration. Garnet Peak's summit is crowned by a jagged cluster of layered, tan-colored metasedimentary rock, the type seen along much of the Laguna escarpment. The peak falls away abruptly to the east and south, revealing a vertiginous panorama of Storm Canyon and its distant alluvial fan. Along the horizon lie the Salton Sea and Baja's Laguna Salada, both desert sinks. To the south and west, the Laguna crest, dusky with patches of pine and oak trees and chaparral, seems to roll like a frozen wave to the edge of the escarpment.

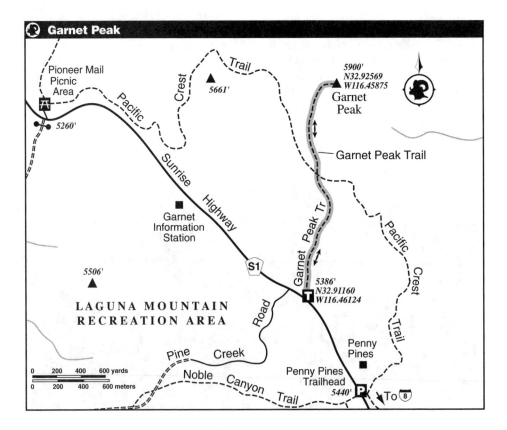

HIKE 92

Sunset Trail

Location	Laguna Mountains
Highlight	Colorful spring and autumn vegetation and views
Distance	7 miles (loop)
Total Elevation Gain/Loss	700'/700'
Hiking Time	3½ hours
Optional Maps	Laguna Mountain Recreation Area map, Tom Harrison Maps San Diego Backcountry, or USGS 7.5-minute *Monument Peak* and *Mount Laguna*
Best Times	September–June
Agency	CNF/DD
Difficulty	Moderately strenuous
Trail Use	Good for kids, dogs allowed

The Sunset Trail, opened in 1993, permits easy access by foot along the west rim of the high Laguna Mountain plateau. Like its analogue a few miles east, the sunrise-facing Pacific Crest Trail, the Sunset Trail offers fine panoramas, but on the sunset side of the mountain. Early mornings are by far best (certainly during the warm summer season) to take advantage of cool temperatures and clear, tangy air. In the hour or two after sunrise, you can often look down upon a white and frothy ocean of stratus clouds hugging a hundred-mile strip of coastline.

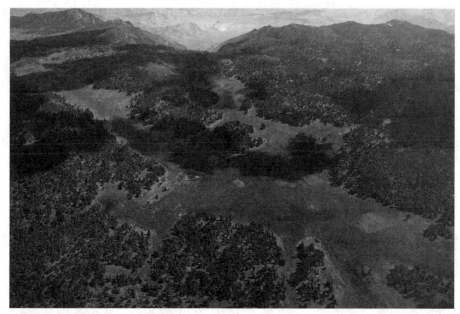

Aerial view of Big Laguna Meadow

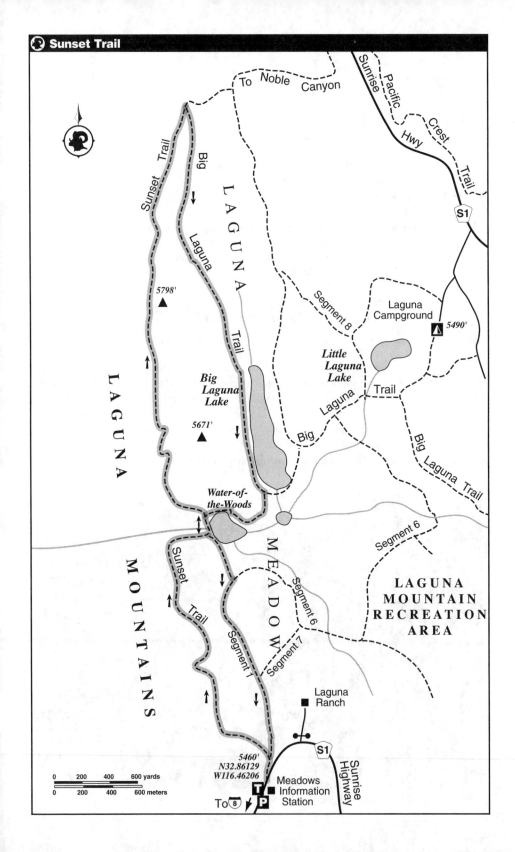

To Noble Canyon

Sunrise

Pacific

Crest

Trail

Hwy

S1

Sunset Trail

Big

Laguna

Trail

L A G U N A

Segment 8

Laguna
Campground

△ 5490'

5798'
▲

*Little
Laguna
Lake*

L A G U N A

*Big
Laguna
Lake*

5671'
▲

Trail

Big

Laguna

Big Laguna Trail

*Water-of-
the-Woods*

M O U N T A I N S

Sunset

Trail

M E A D O W

Segment 6

**L A G U N A
M O U N T A I N
R E C R E A T I O N
A R E A**

Segment 6

Segment 7

Segment 1

Laguna
Ranch

■

5460'
N32.86129
W116.46206

S1

Sunrise
Highway

Meadows
Information
Station

T ■
P

To ⑧

0   200   400   600 yards

0   200   400   600 meters

To Reach the Trailhead: From I-8 just east of Pine Valley, drive about 5 miles uphill along Sunrise Highway. At or near the Meadows Information Station, mile 19.1, park along the highway shoulder, which is wide enough in this area to accommodate parking by visitors who come up by the hundreds in winter to play in the snow.

Description: From the information station, walk a little way uphill along the highway shoulder to reach the trailhead, marked by a wooden sign. Stay left on the main trail at an unmarked fork in 80 yards. In 0.1 mile, stay left again at a junction with the Big Laguna Trail. You will loop back to this junction when you return.

Gradually climb toward a gently undulating ridge crest dotted with vanilla-scented Jeffrey pines and black oaks. After nearly a mile, the trail suddenly veers left to circle a rocky outcrop. There, a view opens of velvet-smooth Crouch Valley, some 500 feet below, and much of coastal San Diego County whenever clear air prevails at lower altitudes. The view is certainly worth the trivial effort you have invested so far.

Onward, you descend gradually for a while, then rise again, reaching (at 1.7 miles) the lowermost edge of Laguna Meadow and a beautiful pond called Water-of-the-Woods. Veering left, the Sunset Trail follows the edge of the pond for a short while and then slants up the ridge to the left (northwest).

You climb back up to the viewful crest, with more opportunities to scan the broad western horizon including Cuyamaca and Stonewall Peaks. Farther north, you pass over a hilltop with views to Garnet Peak, Toro Peak, San Jacinto, and San Gorgonio. Descend to the northernmost arm of Laguna Meadow. Turning east, the trail meets, at 3.7 miles, the Big Laguna Trail. Beware that the Big Laguna Trail is not a single path but actually a complex network of trails in the vicinity of Laguna Meadow. Pay attention to the map to take the proper forks.

Turn right on the Big Laguna Trail, and follow it south about 1.5 miles to Big Laguna Lake, the biggest of several shallow, ephemeral lakes in the meadow. In an average rainy season, these lakes begin to fill with water or snow by December or January. By April or May, as the meadow dries, carpets of wildflowers—tidy tips, buttercups, goldfields, dandelions, wild onions, and western irises—begin to appear. Summer heat causes water levels in the lakes to decline rapidly.

Just past Big Laguna Lake the Big Laguna Trail forks. The left fork leads to the far side of the lake, but you continue straight on the path that returns to Water-of-the-Woods. At the southwest corner of the lake where you originally arrived by the Sunset Trail, turn left on an unsigned segment of the Big Laguna Trail.

When you reach the south end of the meadow, the Big Laguna Trail forks again. Segment 6 leads left (east), but you continue straight on Segment 1 toward Sunrise Highway. Continue straight again at another fork where Segment 7 turns left. Soon you will arrive back at the junction with the Sunset Trail near where you began your hike.

HIKE 93

Culp Valley

Location	Northern Anza-Borrego Desert State Park
Highlights	Secluded, oasislike spring and desert views
Distance	1.7 miles (loop)
Total Elevation Gain/Loss	300'/300'
Hiking Time	1 hour
Optional Map	USGS 7.5-minute *Tubb Canyon*
Best Times	September–June
Agency	ABDSP
Difficulty	Easy
Trail Use	Good for kids

While the low desert swelters, the temperature hovers within a more moderate register at Culp Valley, 3,000 feet higher, the only designated camping area in the Anza-Borrego Desert where the heat on the cooler days of May, June, or September is bearable. July and August daytime temperatures there, typically in the 90s and 100s, are probably too warm for most people's tastes.

Stark, gray boulders are piled up all around the floor of Culp Valley, thrusting upward into an azure sky. The west wind blows capriciously, often whistling eerily through the rocks. Nearby, out of sight from the valley, is a hillside spring surrounded by an oasis of green grass and shrubs. It's this kind of contrast that makes hiking here especially rewarding.

To Reach the Starting Point: About 4 miles east of Ranchita or 9 miles west of Borrego Springs, drive to mile 9.2 (according to the green mileage signs posted every half mile) on County Route S22, Montezuma Highway. Turn north onto the unpaved entrance road leading into the no-frills Culp Valley Campground. The campground is free, with restrooms and several scattered open spaces where you can park your car or small RV, day or night.

Description: On foot from the campground head back toward the highway, and take the road branching west toward Pena Spring. After a few minutes, the road surmounts a crest and then ends. A sign at the far end of the lot indicates the start of the California Riding and Hiking Trail (CRHT) and the path to Pena Spring.

The start of the trail is confusing. You may see a clear path on the left and a less well-defined path going down a shallow ravine to the right. Take the ravine trail. If your trail turns left and begins climbing, you are on the westbound CRHT, which is the wrong path.

In 0.1 mile, reach an unmarked junction where the eastbound CRHT veers right and begins climbing, but you stay left and continue down the sandy ravine. Note this intersection; you will return here after you visit the spring.

Going downhill for 0.2 mile, you pass into the burn zone of the August 2002 Pines Fire, which managed to lick its way northeast into the remote Hellhole and Borrego Palm Canyons farther northeast before dying out due to lack of anything further to burn.

On the hillside to the left look for Pena Spring, an oozing acre or so nourishing a verdant patch of green grass and fire-following vegetation. The spring is a nocturnal mecca for rabbits, coyotes, deer, bighorn sheep, and other animals partaking of the clear, cold groundwater reaching the surface here. Nearby, look for a large, flat boulder pocked with several deep *morteros*, or American Indian grinding holes.

After visiting the spring, backtrack up the road 0.2 mile to the CRHT. Turn left (east) on this trail, climbing up and then along a flattish ridge that offers good views of nearby Culp Valley on the right and tantalizing glimpses of the deep gorge on the left, Hellhole Canyon. The ridge hasn't burned recently, so you'll find juniper, cat's claw acacia, desert apricot, buckwheat, white sage, Gander and prickly pear cacti, and Mojave and Lord's candle yucca—collectively representing a transition zone between montane chaparral and high-desert scrub.

After 0.4 mile on the CRHT, you come to a trail junction in a saddle. To return to Culp Valley, veer right and continue 0.3 mile south into the campground. Before doing that, it's worth the 75-yard detour to a scenic outlook on the left, where you get a jaw-dropping view of the Hellhole Canyon gorge, Borrego Valley, and the towering Santa Rosa Mountains. About 0.2 mile farther southeast a slightly higher vista point on a hilltop offers a better panorama.

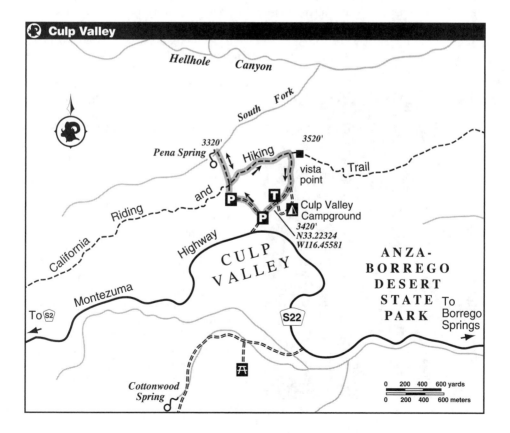

HIKE 94

Hellhole Canyon

Location	Northern Anza-Borrego Desert State Park
Highlight	Hidden waterfall in desert canyon
Distance	5.0 miles (out-and-back)
Total Elevation Gain/Loss	900'/900'
Hiking Time	3½ hours
Optional Map	USGS 7.5-minute *Tubb Canyon*
Best Times	December–May
Agency	ABDSP
Difficulty	Moderately strenuous
Trail Use	Suitable for backpacking, good for kids

In the midst of one of the hottest and driest deserts in the United States, it feels surprising to find a place where mosses, ferns, sycamores, and cottonwoods flourish around a sparkling waterfall in a palm oasis. Maidenhair Falls is such a place, and it lies not far from Borrego Springs and the popular Anza-Borrego Desert State Park Visitor Center.

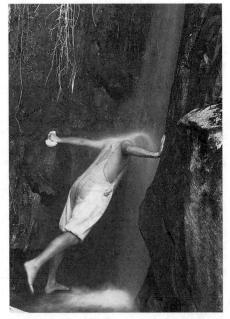

Maidenhair Falls cool-off

To Reach the Trailhead: From Christmas Circle (the traffic circle in the center of Borrego Springs), drive 1.3 miles west on Palm Canyon Drive to Montezuma Highway (County Route S22), and go south 0.7 mile to the large trailhead parking area on the west side of Montezuma Highway.

Description: From the parking lot, head west on a wide trail (an old roadbed) straight across and up an alluvial fan toward the gaping mouth of Hellhole Canyon. In 0.2 mile, pass a four-way junction. The California Riding and Hiking Trail goes left toward Culp Valley, and a 0.8-mile trail goes right to the visitors center. The sandy surface of the fan supports a variety of vegetation, stratified according to elevation. Indigo bush, chuparosa, cheesebush, burroweed, creosote bush, desert lavender, and Gander cholla are the common plant species of the lower fan. They're largely replaced by jojoba, brittlebush, ocotillo, and teddybear cholla on the upper fan. Everywhere, jackrabbits flit among the bushes, startled by your approach. Families with children should be especially cautious around the cholla, whose fallen segments seem to jump from the ground and latch on to careless passersby!

As you approach the canyon mouth, a mile from the trailhead, you may hear (in a wet year at least) the sound of flowing water. Usually the water doesn't get very far on the surface; it quickly sinks into porous sand as it spreads out and slows on the fan below. At 1.6 miles, cross the wash for the second time where the canyon walls pinch in. You soon find yourself threading a path near the flowing water. This route once involved difficult scrambling over large boulders and fallen trees, but a decent trail has formed thanks to heavy use in recent years. Watch for cat's claw acacia that still grows close to the path. Fan palms—the signature tree of the Anza-Borrego Desert—begin to appear. Watch for a deep *mortero* (a grinding hole used by the American Indians) in a granite boulder on the trail near the first palms.

In another 0.5 mile, reach the main palm grove in the Hellhole Canyon oasis. About 200 yards past a dense cluster of palms, the canyon walls pinch in really tight and rock scrambling becomes inevitable. Tucked away in a corner of the canyon bottom—hard to find—you'll discover the grotto containing Maidenhair Falls. The falls plunge about 25 feet into a shallow pool. Tiers of maidenhair fern adorn the grotto, and sopping wet mosses cover the places the ferns don't.

Traveling up-canyon from Maidenhair Falls involves battling with boulders and the underbrush—slow going on a day hike and slower if you're carrying a backpack. Ambitious hikers can explore the canyon's remote higher reaches. Some hikers have traveled up the canyon's South Fork tributary, which leads to Pena Spring near Culp Valley.

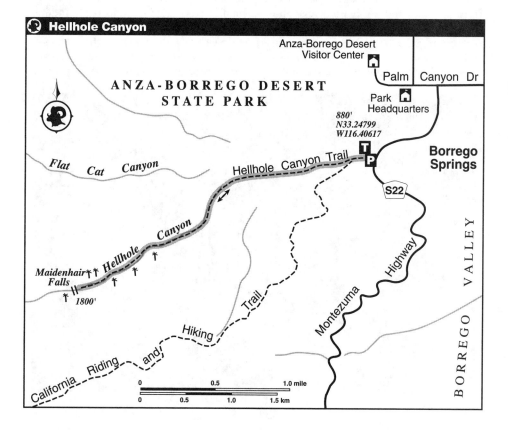

HIKE 95

Borrego Palm Canyon

Location	Northern Anza-Borrego Desert State Park
Highlights	Spring wildflowers and most dramatic display of native palms in California
Distance	2.9 miles (out-and-back)
Total Elevation Gain/Loss	450'/450'
Hiking Time	1½ hours
Optional Maps	Tom Harrison Maps San Diego Backcountry or USGS 7.5-minute *Borrego Palm Canyon*
Best Times	October–May
Agency	ABDSP
Difficulty	Easy
Trail Use	Good for kids

Borrego Palm Canyon has long been famous for harboring many hundreds of native palm trees in an otherwise austere setting of rock and sun-blasted vegetation. Perhaps 80% of these palms, which have surprised and delighted thousands of visitors over several decades, were summarily evicted from the canyon at 4:45 p.m. on September 10, 2004. On that afternoon an isolated, intense summer thunderstorm dumped buckets of rain over a relatively small area of the San Ysidro Mountains above. Sheets of water falling down the steep slopes gathered strength and speed as they joined forces in the narrow constriction of the canyon. A wall of water

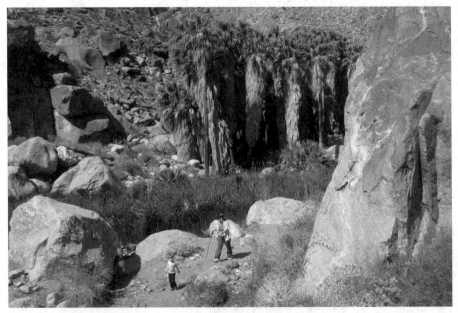

First Grove

perhaps 30 feet high tore away nearly everything in its path.

Borrego Palm Canyon Campground was hit soon after with a roiling mass of muddy water, carrying palm trunks and other debris, about 100 feet wide and moving at least 40 miles per hour. Witnesses ran for higher ground or escaped down the campground's entrance road in speeding cars. Ironically, not a drop of rain fell that day in Borrego Springs, just 3 miles away.

Dubbed a hundred-year flash flood by some, the event was a rare occurrence for that particular location in the Anza-Borrego Desert, but it was not unusual for the geographical region as a whole. Isolated and locally intense thunderstorms commonly strike the Anza-Borrego and Colorado Deserts from mid-July through mid-September, during the "monsoon" season.

Since the 2004 flash flood, Borrego Palm Canyon Campground's facilities have been repaired, and hikers are again making their way up the Borrego Palm Canyon Nature Trail to what remains of the First Palm Grove just inside the canyon's lower portal. You can learn more about California desert flora on that trail than anywhere else around Anza-Borrego. Be sure to pick up the interpretive leaflet for the trail at the Anza-Borrego Visitor Center or when you enter Borrego Palm Canyon Campground. The nature trail begins at the far end of the campground.

To Reach the Trailhead: From Christmas Circle (the traffic circle in the center of Borrego Springs), drive 1.4 miles west on Palm Canyon Drive toward the Anza-Borrego Visitor Center. Just before reaching the visitor center, turn right on the access road leading into Borrego Palm Canyon Campground. At the gate, pay the day-use or camping fee; then proceed to the Borrego Palm Canyon Trailhead at far west end of the campground. Next to the trailhead are restrooms, a drinking fountain, and a pond holding transplanted desert pupfish.

Description: Pick up a brochure at the trailhead with the key to the numbered interpretive markers lining the main nature trail, which roughly parallels the canyon bottom and measures about 1.5 miles along its revised alignment. Also, bring plenty of water; the trail is continuously exposed to the sun.

The main trail's initial crossing of canyon bottom lets you inspect the flood-torn riverbed, which may be wet or dry, depending on recent rainfall. You then ascend moderately on the rocky alluvial fan toward the canyon's mouth. Huge palm logs lay scattered across the canyon where they were left by the torrent. You'll see mesquite, sage, cat's claw acacia, indigo bush, desert lavender, creosote bush, brittlebush, ocotillo, desert-willow, chuparosa, and beavertail, Gander, and barrel cactus. This vegetation looks drab most of the year, but it really lights up in a rainbow of colors by March in a wet year. In the past couple of decades, the native bighorn sheep that frequent the canyon have become quite accustomed to passing hikers. Sometimes they may graze contentedly only a stone's throw from the trail.

As you approach the canyon's narrow mouth, desert-varnished rock walls soar dramatically 3,000 feet upward on both sides. Cross to the south side of the creek, where you find a junction with an alternate trail. Stay out of the alluring creekbed to give the vegetation a chance to regenerate. The trail climbs some steps (believed to have been built in the 1930s by the Civilian Conservation Corps), crosses the creek twice more, and arrives at First Grove. Although a ghost of its former self, it remains quite attractive, with a cluster of large palms and many young ones sprouting nearby. They are of one variety, *Washingtonia filifera*, the only palm indigenous to California.

The Borrego Palm Canyon Nature Trail ends at First Grove. Further exploration of canyon ahead is not for casual tourists. The game is to work your way upward on sketchy paths high above the canyon bed or more often along the flood-scoured bed itself, which is paved unevenly with sand and flood-tossed rocks and granitic or metamorphic bedrock slabs. As riparian vegetation returns to the canyon bottom in the years to come, it will increasingly slow the pace of intrepid hikers.

At 3.3 miles from the trailhead, the South Fork of Borrego Palm Canyon branches obviously to the left (southwest), its discharge of water less than that of the main fork. A spectacular double-cascade of water lies 0.4 mile ahead up this rough gorge and makes a worthy destination for motivated hikers willing to clamber over angular rocks.

On your return, you might choose to take the alternate trail, which follows the ocotillo-dotted slopes above the wash. The rocky route is recommended only for those enjoy some boulder-hopping.

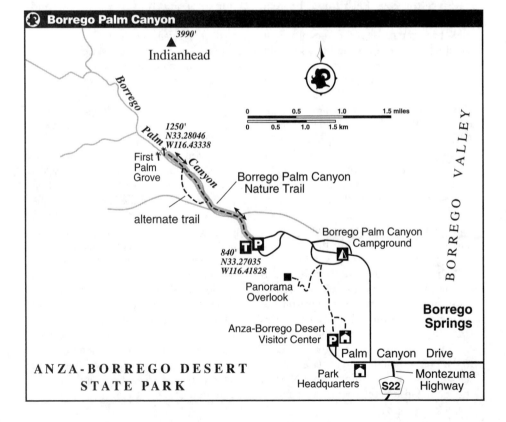

HIKE 96

Villager Peak

Location	Northern Anza-Borrego Desert State Park
Highlights	Ever-present dramatic views
Distance	13 miles (out-and-back)
Total Elevation Gain/Loss	5,000'/5,000'
Hiking Time	11 hours
Recommended Maps	USGS 7.5-minute *Fonts Point* and *Rabbit Peak*
Best Times	October–May
Agency	ABDSP
Difficulty	Very strenuous
Trail Use	Suitable for backpacking

Despite its remoteness, Villager Peak is one of the more popular destinations for "serious" Southern California peak baggers. More than a hundred people every year reach the summit, and the box containing the peak register is often overflowing with business cards and other mementos. Many people backpack the route, but others, who must start at or before sunrise, manage to complete the round-trip as a day hike. The importance of taking plenty of water on this waterless route cannot be overemphasized.

The approach to Villager Peak is straightforwardly up, using a single north-trending ridge of the Santa Rosa Mountains. One or more paralleling trails follow this ridge—the result of recent use by hikers, prehistoric use by desert-dwelling American Indians, and more or less continual use by bighorn sheep. On the way down, however, you may encounter navigational difficulties where watershed divides split and go their separate ways. Bighorn sheep don't necessarily stick to the main route, and their trails may lure you off the main ridge onto some steeply plunging side ridge. Get a good sense of your surroundings at the trailhead or bring a GPS receiver because it can be difficult to find your way back cross-country if you are caught out past dark.

To Reach the Trailhead: From Borrego Springs, drive 13 miles northeast on Borrego Salton Seaway (County Route S22). Park in the northside turnout at mile 31.8.

Description: On foot, proceed north toward the east end of a long, sandy ridge 0.5 mile away. The north face of this ridge is a huge scarp along the San Jacinto Fault—said to be one of the largest fault scarps in unconsolidated earth material in North America. North of this ridge, flash floods exiting from Rattlesnake Canyon have cut a series of braided washes in a swath about 0.6 mile wide. A faint path marked by cairns (small piles of stones) takes you over this dissected terrain to the

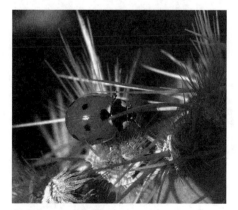
Ladybug on prickly pear cactus

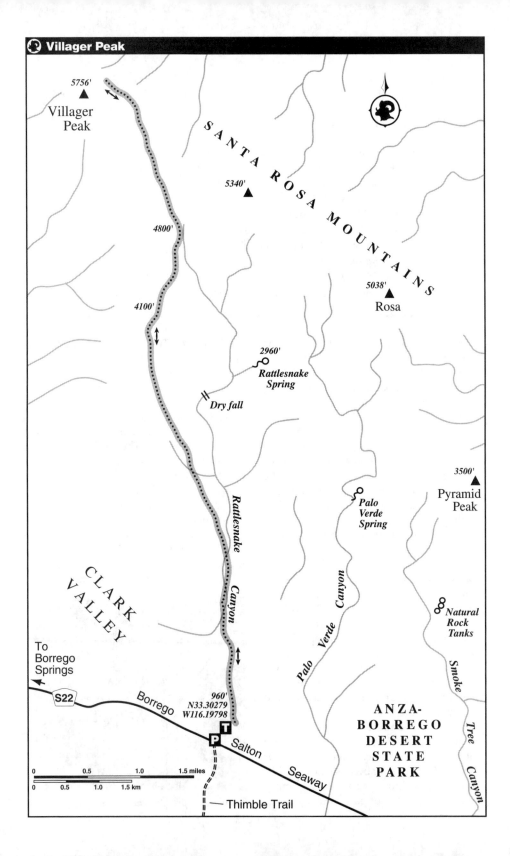

5756'
▲
Villager
Peak

S A N T A   R O S A   M O U N T A I N S

5340'
▲

4800'

4100'

5038'
▲
Rosa

2960'
○
*Rattlesnake
Spring*

Dry fall

3500'
▲
Pyramid
Peak

○
*Palo
Verde
Spring*

Rattlesnake

Canyon

○
*Natural
Rock
Tanks*

C L A R K
VALLEY

Palo   Verde   Canyon

Smoke

To
Borrego
Springs

A N Z A-
B O R R E G O
D E S E R T
S T A T E
P A R K

S22

Borrego

960'
N33.30279
W116.19798

T
P
Salton

Seaway

Tree

Canyon

0	0.5	1.0	1.5 miles
0	0.5	1.0	1.5 km

Thimble Trail

base of the long, ramplike ridge leading to Villager Peak.

The initial climb is very steep, but the route soon levels off to a rather steady gradient averaging about 1,000 feet per mile. Stay on the highest part of the ridge to remain on route. Creosote bush, ocotillo, and glistening specimens of barrel cactus, hedgehog cactus, and silver, golden, and teddy-bear cholla cactus grace the slopes below 3,000 feet. Dense thickets of wicked-looking agave at 3,000–4,000 feet will slow you down. At times, you feel as if you were threading a spiny gauntlet.

Along the lower part of the ridge you will come upon several American Indian sleeping circles, which may have been used as windbreaks or to anchor shelters made from local vegetation. At about the 3,000-foot level and 3.0 miles a green patch marking Rattlesnake Spring comes into view in a tributary canyon of Rattlesnake Canyon, about 1.5 miles east.

At 4,100 feet and 4.3 miles, you pass along the edge of a spectacular dropoff overlooking Clark Valley. The white band of rock prominently displayed along the face of this escarpment is marble, metamorphosed limestone. Thought to be some of the oldest rock exposed in San Diego County, it originated from ocean-floor sediments deposited about a half billion years ago. Just beyond the 4,800-foot contour (at 5.0 miles), the ridge descends a little to a small, exposed campsite with airy views both east and west.

In the next mile the ridgeline becomes quite jagged. Pinyon, juniper, and nolina (a cousin of the yucca) now dominate. At 6.5 miles, you reach the rounded, 5,756-foot summit of Villager Peak, offering good campsites amid a sparse forest of weather-beaten pinyon pines. The views are practically aerial all around the compass. A clear, calm, moonless night spent here is an unforgettable experience. Despite the horizon glows of cities from Los Angeles to Mexicali, the stars above shine fiercely in a charcoal sky. At dawn, the silvery surface of the Salton Sea mirrors the red glow spreading across the east horizon.

Those looking for an even more grueling expedition have been known to continue on along the undulating ridge to Rabbit Peak, the 6,640-foot hogback looming to the north. This monster climb involves a total of 21 miles and 7,900 feet of elevation gain.

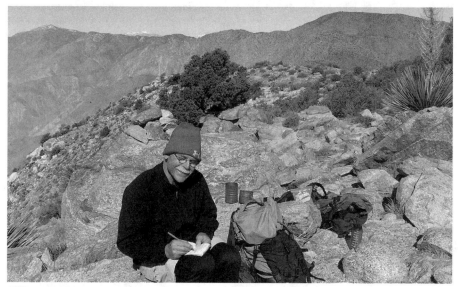

Villager Peak

HIKE 97

Calcite Mine

Location	Northern Anza-Borrego Desert State Park
Highlights	Slot canyons and historically interesting
Distance	4.2 miles (loop)
Total Elevation Gain/Loss	800'/800'
Hiking Time	2 hours
Optional Maps	Tom Harrison Maps San Diego Backcountry or USGS 7.5-minute *Seventeen Palms*
Best Times	November–April
Agency	ABDSP
Difficulty	Moderate
Trail Use	Good for kids, suitable for mountain biking

Thousands of years of cutting and polishing by water and wind erosion have produced the chaotic rock formations and slotlike ravines you'll discover in the Calcite Mine area. The highlight of this hike is, of course, the mine itself. During World War II, this was an important site—indeed the only site in the United States—for the extraction of optical-grade calcite crystals for use in gunsights. Trench-mining operations throughout the area left deep scars upon the earth, seemingly as fresh today as when they were made. The road to the mine is still passable by jeeps and other high-clearance four-wheel-drive vehicles, so you may encounter occasional traffic on your hike.

To Reach the Trailhead: From Borrego Springs, drive 13 miles northeast on Borrego-Salton Seaway (County Highway S22). Park in the roadside turnout at mile 38.0.

Description: From the turnout, walk 0.1 mile east to the Calcite jeep road intersection. An interpretive panel here gives some details about the history of the mine. Follow the jeep road as it dips into and out of South Fork Palm Wash, and continues northwest toward the southern spurs of the Santa Rosa Mountains. Ahead you will see an intricately honeycombed whitish slab of sandstone, called Locomotive Rock, which lies behind (northeast of) the mine area.

About 1.4 miles from S22, the road dips sharply to cross a deep ravine. You'll have the option of exploring it on your way back. At the road's end you may find

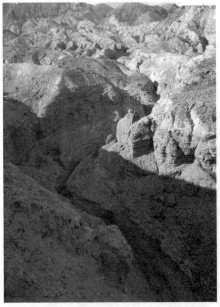

Palm Wash

bits of calcite crystal strewn about on the ground, glittering in the sunlight. You could spend a lot of time exploring the mining trenches and the pocked slabs of sandstone nearby. Palm Wash, a frightening gash in the earth, precludes travel to the east.

Adventurous hikers may enjoy making a partial loop back through the ravine, which contains one of the best slot canyons in Anza Borrego. From the upper trench of the mine, look for a use trail curving left and down toward a canyon. The canyon is deep with vertical walls, but look for a trench slicing down a weakness offering a way to scramble to the bottom. If you turn right, you will soon find the canyon blocked by a 20-foot drop jammed with two huge chockstones; only

technical climbers with proper gear could head that way. But instead, turn left and walk down the canyon. You will have to scramble down two interesting drops and several more easy ones while descending the gorgeous slot to rejoin the jeep road.

Whether you explored the upper ravine or backtracked on the road, you'll likely enjoy leaving the road here and descending the lower portion of the ravine. As you pass through deeper and deeper layers of sandstone strata, the ravine narrows until it allows only one person at a time to pass. When you reach the jumbled blocks of sandstone in Palm Wash at the bottom of the ravine, turn right, walk 0.3 mile downstream, and exit the canyon via a short link of jeep trail that leads back up to the Calcite road.

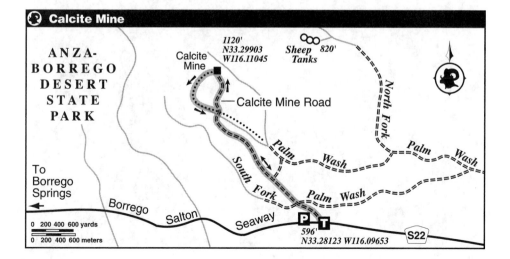

HIKE 98

Ghost Mountain

Location	Southern Anza-Borrego Desert State Park
Highlight	Historically interesting
Distance	1.2 miles (out-and-back)
Total Elevation Gain/Loss	450'/450'
Hiking Time	1½ hours
Optional Maps	Tom Harrison Maps San Diego Backcountry or USGS 7.5-minute *Earthquake Valley*
Best Times	October–May
Agency	ABDSP
Difficulty	Moderate
Trail Use	Good for kids

The California desert has been home to many an eccentric person, but possibly none so audacious as Marshal South. From 1931 until the mid-1940s, Marshal and his poet wife, Tanya, lived atop Ghost Mountain, a rock-strewn, remote mountaintop in the Anza-Borrego Desert, depending in large part on local resources for food, water, and shelter.

There, they built an adobe cabin that they called Yaquitepec, fashioned an ingenious rainwater collection system, raised three children, and tried to emulate, to one degree or another, the life of the prehistoric American Indians.

The ruins of Yaquitepec are one of Anza-Borrego's noted attractions—and quite easy to reach.

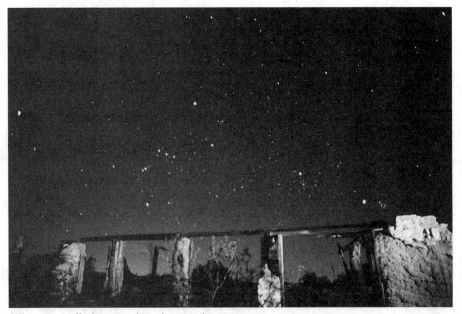

Winter constellations over Yaquitepec ruins

To Reach the Trailhead: From Scissors Crossing (the intersection of CA 78 and County Route S2 on the west edge of Anza-Borrego Desert State Park), drive 5 miles south on Highway S2 to a dirt road on the left (at mile 22.9 according to the green highway mileage markers) into Blair Valley, a large, flat expanse of land spreading east. Take the main dirt road into the valley, following signs for the Marshal South Homesite. Pass around the north and east sides of Blair Valley for 3 miles. On the right is a signed spur road going southwest, leading a quarter mile to a trailhead at the base of Ghost Mountain.

Description: From the parking area at the end of the road a trail switchbacks up the rocky slope, and then it turns east along the ridge to the Yaquitepec site. Little remains of the dwelling except melting mud walls and a water cistern, but the view from the site is impressive.

When not consumed with the business of survival, Marshal South wrote magazine articles detailing the family's experiences on what was then a nearly inaccessible mountaintop. His writings appeared frequently in *Desert Magazine* during the 1940s and are well worth looking up in your local library.

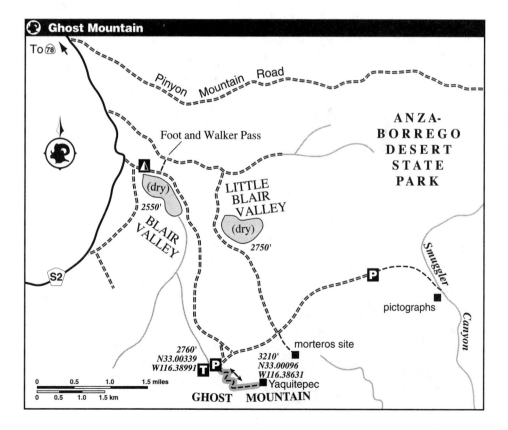

HIKE 99

Moonlight Canyon Loop

Location	Agua Caliente Regional Park (Southern Anza-Borrego)
Highlights	Desert views and geologically interesting
Distance	1.5 miles (loop)
Total Elevation Gain/Loss	350'/350'
Hiking Time	1 hour
Optional Map	USGS 7.5-minute *Agua Caliente Springs*
Best Times	October–May
Agency	SDCP
Difficulty	Easy
Trail Use	Good for kids

Take in a deep breath of clean, dry air. Bask in the larger-than-life brilliance of the desert sun. Sink into the womblike comfort of warm spring water. At Agua Caliente Springs you can have your cake and eat it too—hike first, then enjoy a relaxing soak in the hot springs. A San Diego County park has been established here in the midst of state park lands at the foot of the Tierra Blanca Mountains.

A splinter of the Elsinore Fault is responsible for the upwelling of warm,

mineral-rich water here. The same fault passes through the Lake Elsinore area and Warner Springs, where hot springs are also found. You have two options for soaking at Agua Caliente Springs: a shallow outdoor pool with spring water flowing through at an ambient temperature of about 95°F, and a large indoor jacuzzi pool where the water's temperature is boosted to more than 100°F. The pools are open 9:30 a.m.–5 p.m., and there is a small fee for day use. Overnight campers should make reservations well in advance for the popular sites.

To Reach the Trailhead: You'll find Agua Caliente along County Highway S2, 27 miles northwest of I-8 at Ocotillo, and 22 miles southeast of CA 78 at Scissors Crossing. Currently, the park is open September through May and closed during the hot summer months.

Description: As for hiking, the Moonlight Canyon Trail (one of several short trails in the area) is a good one to start on. This well-marked but somewhat steep and rugged trail starts at the south end of the campground, climbs over a rock-strewn saddle, drops into a small wash mysteriously named Moonlight Canyon, descends past some seeps and a little

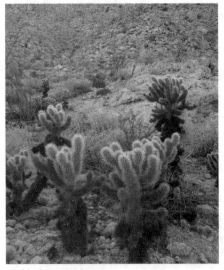

Teddy bear cacti

oasis of willows in the wash bottom, and finally circles back to campground. Kids will enjoy scrambling up the rocks. The canyon is rich with spiky desert vegetation, including barrel and teddy-bear cholla cactus, desert agave, and ocotillo. Bighorn sheep roam the area; scan the ridgetops near the canyon mouth for the well-camouflaged animals. Although moonlight treks around this trail are possible, a good flashlight wouldn't hurt after dark.

True to their name, the Tierra Blanca ("white earth") Mountains are composed of light-colored granitic rock. In some areas this type of rock gradually acquires a patina of oxidized iron and manganese called desert varnish. Right here, however,

the rock has been pounded and fractured by movements along the Elsinore Fault. It easily decomposes into the light-colored mineral crystals that make up the coarse sand you are walking on.

From the high point on the Moonlight Canyon Trail, 300 feet above the campground, you can climb off-trail an additional 250 feet to reach Peak 1882, which offers a superb view of Carrizo Valley and the Vallecito Mountains, including Whale Peak. If you would like, you could take on another, longer side trip, again cross-country, up-canyon (south) in Moonlight Canyon to a point overlooking the Inner Pasture, an isolated valley ringed by the boulder-punctuated Tierra Blanca and Sawtooth Mountains.

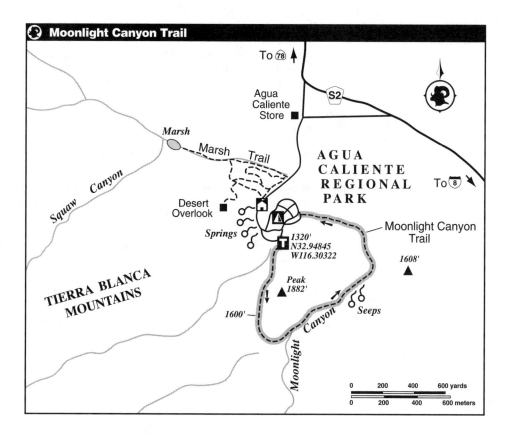

HIKE 100

Mountain Palm Springs

Location	Southern Anza-Borrego Desert State Park
Highlights	Groves of native palms
Distance	2.1 miles (loop)
Total Elevation Gain/Loss	350'/350'
Hiking Time	1½ hours
Optional Maps	Tom Harrison San Diego Backcountry or USGS 7.5-minute *Sweeney Pass*
Best Times	October–May
Agency	ABDSP
Difficulty	Moderate
Trail Use	Good for kids

If you like the contrast between palm-tree oases and a raw landscape of sand and eroded rock, you'll love Mountain Palm Springs. The palms here are gregarious, growing in dense clusters, often with pools of water at their feet. Some have never been burned: they still hold full skirts of dead fronds around their trunks, the better to serve the local population of rodents and snakes. In late fall and early winter, the sticky, sweet fruit of the palms hangs in great swaying clusters, sought after by birds and the sleek coyotes that prowl up and down the washes. The palm groves are distributed along several small washes that drain roughly a square-mile area on the east side of the Tierra Blanca Mountains near the south end of Anza-Borrego Desert State Park.

The trails in this area are often faint and unsigned. Don't hike here unless you have a good sense of direction, and pay close attention to your surroundings. When a trail becomes faint, watch for cairns marking the way. Consider the loop hike described here as a fairly complete tour of the area, but be enticed to extend your explorations in the form of side trips or extended loop trips if the spirit moves you.

To Reach the Trailhead: At a point 20 miles northwest of I-8 at Ocotillo, and 29 miles southeast of CA 78 at Scissors Crossing (mile 47.1 on County Highway S2 according to the green roadside mile markers), take the dirt road going 0.7 mile west, passing the Mountain Palm Springs primitive camping area and ending at a bowl at the foot of the mountain range.

Description: Two canyon mouths open near the road's end. Start up the small canyon to the left (southwest) behind an interpretive panel. Past some small seeps you'll come upon the first groups of palms, Pygmy Grove. Some of these smaller but statuesque palms grow out of nothing more than rock piles.

Follow the canyon as it veers left, then follow the trail onto the low ridge to the left where you reach a junction with a trail coming up from Bow Willow Campground. Continue west on the ridge to Southwest Grove, a restful retreat shaded by a vaulted canopy of shimmering fronds. A rock-lined catch basin fashioned for the benefit of the local wildlife mirrors the silhouettes of the palms. A couple of elephant trees cling to the slopes just above the grove, but for a better look at these curious plants, you can climb a spur trail to Torote Bowl, which has a larger group of elephant trees.

From Southwest Grove, pick up the well-worn but obscure trail that leads north over a rock-strewn ridge to Surprise Canyon Grove in Surprise Canyon. Up-canyon from this small grove lies Palm Bowl, filled with tangled patches of mesquite and fringed on its western edge by more than 100 tall palms. On warm winter days, the molasses-like odor of ripe palm fruit wafts upon the breeze,

and phainopepla hoot and flit among the palm crowns, their white wing patches flashing.

North of Palm Bowl Grove, an old American Indian pathway leads over a low pass to Indian Gorge and Torote Canyon, where many more elephant trees thrive—another possible diversion. To conclude your loop, however, return to Surprise Canyon Grove and continue down-canyon to the campground. On the way, you pass North Grove, hidden in a side drainage on the left.

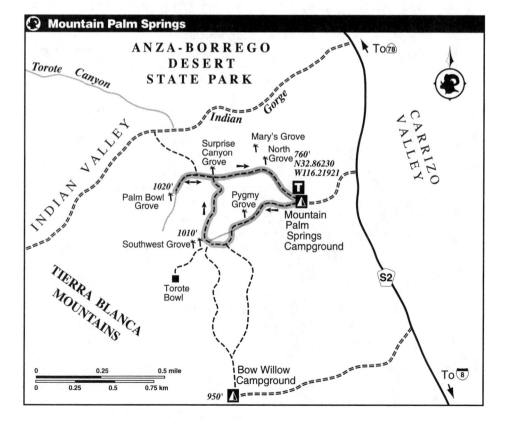

HIKE 101

Mortero Palms to Goat Canyon

Location	Southern Anza-Borrego Desert State Park
Highlights	Rugged, palm-filled canyon and a view of a historic railroad
Distance	6 miles (out-and-back)
Total Elevation Gain/Loss	2,400'/2,400'
Hiking Time	5 hours
Recommended Map	USGS 7.5-minute *Jacumba*
Best Times	November–April
Agency	ABDSP
Difficulty	Moderately strenuous
Trail Use	Suitable for backpacking

The 200-foot-high, 600-foot-long trestle over Goat Canyon on the San Diego & Arizona Eastern rail line is revered among railroad buffs everywhere. It has been called the longest curved railroad trestle and is one of the highest wooden trestles in the world.

Dubbed the impossible railroad, the San Diego & Arizona Eastern tracks were

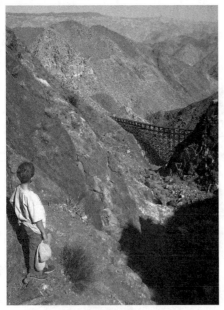

Goat Canyon trestle overlook

laid through southern Anza-Borrego's Carrizo Gorge in the second decade of the 20th century. Starting in 1919, the railroad carried freight, and for a time passengers, between San Diego and the Imperial Valley. The gorge section features 11 miles of twisting track, 17 tunnels, and numerous trestles. The current Goat Canyon trestle, built over a tributary of Carrizo Gorge, was completed in 1933 as part of a realignment of the original route. In 1976 Hurricane Kathleen churned northward up along the Gulf of California, dropped about 10 inches of rain on southern Anza-Borrego, and severely mangled the gorge section of the railroad—rendering it impassable for almost five years. After reopening in 1981, the line was quickly severed again, this time by a fire that burned several trestles. The line did not open again until 2004, and even then it was restricted to limited freight service, and at the time of this writing, it is inactive yet again.

Walking the tracks is expressly forbidden. This hike makes a beeline approach over rough terrain to get a fine view of the magnificent Goat Canyon trestle, which lies in the middle and most remote section of Carrizo Gorge. This is a trip for those who enjoy rock-hopping and cross-country navigation; it is not for the faint of heart.

To Reach the Trailhead: Reaching the remote trailhead is an adventure in itself. A high-clearance vehicle is required, but when the road is in good shape, four-wheel-drive is not essential. These directions assume you have a detailed topographic map of the area. You start hiking at the Mortero Palms Trailhead, close to the rock outcrop known as Dos Cabezos ("two heads"). To get there from I-8 at Ocotillo, proceed north and west on County Route S2 for 4.1 miles to Dos Cabezos Road on the left. This major but unsigned dirt road leads past some buildings servicing the Ocotillo Wind Energy Facility, a 315-megawatt energy project. The wind farm is under development; expect to see changes to the mazelike network of roads.

In 1.1 miles, stay right. The road is now signed EC158. Continue west for another 4.6 miles, passing many intersections on the wind farm, some of which are confusing. Turn left across the railroad tracks on a paved crossover. Go right, continue another 0.1 mile, then veer left, away from the tracks. Go another 0.9 mile to a Y-junction at a sign for Piedras Grandes Cultural Preserve, where you stay left. Cross Palm Canyon Wash and pass spurs on both sides. In 0.7 mile, go right at a second signed Y-junction and reach the end of the road in 0.4 mile, where you can park or camp.

Description: A wide wash lies below the road's end. The Mortero Palms grove, your first destination, is hidden in Palm canyon to the west (not the narrower canyon to the south). So, head northwest along the south side of that west-trending canyon for a

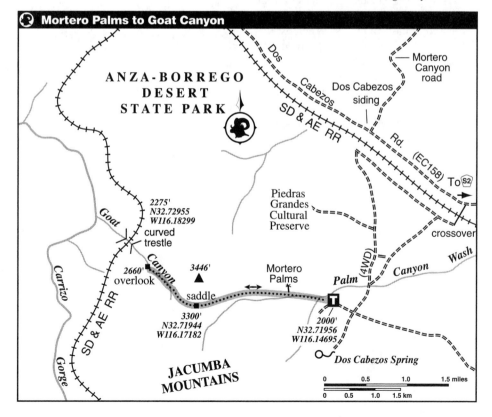

while, avoiding the vegetation-choked streambed. This part of the Jacumba Mountains is home to all things sharp and thorny, including at least six species of cactus, cat's claw acacia, honey mesquite, Mojave yucca, nolina, desert agave, and ocotillo. Don't stumble! Late April is a promising time to see cacti, agave, and ocotillo in bloom.

In 0.3 mile, you may notice a concrete guzzler on the right. Beware of a trail marked by cairns that may tempt you to veer north; instead, continue straight west up the bouldery canyon, watching for a use trail on the north side. After you've climbed the steep slope, look for a half-dozen *morteros* (American Indian mortars), namesakes of the palm grove, in the center of the drainage 100 yards below the lower end of the grove.

Groundwater close to the surface supports the dense cluster of palms amid an otherwise dramatically desolate scene of rounded granitic boulders set against the deep blue sky. On warm days the grove is a seductively cool spot, and it takes some willpower to get moving again to tackle the short but steep stretch of canyon ahead. Traverse left or right, or climb the water-polished rocks directly if you're a real daredevil. Any way you choose you'll get briefly involved in at least one difficult rock-climbing maneuver.

Watch for cairns and a surprisingly good use trail heading up the canyon. At the 2,400-foot contour it's easier to leave the watercourse temporarily and go up on the slope to the north through stands of cholla and Mojave yucca. Drop back in at about 2,750 feet, but leave the wash again at the 2,840-foot contour. Proceed west and southwest across a small saddle, and continue west over a divide into the Goat Canyon drainage, 2.0 miles from the start.

Descend to a delightful, juniper-dotted bowl at about 3,200 feet, a pleasant spot to spend the night if you are backpacking. Goat Canyon descends steeply farther west of here. Down at about 2,700 feet in the canyon where you reach a sudden drop (1.0 mile from the divide), there's an excellent, though somewhat distant, view of the curved trestle, framed by the steep walls of the canyon. If you don't mind more steep rock scrambling, you can descend the steep slopes to the left of the dry waterfall and pick a path another 0.3 mile down to the trestle, which is bracketed by tunnels at both ends.

Further exploration in the area might include a visit to 4,512-foot Jacumba Peak, the high point of the Jacumba Mountains, which lies some 2 miles south.

Recommended Reading

Anderson, Kristi, and Tavernier, Arleen (eds.), *Wilderness Basics,* 3rd edition, The Mountaineers Books, 2004.

Bakker, Elna, *An Island Called California,* 2nd edition, University of California Press, 1984.

Belzer, Thomas J., *Roadside Plants of Southern California,* Mountain Press Publishing Company, 1984.

California Coastal Commission, *California Coastal Access Guide,* 6th edition, Berkeley: University of California Press, 2003.

Clarke, Herbert, *An Introduction to Southern California Birds,* Mountain Press Publishing Company, 1989.

Dale, Nancy, *Flowering Plants: The Santa Monica Mountains, Coastal and Chaparral Regions of Southern California,* Consortium Book Sales and Distributing, 1986.

Ferranti, Philip, *Great Hikes in and near Palm Springs,* Westcliffe Publishers, 2009.

Furbush, Patty A., *On Foot in Joshua Tree National Park: A Comprehensive Hiking Guide,* 5th edition, M. I. Adventure Publications, 2005.

Lightner, James, *San Diego County Native Plants,* 3rd edition, San Diego Flora, 2011.

Lindsay, Diana, and Lowell Lindsay, *The Anza-Borrego Desert Region,* 5th edition, Wilderness Press, 2006.

McAuley, Milt, *Hiking Trails of the Santa Monica Mountains,* Canyon Publishing Company, 1987.

Munz, Philip A., *Introduction to California Desert Wildflowers,* University of California Press, 2004.

————, *Introduction to California Mountain Wildflowers,* University of California Press, 2003.

————, *Introduction to California Spring Wildflowers of the Foothills, Valleys, and Coast,* University of California Press, 2004.

Peterson, P. Victor, *Native Trees of Southern California,* University of California Press, 1966.

Raven, Peter H., *Native Shrubs of Southern California*, University of California Press, 1974.

Robinson, John W., with David Money Harris, *San Bernardino Mountain Trails*, 6th edition, Wilderness Press, 2006.

Robinson, John W., with Doug Christiansen, *Trails of the Angeles*, 8th edition, Wilderness Press, 2005.

Schad, Jerry, *Afoot and Afield in Los Angeles County*, 3rd edition, Wilderness Press, 2009.

———. *Afoot and Afield in Orange County*, 3rd edition, Wilderness Press, 2006.

———. *Afoot and Afield in San Diego County*, 4th edition, Wilderness Press, 2007.

Schaffer, Jeffrey P. et al., *The Pacific Crest Trail: Southern California*, 6th edition, Wilderness Press, 2003.

Schoenherr, Allan A., *A Natural History of California*, University of California Press, 1995.

Sharp, Robert P., and Allen F. Glazner, *Geology Underfoot in Southern California*, Mountain Press Publishing Company, 1993.

Tway, Linda, *Tidepools of Southern California: An Guide to 92 Locations from Point Conception to Mexico*, 2nd edition, Wilderness Press, 2011.

Agencies and Information Sources

Agua Caliente Band of Cahuilla Indians (**ACBCI**)
760-416-7044

Angeles National Forest
Los Angeles River District (**ANF/LARD**)
12371 N. Little Tujunga Rd.
San Fernando, CA 91341
818-899-1900

San Gabriel River District (**ANF/SGRD**)
110 N. Wabash Ave.
Glendora, CA 91741
626-335-1251

Santa Clara/Mojave Rivers District (**ANF/SCMRD**)
28245 Avenue Crocker, Ste. 220
Valencia, CA 91355
661-296-9710

Anza-Borrego Desert State Park (**ABDSP**)
P.O. Box 299
Borrego Springs, CA 92004
760-767-4684 *(recording)*
760-767-4205 *(visitor center)*
760-767-5311 *(administration)*

Big Morongo Canyon Preserve (**BMCP**)
760-363-7190

Blue Sky Ecological Reserve (**BSER**)
858-668-4781

Bureau of Land Management, Palm Springs (**BLM/PS**)
760-251-4800

Caspers Wilderness Park (**CWP**)
949-923-2210

Catalina Island Conservancy (**CIC**)
310-510-2595

Charmlee Wilderness Park (**CW**)
310-457-7247

Chino Hills State Park (**CHSP**)
951-780-6222

City of Riverside Parks and Recreation (**CRPR**)
951-826-2000

Cleveland National Forest
Descanso District (**CNF/DD**)
3348 Alpine Blvd.
Alpine, CA 91901
619-445-6235

Palomar District (**CNF/PD**)
1634 Black Canyon Rd.
Ramona, CA 92065
760-788-0250

Trabuco District (**CNF/TD**)
1147 E. Sixth St.
Corona, CA 92879
951-736-1811

Coachella Valley Preserve (**CVP**)
760-343-1234

Conejo Recreation and Park District (**CRPD**)
805-495-6471

Crystal Cove State Park (**CCSP**)
949-494-3539

Cuyamaca Rancho State Park (**CRSP**)
760-765-0755

Devil's Punchbowl Natural Area (**DPNA**)
661-944-2743

Eaton Canyon Natural Area (**ECNA**)
626-398-5420

Glendale Parks and Recreation (**GPR**)
818-548-2000

Griffith Park (**GP**)
323-913-4688

Joshua Tree National Park (**JTNP**)
74485 National Park Dr.
Twentynine Palms, CA 92277
760-367-5500

Lake Poway Recreation Area (**LPRA**)
858-668-4770

Los Penasquitos Canyon Preserve (**LPCP**)
619-484-7504

Mission Trails Regional Park (**MTRP**)
619-668-3281

Mt. San Jacinto State Wilderness (**MSJSW**)
951-659-2607

Orange County Parks (**OCP**)
949-923-2245

Palomar Mountain State Park (**PSP**)
760-742-3462

Palos Verdes Estates Shoreline Preserve
(**PVESP**)
310-378-0383

Placerita Canyon Park (**PCP**)
661-259-7721

Point Mugu State Park (**PMSP**)
818-880-0363

San Bernardino National Forest
  Arrowhead District (**SBNF/AD**)
  28104 Highway 18
  Skyforest, CA 92385
  909-382-2782

  Big Bear District (**SBNF/BBD**)
  North Shore Dr., Highway 38
  Fawnskin, CA 92333
  909-382-2790

San Gorgonio District (**SBNF/SGD**)
34701 Mill Creek Rd.
Mentone, CA 92359
909-382-2881

San Jacinto District (**SBNF/SJD**)
54270 Pinecrest
Idyllwild, CA 92549
909-382-2921

San Diego County Parks and Recreation
Department (**SDCP**)
858-694-3049

San Dieguito River Park (**SDRP**)
858-674-2270

Santa Monica Mountains Conservancy
(**SMMC**)
310-858-7272

Santa Monica Mountains National
Recreation Area (**SMMNRA**)
401 W. Hillcrest Dr.
Thousand Oaks, CA 91360
805-370-2301

Santa Rosa and San Jacinto Mountains
National Monument (**SRSJMNM**)
760-862-9984

Santa Rosa Plateau Ecological Reserve
(**SRPER**)
951-677-6951

Santiago Oaks Regional Park (**SORP**)
714-973-6620

Torrey Pines State Reserve (**TPSR**)
858-755-2063

Wildlands Conservancy Whitewater
Preserve (**WCWP**)
760-325-7222

Will Rogers State Historic Park (**WRSHP**)
310-454-8212

Index

About the Authors

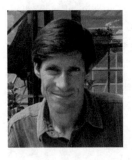

Jerry Schad (1949–2011) was Southern California's leading outdoors writer. His 16 guidebooks, including the popular and comprehensive Afoot & Afield series, and his "Roam-O-Rama" column in the *San Diego Reader* have helped thousands of hikers discover the region's diverse wild places. Schad ran or hiked many thousands of miles of distinct trails throughout California, in the Southwest, and in Mexico. He was a sub-24-hour finisher of Northern California's 100-mile Western States Endurance Run and served in a leadership capacity for outdoor excursions around the world. He taught astronomy and physical science at San Diego Mesa College and chaired the Physical Sciences Department from 1999 until 2011. His sudden and untimely death from kidney cancer shocked and saddened the community.

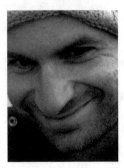

David Money Harris is a professor of engineering at Harvey Mudd College. He is the author or coauthor of five hiking guidebooks and four engineering textbooks. David grew up rambling about the Desolation Wilderness as a toddler in his father's pack and later roamed the High Sierra as a Boy Scout. As a Sierra Club trip leader, he organized mountaineering trips throughout the Sierra Nevada. Since 1999, he has been exploring the mountains and deserts of Southern California. He lives with his wife and three sons in Upland, California, and delights in sharing his love of the outdoors with their boys.

Other Wilderness Press Titles by Jerry Schad

Afoot & Afield Los Angeles County

Covering all the best L.A. adventures, from strolling along at Malibu Lagoon
State Beach to trekking up a mountain on Catalina Island. The more than 200
trips explore the City of Angels' own backyard, traveling through a variety of
climate zones and revealing a diverse array of plant and animal life.

ISBN 978-0-89997-499-6

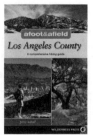

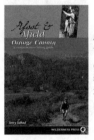

Afoot & Afield Orange County

Whether you're up for exploring marine life at the Bolsa Chica Reserve,
climbing Santiago Peak in the Santa Anas, or anything in between, this guide
shows the way. Details 87 salubrious outings in every kind of natural environ-
ment, from teeming tidepools to windswept mountaintops.

ISBN 978-0-89997-397-5

Afoot & Afield San Diego County

San Diego's best-selling comprehensive hiking guidebook, featuring 250 detailed descriptions of every trail worth hiking in the county. Catalogs the best
trips along the beaches, the bays, over the foothills, to the mountains, and out
to the desert.

ISBN 978-0-89997-428-6

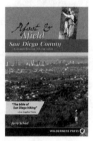

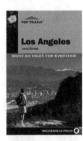

Top Trails: Los Angeles

A succinct and portable guide to the 57 must-do hikes in the greater L.A.
area. Get going fast with the "don't-get-lost" trail milestones, innovative trail-
feature tables, and more of Schad's insight and insider's knowledge of the best
trails in the Southland.

ISBN 978-0-89997-627-3

Trail Runner's Guide: San Diego

A comprehensive guide to running the myriad trails of sun-soaked San Diego, from the beach at La Jolla to the summit of Palomar Mountain. Runners
and hikers alike will appreciate the detailed descriptions of 50 exhilarating
routes. Includes climate and topography tips, maps, photos, and more.

ISBN 978-0-89997-308-1

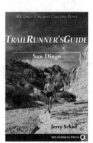

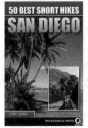

50 Best Short Hikes: San Diego

Diverse routes in Southern California's showpiece city for a year of weekly
hikes. From sidewalk strolls and historic neighborhoods, to wildflowers and
waterfalls, pleasant pastimes and panoramic vistas unfold in this handy guidebook. All routes range 1–8 miles and lie within 30 miles of San Diego's central
core. Includes climate and topography tips, maps, photos, and more.

ISBN 978-0-89997-629-7

Other Wilderness Press Titles by David Money Harris

Afoot & Afield Inland Empire

David and Jennifer Money Harris

Riverside and San Bernardino Counties are a hiker's paradise, with Joshua Tree National Park, the Santa Rosa and San Jacinto Mountains National Monument, Mojave National Preserve, and the three tallest peaks in Southern California. This guide spans more than 200 hikes in the desert, mountains, and urban parks.

ISBN 978-0-89997-462-0

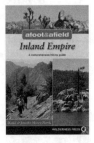

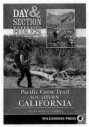

Day & Section Hikes: Pacific Crest Trail Southern California

The world-famous Pacific Crest Trail runs 2,650 miles from Mexico to Canada. This book describes 31 of the best day hikes and moderate overnight hikes on the PCT in the San Diego backcountry, the San Jacinto Mountains, the San Bernardino Mountains, the San Gabriel Mountains, and the Southern Sierra Nevada Mountains.

ISBN 978-0-89997-684-6

San Bernardino Mountain Trails

John Robinson with David Money Harris

100 hikes in and near the San Bernardino National Forest, including Lake Arrowhead, Big Bear Lake, the San Gorgonio Wilderness, the San Jacinto Wilderness, and the Santa Rosa Mountains near Palm Springs. In print for more than 30 years.

ISBN 978-0-89997-409-5

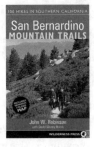

For ordering information, contact your local bookseller or Wilderness Press at **wildernesspress.com.**